WEIGHT SUCCESS FOR A LIFETIME

WEIGHT SUCCESS FOR A LIFETIME

CAROL SIMONTACCHI, C.C.N., M.S.

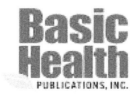

Basic
Health
PUBLICATIONS, INC.

The information contained in this book is based upon the research and personal and professional experiences of the author. It is not intended as a substitute for consulting with your physician or other healthcare provider. Any attempt to diagnose and treat an illness should be done under the direction of a healthcare professional.

The publisher does not advocate the use of any particular healthcare protocol but believes the information in this book should be available to the public. The publisher and author are not responsible for any adverse effects or consequences resulting from the use of the suggestions, preparations, or procedures discussed in this book. Should the reader have any questions concerning the appropriateness of any procedures or preparation mentioned, the author and the publisher strongly suggest consulting a professional healthcare advisor.

The author of this book has a financial interest in the products Wings Breakfast Drink, Wings Klean Tea, Wings Healing Tea, and Wings educational materials. This does not constitute an endorsement by Basic Health Publications, Inc.

Basic Health Publications, Inc.

Library of Congress Cataloging-in-Publication Data

Simontacchi, Carol N.

   Weight success for a lifetime / Carol Simontacchi.
     p. cm.
   Includes bibliographical references and index.
   ISBN: 978-1-68336-686-7 (Pbk.)
   ISBN: 978-1-68162-890-5 (Hardcover)

  1. Weight loss. I. Title.
RM222.2.S554197   2005
613.2'5—dc22

                                        2005006607

Editor: Kate Johnson
Typesetting/Book design: Gary A. Rosenberg
Cover design: Mike Stromberg

Contents

Introduction, 1

To my four daughters,
Caryl Anne, Bobbie Anne, Melissa Anne, and Laurie Anne:
You are the loves of my life.
You make me proud to be your mom.

To my sisters and daughters everywhere:

"I pray that you may enjoy good health
and that all may go well with you,
even as your soul is getting along well."

(III John 12)

Introduction

There is certainly no shortage of weight-loss ideas in this country. Every year, new diet and weight-loss books sprout on bookstore shelves like weeds in an untended garden. Some promise a balanced diet; that is, they stress the importance of including generous amounts of vegetables, fruits, nuts, and seeds, and some animal protein, and tout the benefits of essential fatty acids that are healthful to the body and assist in weight loss. But for the most part, the mainstream press promotes diets that actually increase your risk of gaining weight, or that make it virtually impossible to keep the extra weight off if the diets are followed over the long term. The failure rate of the weight-loss industry to succeed in its purpose is a staggering 92 percent.

That is not good news for the dieter. Even worse, the mainstream press addresses the diverse issues of unwanted weight gain from one of two perspectives: you eat too much—or you don't exercise enough. The common understanding of weight management is that it is a simple matter of taking in fewer calories than you expend; for most people, however, that simply isn't true. The management of caloric resources is governed by virtually every organ system of the body, and, to further complicate matters, is influenced by food and environmental allergies, prescription medications, environmental toxins, past sexual, emotional, and/or physical abuse, and many other factors.

Weight management is, therefore, a very complex issue, as you will learn in this book. Laying the blame for weight failure at the feet of diet or exercise alone often leaves the real source of the problem untouched. The diet industry itself is simply making us fatter, less healthy, and terribly bewildered.

YOU KNOW HOW TO DIET— AND YOU'RE STARVING

If you are like most Americans, you've been introduced to dietary restriction and self-control. You've been trained to calculate calories, fat grams, and car-bohydrate grams. You know how to go to sleep hungry and wake up hungry. You can flip through a cookbook and ignore your growling stomach without even twitching an eyelid. You've probably memorized an impressive list of weight-loss tips: Don't eat standing up. Don't eat in front of the refrigerator. Tape a picture of your ideal figure to the bathroom mirror. Take tiny bites and chew thoroughly. Drink lots of water. Throw away your "fat clothes." Brush your teeth after each meal and again when you feel hungry. Eat lots of lettuce.

But if you really want to lose weight and keep it off, if you want to regain your health and vitality and turn the clock back on the aging process, you're going to have to go beyond simple dietary restriction and "fix" your body and your relationship with food. You will have to do things differently. Years of dieting, *unless* based on a diversity of nutrient-dense foods, may have set up metabolic responses that can be difficult to overcome. If you have dieted frequently or over a long period of time, it is likely that your body has shifted into "preservation and starvation mode" and that your metabolic rate is too low to sustain weight-loss goals. You're probably slowly starving to death!

The Diet Mentality in Western Culture

The flourishing diet mentality in our culture is not based on good science or clinical nutrition research but on a dogmatic and largely unfounded belief system. Everyone who has an opinion has become a nutrition expert—but opinions are frequently incorrect. As one wag put it, "It isn't that we don't know enough. The problem is that so much of what we know is wrong."

Things might have gone differently if the diet industry, with its amazing variety of pseudo-foods and malnutrition-based programs, had emerged in a relatively well-nourished society. Unfortunately, the diet industry and the epidemic of excess weight both emerged within a society that was already struggling with diverse manifestations of undernutrition and malnutrition. We in Western culture have been hungry for decades, so we eat huge quantities of pseudo-foods to try to stanch the hunger pangs; but artificial foods cause chronic hunger, no matter how much food is eaten. We just keep getting hungrier—and fatter.

Excess Weight as a Symptom and a Syndrome

Excess weight is not a disease but a symptom, a sign that the body's own homeostatic (self-balancing) mechanisms have failed. Excess weight indicates that the body is no longer able to appropriate its caloric resources wisely: it has lost part of its innate ability to burn excess calories, to maintain appropriate stores of excess energy and "waste" other calories, and to use hunger solely to satisfy the body's nutrient and energetic needs.

Hunger is likewise a symptom, and we're missing its message. A normal, healthy body will eat when it is hungry, eat just the type and amount of food needed to meet basic requirements, and stop eating when satisfied. As you will see in Lessons I-4 and II-11, hunger is not an enemy to be vanquished; it is an important biological signal that our bodies need to be fed.

Much of our normal hunger response has been overpowered by pseudo-foods that artificially stimulate our desire to eat. Remember the potato-chip commercial that taunted, "You can't eat just one . . . "? Why do we just keep eating potato chips? Or candy, or sugary breakfast cereals? Our insatiable appetites have nothing to do with the number of calories consumed, and everything to do with physiological addiction and hunger. We eat the wrong foods—for all the wrong reasons.

Excess weight is rarely a simple dietary or activity issue; rather, it is a complex issue involving the digestive system, endocrine system, nervous system, and more. It may be a genetic or even a childhood issue. Being overweight is a syndrome, a collection of symptoms or conditions, showing that one or several of these organ systems is not functioning correctly and is asking for adjustments to be made. Adjustments may indeed be necessary in the appetite or in the selection of different foods, but not so much to correct for caloric intake as to meet the underlying metabolic needs of the body.

Unwanted weight gain is often only one coil in the downward health spiral generated by the consumption of processed, nutrient-poor food. You will learn how the current diet mentality leads to chronic dysregulation of several body systems, and how dys-regulation then leads to further weight gain and poor health. For example, hypothyroidism can hinder digestion, slow the metabolic rate, and cause a baffling variety of symptoms. If digestion is impaired, food allergies often develop, leading to myriad symptoms including excess weight. Stress can compound problems of the thyroid gland or pancreas, which may then lead to problems with the female hormone system or with blood sugar levels. As you will see, weight-management issues generally come in clusters, and people usually struggle with more than one. It is not a simple problem!

Seldom can permanent, healthful weight loss occur through dietary changes alone. The other needs of the body—the whole syndrome of excess weight and poor health—must be addressed. And that is why you're reading this book.

WHY TRY THE WINGS PROGRAM?

Failure to recognize the complexity of weight management is one of the biggest reasons that Americans have not been successful with their weight despite their penchant for diet books and plans, surgery, exercise equipment, pills, potions, and even lotions. They haven't understood the language of the body. An overweight body will not drop excess pounds until the needs of that body have been met, until the language of the body has been decoded—until the body has been fed.

The Wings Program is not a quick fix or a fad. It is not designed to help you drop a lot of weight at first, only to regain it later. It is a long-term program based on solid science and practical clinical experience. In this training course, you will learn to understand the language of the body. You will learn the diverse reasons why the body becomes overweight, and how to address them. You will learn about your homeostatic regulatory mechanisms and how to accommodate your body's needs. Some of the information may be new to you; perhaps you have never heard of these correlations with weight disorders. Some of the information you may have heard before, but now you are hearing it in the context of weight management. You will find that Wings is a very comprehensive program—and there's really nothing like it on the market.

An Overview of the Wings Program

The Wings Program is a curriculum of forty-nine weeks divided into four modules. Each module contains ten to fourteen lessons on thematically grouped topics, as follows.

- Module I, Living Successfully with Food: food issues, diet issues, cravings, binge eating, allergies, family-food preparation, handling special occasions, and so on.

- Module II, Getting the Body Back into Shape: exercise, shift work and other special problems, body cleansing, digestion, constipation, and so on.

- Module III, Hidden Issues of Weight Management: depression, prescription medications, hormonal dysregulation, thyroid dysfunction, brown fat thermogenesis, Syndrome X, and other health conditions and medical issues.

- Module IV, Healing the Heart and the Mind: fear of success, abuse issues, body image, putting the fun back in food, and so on.

I'll say it often: Weight management is not a simple matter of dietary control; it involves the whole organism, the whole body. So I'll address the whole body! And that is what distinguishes Wings from every other program on the market today. I want to build your health from your head to your toes, from the inside out! You'll learn to love the special whole-body focus of this program because for the first time in your life, you will truly satisfy the needs of your body and achieve total body health.

HOW TO USE THIS BOOK

The Wings Program is a journey toward health and weight management, and this is your guide and textbook. It is designed to be a "consumable" workbook, with space for taking notes, recording information, and doing written assignments. Don't think that you will meet your weight-loss goals more quickly if you race through the material. Study the lessons carefully, spending one week on each. Do your assignments and stay on task. Get someone to walk through the material with you and hold you accountable.

Each lesson begins with an introductory question. Take time to ponder it and answer carefully. The questions are designed to introduce the material and make it personally relevant to you. The study guides and assignments that accompany the lessons will help you discover your unique weight-management challenges and develop strategies for meeting and resolving them. So don't just read about it: do it! (In discussing the emotional and spiritual issues associated with physical health and weight management, I make occasional references to Judeo-Christian religious tradition. If you feel uncomfortable with those,

please substitute any alternative wording with which you are comfortable.)

One of my goals is to help you take responsibility for your own good health, so each lesson ends with a Health Tip. Using these tips is an excellent way to learn about natural holistic health care. (For more information, see the Resource Guide, which provides sources for natural healthcare products and lists some of the wonderful books available for your self-education; start building your health library!) Sometimes, of course, you will require the aid of a physician; don't hesitate to consult your physician if you need medical intervention. Much of the time, however, you can prevent illness by learning how to care for yourself.

Starting with the first lesson, all four modules are coordinated with the healthful eating plan that is integral to the Wings Program. The eating plan, detailed in the Menus and Recipes section of this book, is based on nutrient-dense, whole foods that are (for the most part) available at your local supermarket, health food store, or farm stand. Check out local organic growers, family farms, and community sponsored agriculture (CSA) farms in your area—purchasing their healthful products is a wonderful way to support our neighbors and help heal our Earth. As you follow the Wings Program eating plan, you'll relearn how to select, cook, eat, and enjoy food.

Please keep a Food Diary throughout the program, and keep an Exercise Diary as well (forms for these are provided in Appendices 1 and 2). Although you won't learn why this record keeping is so important until Lesson I-3, start your Food Diary with Lesson I-1, on faith that you'll understand soon enough.

PEOPLE AND PRODUCTS TO SUPPORT YOU

One of the most significant features of the Wings Program is that it is designed to be personally tailored for the individual. You may be wondering, "Why is that necessary, or even beneficial, in weight management?" Because the specific needs and issues for each person are different. Some people struggle with eating, some with exercise, others with stress; some have thyroid trouble, hormone imbalances, food allergies, or other medical conditions. Given that, you may then wonder, "How can it be possible for one program to meet such an array of individual needs?"

By reading this book and doing the assignments in each lesson, you will learn a great deal about how your own body works. I also urge you to take full advantage of the supporting materials that Wings offers. Some people are auditory learners; that is, they learn better by hearing. For this reason, all four modules of the program have been videotaped for optional use along with this workbook. Each videotaped module contains the complete set of lessons (with even more information than is contained in the book), plus a Wings Student Manual.

When you purchase a videotaped module, you automatically receive (at no additional cost) the on-line *Wings Newsletter*. This monthly newsletter provides "hot-off-the-press" research material on health and weight that is too new to have already been included in the program. Each edition also contains a "chat" from program author and designer Carol Simontacchi (that's me), new recipes and menus to add to the food plan, and other valuable information. You can also subscribe to the *Wings Newsletter* without purchasing a videotaped module (see the Resource Guide for contact information).

A key form of support in the course of your program is the personalized nutrition counseling that Wings provides to identify your specific needs and help you with the food plan (visit the Wings website www.flywithwings.com/pnc.html and click on the link MyProConnect for a consultation). To further support your weight-management and health goals, our on-staff clinical nutritionist may also recommend products that are particularly suited to your personal biochemistry—for example, herbal supplements that help against depression and its accompanying eating behaviors; or, natural anti-inflammatories that are effective against pain and allergy but don't cause weight gain. Other natural products can improve energy, cleanse the body, reduce cravings for sweets, and balance blood sugar. In cases of possible food or environmental allergies or other medical conditions, she will put you in touch with a local holistic physician who can prescribe the appropriate testing.

From many natural products on the market today, I've selected professional, quality-guaranteed products that have been formulated specifically to meet the needs of the American malnourished population. Some are only supplied through Wings, but most are available at local health food stores and supermarkets. I suggest that everyone on this program start with the Wings Breakfast Drink and a good companion multivitamin and mineral supplement (see the Resource Guide). As you proceed through the material, I will suggest specific dietary supplements to help assure your weight and health success.

A note about Wings products and alternatives: The Wings Breakfast Drink is a unique blend of rice-based protein, amino acids that aid in physiological functions including detoxification, and additional nutrients that promote the health of the digestive tract. Similarly, Wings Klean Tea and Wings Healing Tea are unique herbal blends formulated for internal cleansing and intestinal healing. If desired, however, you may substitute another rice-based protein powder (manufactured by companies such as Nutribiotics) for the Wings Breakfast Drink; other natural digestive products available at the health food store can also be substituted for the Wings teas.

WHAT TO EXPECT FROM YOUR WINGS PROGRAM

As you begin to understand how very complex weight management is, you will look at yourself with new understanding, with new compassion. You'll give yourself more grace. You'll lose your fear of food, and be delighted with new sensual pleasure in your meals. You won't be hungry again; you'll feel deeply satisfied. Your eyes will take on a new sparkle; your hair will achieve a new luster; your skin will stop wrinkling and feel soft to the touch. Your energy level will soar, you'll feel like working and exercising—and best of all, you'll lose your excess weight!

If you continue on this program through the entire forty-nine weeks, you will develop lifelong good nutritional habits. You will learn how to eat forever—because this is a permanent, "forever" type of program. After you have successfully completed your Wings Program, you will not ever need to purchase or read another weight-loss book or article.

GETTING STARTED

You will be asked to use the Wings Breakfast Drink (or your chosen alternative) for the first meal of the day from the very beginning of your program (see the Resource Guide for ordering information). Starting with the first lesson, you will also be asked to check the pH of your urine on a regular basis, for which you need strips of pH-testing paper; if you can't obtain them through your local pharmacy, call the company Thinking of You at 1-800-806-8671 (please make reference to this book when you call). Once you've gotten your supplies (and your motivation) together, turn the page to Lesson I-1.

Are you ready to begin this journey? Let's get started. . . .

MODULE I
Living Successfully with Food

You have read diet books. You have followed dieting programs. You speak the language of a seasoned dieter. You know about high-protein, high-carbohydrate, low-calorie, and low-fat regimens. You know how to "bust your buns" at the gym. Frankly, you are tired of "doing it right" but feeling like a failure. You need a new approach.

You need Wings!

The book you are holding in your hands is not "just another diet book." It is a guide, a map, and a path. Where are you going with it? You are beginning a journey through the complex issues that have made it difficult to achieve "weight success." This book will teach you about those issues and help you design your own personal solutions on your journey toward health.

Module I covers the first few steps, and it is designed to restore your pleasure in food. No more deprivation! No more unsatisfied hunger! No more cravings! Just delightful food that nourishes the body and the soul.

When you embark on a journey, you don't always have to race through to the end. You can stop and enjoy the scenery along the way—and that's how to take your Wings journey. Don't read and read and read to get to the end of each section as soon as you can. Take your time. Enjoy each lesson and do the tasks requested of you. Let the lesson "soak in," and make it part of your new life, because if you take the time and do the work, you will establish new habits of health to enjoy for the rest of your life.

Lesson I-1. Welcome to Wings!

There is a great deal of confusion about what really constitutes a healthful diet. Is it low-fat? Is it fat-free? Low-calorie? High-carbohydrate? Vegetarian, or meat-based? You may have come to feel that you need to check with your cardiologist or family doctor before you consult a cookbook for dinner plans. Deciding what to prepare for a meal should not be so complicated! Food was lovingly created to support abundant, vibrant health. Food should be celebrated, not feared.

❓ TODAY'S QUESTION

Why did you "join" the Wings Program?

_____

_____

_____

_____

The Wings Program is not a temporary "fix" while you lose 10 or 15 pounds. As described in the introduction to this book, the comprehensive Wings curriculum is designed to teach the concepts of holistic weight management and provide a support network to assist you in making permanent lifestyle changes. You'll hear those words often throughout the program because I really mean them. Permanent! Lifestyle!

I am interested in promoting total body health. Wings is intended, in fact, to help you maintain and improve your health in every area of your life—to heighten and support your desire to be physically, spiritually, and emotionally healthy. The program emphasizes natural healing to increase well-being and self-worth and to help you take responsibility for your own good health. Weight loss is one of the goals to that end—and weight loss occurs as a natural consequence of the "get healthy" program. When you think of Wings, think natural, holistic, comprehensive, delicious, and permanent!

THE WINGS CONCEPT OF A HEALTHFUL DIET

The meals on the Wings Program food plan are so delicious that you will not feel deprived. In fact, you will probably feel that a whole new world of culinary delight has been opened up to you! You'll find that food can be delicious and "dietary" at the same time. The Wings recipes and meals were designed with the following criteria in mind:

- Recipes are easy to follow and delicious for the entire family.

- Recipes use whole foods, as close as possible to the way they are provided in nature. ("Real" and "unreal" foods will be discussed in Lessons I-5 and I-7.)

- Meals contain a balance of essential nutrients, including protein, fats, carbohydrates, fiber, vitamins, and minerals. (These nutrients and their balance will be discussed in Lesson I-2.) The beverage, at meals and otherwise, must be pure water, herbal tea, or—as a special treat—juice.

- Meals are supplemented with a high-quality multivitamin-mineral product to help make up for longstanding nutrient deficiencies.

- Meals are low in common allergenic foods such as

✒ NOTES

_____

_____

_____

_____

_____

_____

wheat, corn, and dairy products. (Food allergy and food intolerance will be discussed in Lesson I-10.)

For daily multivitamin-mineral supplementation, you may use a high-quality supplement of your choice from a health food store, or ask your Wings nutritionist to recommend a supplement specifically geared to your needs (go to the website www.flywith wings.com/pnc.html and click on MyProConnect). A good companion multivitamin-mineral is a professional supplement called Optimum 6 (see the Resource Guide). This excellent product is rich in nutrients that are known to reduce food cravings and make up for years of malnutrition-based dieting.

It is nearly impossible for most people to prepare a healthful, well-balanced breakfast that does not consist of highly allergenic foods like cereal, milk, and eggs. I advise, instead, that you enjoy the Wings Breakfast Drink each morning (with occasional exceptions, which you'll encounter from time to time in the food plan). The Breakfast Drink, which has a hypoallergenic rice-protein base combined with nutrients for additional digestive support, can be prepared quickly and simply and in delicious variations (see page 236). The Wings Breakfast Drink works marvelously to balance blood sugar and reduce hunger throughout the day. (The drink does not contain added vitamins and minerals because these can alter the taste, and sweeteners and/or other flavoring agents would need to be added to mask the effect.)

Sound good so far? It is!

For the first eight lessons of your Wings Program, you are to follow the recipes and menus provided for each lesson as closely as possible, starting tomorrow morning. The menus are designed to provide the following benefits:

- Blood sugar balance, so your energy will remain steady throughout the day

- Adequate amounts of protein, fats, and carbohydrates evenly spaced throughout the day

- Hunger satisfaction, so you will not feel deprived

- Sensory pleasure, so you will truly enjoy your food—and not feel guilty eating it

Don't try to figure it out for yourself until Lesson I-9, when you will have more latitude in designing your own meals. Not that you won't still need "supervision"—the human tendency is to start slipping, and you can veer wildly off course within a short period of time. You may need an accountability partner to keep you on track (Lesson I-3). But by Lesson I-9, you will understand the principles of healthful eating more clearly and will be able to design your own meals and menus that are faithful to the concepts contained in this program.

YOUR ACID/ALKALINE BALANCE

Today's lesson kicks things off by introducing a topic that will be carried thematically throughout the entire Wings Program: the acid/alkaline balance, or pH, of the body. In today's assignments, you are asked to work toward achieving your body's proper pH over the course of this week. As you continue through the program, you will be reminded periodically to recheck the pH of your urine to monitor your body's acid/alkaline balance. The food plan outlined in the Menus and Recipes section is also geared toward helping you maintain a healthful internal pH.

This discussion borrows heavily from a highly respected, holistically trained medical doctor and well-known lecturer, Russell Jaffe, M.D., Ph.D., C.C.N., author of *The Alkaline Way* (published by ELISA/ACT Biotechnologies LLC, available through Perque Laboratories; see the Resource Guide).

You probably already know that a pH value of 7.0 is considered neutral, that is, neither acid nor alkaline. The internal environment of the human body is maintained at a pH between 6.5 and 7.5, a narrow range that is critically important for the functions and reactions of cells. This slightly alkaline internal pH does not remain static: its maintenance is a highly dynamic process that is influenced and controlled by many dietary, environmental, and internal conditions on a moment-to-moment basis.

Unfortunately, the vast majority of foods in the American diet are acid producing. This includes all animal proteins, sugar, some nuts (hazelnuts, walnuts, and Brazil nuts), dairy products, fried foods, most grains, many legumes, and many other foods, including all caffeinated and carbonated beverages. Alkaline-producing foods, on the other hand, include most vegetables and fruits, which we simply do not enjoy as frequently as we should. The consequences of a predominantly acid-producing diet may be considerable, not the least of which are unwanted weight gain and the inability to lose weight easily. Foods are not the only contributor to this problem, as stress, medications, and other lifestyle factors can also acidify the body.

How does the body counteract an unhealthful acidity of its internal environment caused by this mostly non-alkaline, acid-producing diet? Minerals can provide a buffering alkalinity to restore the required pH. The best bodily reservoir of minerals is, of course, the bones. When we overconsume high-acid foods like meats, sugar, and grains and under-consume alkalinizing foods like fresh vegetables and fruits, the body pulls minerals out of the bones. As a result, the bones become porous (osteoporotic) over time. The immune system flares up with food and environmental allergies. Fatigue sets in, and we are set on a downward spiral of poor health.

The Alkaline Way

In *The Alkaline Way,* Dr. Russell Jaffe writes: "When an alkaline environment is maintained in the body, metabolic, enzymatic, immunologic, and repair mechanisms function at their best. The acid-forming metabolics of stress and inflammation and of high fat and high protein foods are adequately and effectively neutralized only when sufficient mineral-buffering reserves are present. Mineral buffering reserves are the gift that alkaline-forming foods give to our body. A diet that is predominantly alkaline forming is essential to the maintenance of sustained health."

Excess acids are also excreted by the body during its resting time overnight. The body's performance of this task is based on its toxic load (that is, amount of toxic materials: environmental pollutants, products of incomplete digestion, and so on), its individual ability to produce cellular energy through its mineral status, and its ability to inactivate and excrete toxins. According to Dr. Jaffe, the pH of the first morning urine is a good indicator of the body's mineral reserves and its acid/alkaline balance.

Checking Your pH

You can follow these simple steps to determine your pH by testing your first morning urine.

1. Obtain a packet of pH test paper with a test range of 5.5–8.0.

2. Before you retire for the night, tear off a two- to three-inch strip of test paper and set it aside with the packet's color chart in the bathroom that you'll use during the night or in the morning.

3. You will test the first urine that you produce after sleeping for at least five hours. If you awaken in the night to urinate after five or more hours of sleep, test that urine by dipping the pH test strip in your urine stream and proceeding to step 4 below. If you sleep through the night and don't awaken until the morning, test that urine by the same procedure.

4. As the test strip is briefly moistened with urine, it will change color. The strip's color (ranging from yellow to dark blue) indicates the urine's acid or alkaline state, as shown by the color chart on the packet of test paper. Compare the test strip to the color chart and jot down the number that corresponds to the color of the test strip. (A pH testing form is provided in Appendix 3.)

5. Any number below the neutral point of 7.0 means that your urine is on the acid side. The lower the number, the more acid it is; for example, a value of 5.0 indicates ten times more acidity than 6.0. Ideally, the pH of your first morning urine should range from 7.0 to 7.5, as the cells of your body work best in this slightly alkaline state.

THE ASCORBIC ACID FLUSH

If you find that your urinary pH does not fall within the desirable range of 7.0–7.5, you may wish to try a technique called an ascorbic acid flush. In a nutshell, "doing the flush" means drinking a solution of ascorbic acid (that is, buffered vitamin C) at fifteen-minute intervals to stimulate the bowels to evacuate completely and eliminate toxins through the digestive system.

Dr. Jaffe believes that doing this flush frequently is one of the best ways to restore proper pH and rebuild health. He recommends using a fully reduced form of ascorbic acid called L-ascorbate, buffered with alkalinizing minerals. For best results, he balances each gram of L-ascorbate with 66 milligrams (mg) of potassium, 16 mg of magnesium, 27 mg of calcium, and 600 micrograms (mcg) of zinc. Each $\frac{1}{2}$ teaspoon of this buffered ascorbate contains 1.5 grams (g) ascorbate, 99 mg potassium, 16 mg magnesium, 40 mg calcium, and 600 mcg zinc. (This mixture, which contains no masking or inert ingredients, is available through Perque Laboratories; see the Resource Guide.) *Caution:* Do not use DL-ascorbate or D-ascorbate, because these forms of ascorbic acid are not absorbed by humans and may irritate the intestinal tract.

Doing the Flush

Although the flush is easy to do, you may wish to stay home the first time you try it. Start early in the morning on an empty stomach and allow ample time (which varies widely from person to person) to finish the flush that day.

1. According to the bulleted list below, dissolve the appropriate amount of fully reduced mineral-buffered L-ascorbate powder in the appropriate amount of room-temperature water, or, if you prefer, juice that has been diluted with water at a ratio of 1:1. Allow the effervescence to abate and then drink the beverage.

   ▪ A healthy person begins with a level ½ teaspoon (1.5 g) of the powder dissolved in 1–2 ounces of water or diluted juice.

   ▪ A moderately healthy person begins with 1 teaspoon (3 g) dissolved in 4 or more ounces of water or diluted juice.

   ▪ A person in ill health begins with 2 teaspoons (6 g) dissolved in 8 or more ounces of water or diluted juice.

2. Repeat the procedure in step 1 three more times, at fifteen-minute intervals. Meanwhile, review "Tips for the Flush." If, after four doses, there is no gurgling or rumbling in your gut, you should double your initial dose and continue every fifteen minutes.

3. Continue the procedure at the proper time intervals until you reach the "flush reaction," which is a watery stool or an enema-like evacuation of liquid from the rectum. *Note:* Do not stop prematurely at the point of loose stool. You want to energize the body to flush out toxins and reduce the risk that they may be reabsorbed back into the body from the colon.

Tips for the Flush

For most people, it takes between 3 and 8 teaspoons of L-ascorbate to complete the full flush reaction. Others may require 15, 20, or more than 50 grams, depending on individual health status and how rapidly the body uses up ascorbate.

▪ Following each dose, be sure to drink plenty of room-temperature water or diluted juice. Some people report gas or fullness while doing the flush, but that is almost always due to inadequate fluid intake or rushing the process. Cramps are also a consequence of drinking too little water.

▪ You may pre-prepare a batch of the beverage for convenience. Dissolve 30 g (10 teaspoons) of the powder in 20–30 ounces of room-temperature liquid. Use a dark, capped bottle to avoid exposing the beverage to air or light. Dissolved ascorbate is stable for a day if the bottle is kept cool and tightly sealed.

▪ Some people report "hot" stools that seem to burn the anus after several evacuations. If this occurs, you can use a natural salve such as calendula ointment to soothe the area.

▪ People who have hemorrhoids, irritable bowel syndrome (see the Health Tip on pages 119–120), or inflammatory bowel disease may find that the ascorbate activates their tissues in the healing process. If you have any of these conditions, you may need to increase your ascorbate and bioflavonoid intake slowly over time before attempting the flush.

▪ You will wish to do the flush on a regular basis, perhaps once per month, to keep your tissues saturated with ascorbic acid and minerals. Between flush days, take a daily dosage of vitamin C that is 75 percent of the amount needed to induce the flush reaction.

Benefits of the Flush

Most people feel better after doing an ascorbic acid flush, with increased energy and a sense of well-being each time they do it. That's great—a sign that the body is in recovery and is cleansing itself! The benefits of the flush include:

▪ Decreased digestive transit time (reduces constipation)

▪ Enhanced detoxification and reduced toxic mineral load

▪ Improved blood vessel and cardiovascular system integrity

▪ Improved hormone balance

▪ Enhanced neurotransmitter and immune system functions

▪ Enhanced repair function and bone formation

▪ Enhanced production of adenosine triphosphate (ATP) for cellular energy

▪ Increased iron uptake and release

▪ Enhanced anticancer surveillance and direct cytolytic (cell-destroying) effects on tumors

▪ Resistance to scurvy (a vitamin C–deficiency disease)

Read Dr. Jaffe's book for more information about the ascorbic acid flush. If you would like to consult a healthcare professional about its appropriateness for you, see the Resource Guide to find a holistic physician in your area.

TODAY'S FIRST ASSIGNMENT

START YOUR NEW FOOD PLAN

Flip to Menus and Recipes in the back of this book, and read through the meal plan for the next seven days. Prepare your shopping list, purchase the ingredients, and start eating on the Wings food plan—now!

TODAY'S SECOND ASSIGNMENT

START YOUR PROGRESS CHART

Weigh yourself, and then take five girth measurements: bust at the largest point, waist at two inches above the navel, hips at the largest point, and right and left thigh circumference at the point where your extended fingertips reach with your arms hanging down at your sides. Record these figures on the Progress Chart provided in Appendix 4a, and calculate your body mass index (BMI) value according to Appendix 4b. There is, intentionally, only enough space on the Progress Chart for you to record this information every four weeks. Resist the urge to re-weigh yourself or take your measurements any more frequently than that! (BMI will be discussed later in the program, in Lessons I-12 and IV-4.)

TODAY'S THIRD ASSIGNMENT

ASSESS YOUR INTERNAL pH

Practice testing your urinary pH today. Then, starting tomorrow morning, start testing your first morning urine regularly. If you find your pH is too acidic, there are a number of things you can do to correct it, such as trying an ascorbic acid flush or making dietary changes to increase your alkalinity. *Note:* Internal pH is seldom too alkaline. An overly alkaline pH over an extended period of time would suggest a metabolic problem that should be addressed by a physician.

If your pH readings commonly fall below 6.5, incorporate the suggestions below into the prescribed daily menus. Remember that alkalinity reflects your body's mineral reserves; if these are very deficient, you must replenish them before you can restore alkalinity to your internal environment. Be patient. It may take several days, or even weeks, to bring your first morning urine up to the desired pH range of 7.0–7.5, but it's important, and you can do it. Following the Wings menus should then keep your pH in proper balance.

- Drink the juice of half a lemon or lime (or 1 teaspoon of apple-cider vinegar) in 8 ounces of water several times per day. Although it is commonly believed that citrus products are acidic, they actually produce an alkaline residue.

- Add a serving of lentils, sweet potatoes, or yams to your daily diet until alkalinity has been restored, and then enjoy a serving of one or more of these vegetables several times per week.

- Include one large serving of dark green vegetables per day. (Enjoy romaine or another dark green variety; iceberg lettuce doesn't count.)

- Enjoy a cup or two of miso soup daily. (Miso is available at health food stores or in supermarkets' whole-foods sections, and miso soup is easily prepared.)

- Enjoy at least two servings of watermelon or other fruits each day.

LESSON I-1 STUDY GUIDE

1. What are your goals for your Wings Program? Make these written goals as specific as you can, and make them very achievable.

2. What are some benefits you should experience within your first few weeks on the program?

3. Describe the guiding concepts of the Wings food plan. What will you eat this week? What foods will be eliminated and why?

4. Review page 236 in the Menus and Recipes section and design your own delicious Wings Breakfast Drink. Even better, share it with Wings by e-mail: Carol@flywithwings.com. Thanks!

_____

_____

_____

 HEALTH TIP

SKIN SUPPORT

Who doesn't want gorgeous, healthy skin?

- When you think of skin health, think of liver health. The skin is a major organ of detoxification, along with the liver, kidneys, colon, and lungs. If the liver is congested, more toxins will need to be eliminated through the skin, so keep the liver clean.

- Enjoy drinking Wings Klean Tea (see page 82) each day for internal cleansing. You may also try a daily cup of burdock tea or some capsules of burdock root. Burdock makes beautiful skin!

- Clean your face each morning and night with a natural cleanser that retains the moisturizing oils on the surface of the skin and doesn't disturb its normal pH. Look for skin-care products that nourish the skin: some of my favorites are made by Aubrey, Annemarie Borlind, and Zia.

✒ ADDITIONAL NOTES

_____

_____

_____

_____

_____

_____

_____

_____

_____

_____

_____

_____

_____

_____

_____

Lesson I-2. Achieve Your Wings Balance

At this point, most people who have been faithful to the Wings Program will have already begun to lose weight. Some will lose 5–10 pounds in the first week or ten days; others will lose just 1–2 pounds. This weight loss is typically water weight and a little fat weight. When you reduce the high-carbohydrate foods in your diet, such as bread and pasta, you often lose excess water. If you are one of the lucky ones who drop a significant amount of weight, good for you—but if not, remember that you're still making good progress.

Rapid weight loss will not usually continue past the two-week mark, however, and your body will settle down into losing fat weight at a slower rate: 1–1½ pounds per week is ideal. Don't get frustrated with losing weight slowly and steadily or be tempted to quit this program and look for some "quick and easy" diet plan. Remember that you didn't gain your weight overnight, so you won't lose it overnight. Slow, steady weight loss helps ensure your long-term, even permanent success.

? TODAY'S QUESTION

How did you do last week?

_____

_____

_____

Now that you've completed the first week of your program, how do you feel? Did you enjoy the new taste sensations in the Wings recipes and menus?

Did you experience any side effects of following this natural diet, or go through withdrawal as you eliminated some of your favorite "food toys"? Perhaps you had symptoms like headache, low energy, irritability, or depressed mood. Don't worry about it; within two or three days, the symptoms will disappear and you will feel wonderful.

Review your Food Diary. Did you fill it out each day and were you totally honest with yourself about what you ate and drank? What areas of your program need tightening up?

Was it difficult to fit these new meals and cooking instructions into your busy schedule? If so, don't be discouraged, because you can design techniques to help incorporate healthful meal planning into your lifestyle. Brainstorm with others about how to make the eating plan work for you.

BALANCED NUTRITION AT ITS BEST

Studying the eating habits of cultures around the world shows that "pre-Westernized" daily diets consisted of natural foods that provided a balance of protein, carbohydrates, fats, fiber, vitamins, and minerals. Although the portions and quantities of these nutrients differed greatly among pre-Western and older Western civilizations, the dietary theme throughout each culture was the consumption of natural foods. They ate "real food." The typical outcome was good health and good weight: obesity (and the health conditions that occur simultaneously with weight problems) was virtually nonexistent.

If we wish to enjoy that same level of health, it's important for us to eat in that same way. The conventional Western food pyramid recommends a diet that

✒ NOTES

_____

_____

_____

_____

_____

_____

is extremely heavy in grains and light in oils—but that isn't the way nature designed our food choices. So forget the food pyramid, unless you wish to be shaped like the food pyramid! What should our diet look like?

Proteins

Protein is an essential part of the diet. It yields some energy but functions primarily as a structural nutrient by providing amino acids, which are the building blocks of all proteins. Our bodies use dietary and endogenous amino acids (those stored or synthesized within the body) to construct muscles, blood vessels, skin, hormones, neurotransmitters, enzymes, and thousands of other tissues and compounds.

Protein must therefore be eaten daily, in amounts spread evenly throughout the day. Men require about 55–75 grams (g) of protein per day and women require about 45–65 g per day. If you are struggling with stress, facing illness, physically working very hard, exercising strenuously, pregnant or breastfeeding, or experiencing other unusual circumstances, you may require extra protein.

Protein is found in animal tissue like beef, fish, chicken, eggs, lamb, and so on, and is also found in nuts and seeds, legumes, tofu, and other vegetables. Animal sources typically provide about 9 g of protein per ounce, whereas the amount of protein in vegetable sources varies greatly. Most vegetable proteins do not provide all of the essential amino acids, that is, those amino acids that cannot be synthesized by the body and must be obtained from food. Many vegetarian sources of protein are also low in sulfur-bearing amino acids like L-cysteine and L-methionine, which are used by the liver in detoxification. (Vegetarianism is discussed in Lesson I-8.)

Carbohydrates

As energy sources for the body and brain, carbohydrates are critically important in the healthful diet. Carbohydrates are converted into blood sugar that is used to maintain cellular energy and to fuel the brain. When the blood sugar level drops too low as a result of dietary inadequacy or metabolic problems, the brain's fuel needs are not met. In response, the adrenal gland produces the hormone cortisol to help pull stored sugars out of the liver for immediate blood sugar elevation. Over time, the body's stress response dysregulates blood sugar and causes other metabolic problems.

Best-selling books have popularized low-carbohydrate diets over the past few years, but even though such diets induce rapid weight loss and little hunger, they are not good for the body or brain, especially when used over a long period of time (Lesson I-8).

Like proteins, carbohydrates must also be eaten daily, in moderate amounts spread throughout the day. The best sources of carbohydrates are vegetables and small amounts of fruit. We should eat seven or eight servings of vegetables per day, particularly non-starchy vegetables like the brightly colored varieties. I recommend limiting daily fruit intake to one serving of raw fresh fruit (but see the Wings Meal Plan, pages 24–25).

Although grains are rich in carbohydrates, I do not recommend using grains as a primary food source, with the exception of brown rice, minimal amounts of white rice, ancient grains like millet or quinoa, and tiny amounts of corn (if allergy is not a problem). You will find that grains appear only sparingly in the Wings recipes. Lesson I-10 discusses why eating grains can be so problematic for individuals who are seeking to improve their health and manage their weight.

Fats

Why did nature provide so much fat in natural foods? Fat is incredibly important in the diet because it contributes to the structure and functionality of every cell in the human body. Fat is wrapped around each nerve cell, protecting its insulating myelin sheath from damage and increasing the electrical potential of the nerve's transmission. Fats are a prime energy source for muscle tissue; fats are used to synthesize female and male hormones; fats keep the skin soft and pliable (wrinkle-resistant); and so on.

Dietary fat also helps keep the metabolism of the body "hot" or burning more calories. So when people embark on a low-fat diet, their metabolic rate quickly drops, making it more difficult to lose weight and keep it off (Lesson I-8).

Fats needn't be, and should not be, severely restricted, as long as they are natural fats found in vegetables, nuts and seeds, and animal protein. Natural fats should be abundantly enjoyed on a daily basis. Rancid or processed fats, however, are to be strictly avoided, as they damage the body and reduce your chances of losing weight. Rancid and processed fats include bacon, margarine, other hydrogenated oils, and foods cooked at high temperatures in fat that has been repeatedly reheated, as well as potato chips and other fatty snack foods.

Include small amounts of butter and lots of olive oil in your daily diet. Enjoy avocados, raw nuts and seeds, and flaxseed oil (in your Breakfast Drink, for example). Eat ocean-raised seafood that's rich in healthful omega-3 fatty acids. Sprinkle an olive-oil-based dressing on your salad each day. Snack on raw almonds or other nuts. Each of these foods is rich in essential fats that promote good health and weight loss.

Vitamins and Minerals

Vitamins and minerals are the micronutrients embedded in natural foods. More than seventy vitamins and minerals are known to be essential to human health. Micronutrients provide the metabolic energy to run the body and are necessary for every enzymatic reaction. They are also used in building structures like bone and muscle and compounds like hormones and neurotransmitters.

Sadly, most Westerners are deficient in many vitamins and minerals, and people who engage in prolonged and frequent dieting are at an even greater risk for nutrient deficiencies. I strongly recommend that you use a high-quality multivitamin-mineral supplement to make up for years of malnutrition or undernutrition, particularly if you have dieted frequently or recently.

Do You Need to Take Nutrient Supplements?

You need a dietary supplement that provides generous amounts of vitamins and minerals if you:

- Have dieted frequently or have embarked on extremely restricted diet plans
- Frequently feel tired
- Are frequently hungry, even after a meal
- Don't sleep well at night
- Have been diagnosed with any type of health condition
- Have weak nails or hair
- Can't lose your extra weight
- Have dry or rough skin
- Get sick frequently
- Are forgetful, depressed, moody, or mentally foggy
- Crave sugars, chocolate, alcoholic beverages, or any other sweet foods
- Crave fatty, salty, crunchy, or "harmful" foods
- Have any other unexplained symptoms

Any of these symptoms can indicate a vitamin and/or mineral deficiency. Ask your Wings nutritionist (go to the website www.flywithwings.com/pnc.html and click on MyProConnect) to recommend a daily supplement that provides an excellent nutrient base, or refer to the Resource Guide in the back of this book for recommendations.

QUESTIONS AND ANSWERS

At this point, people often have questions about how the program is working for them. Here are some common questions and their answers.

■ *I was hungry all week. Can I eat more food?*
If you are hungry, you may need to eat more food. Simply eat larger portions, or have four or five small meals daily, or try the delicious, balanced snacks in the Menus and Recipes section. Or, perhaps you are still eating too many carbohydrates. Carbohydrates stimulate hunger. Make sure you're not sneaking carbohydrate snacks between meals and that you are eating enough of the protein portion of the meal.

Another reason for inappropriate hunger is a food allergy. Lesson I-10 deals with food allergies, so for now, continue to follow the menus in the back of this book. Food addictions also commonly cause "false hunger" for the addictive foods you are no longer consuming; these sensations typically disappear in a few days.

If you're still eating hot or cold cereal, thinking it is a healthful breakfast, please note that cereals often stimulate hunger. You'll feel like eating all day! To solve your hunger problem, make sure your breakfast contains enough protein to balance the carbohydrates. Use the Wings Breakfast Drink for breakfast each morning, as it is an excellent tool for balancing blood sugar.

■ *Will I lose weight quicker if I'm hungry?*
Actually, no! There is no reason to be hungry on the Wings Program, and you will still lose weight.

■ *This is too much food! What if I can't eat this much?*
Simply cut back on your portions. Eat slowly and stop eating just when you are satisfied, not stuffed. But do not skip meals! It is important to keep your blood sugar steady throughout the day. This is best accomplished by eating small but regular meals, which helps your body burn calories more efficiently.

If you are accustomed to someone telling you exactly how much food to eat, forget it! I have no idea how much food you need, because each person is different. Your calorie requirements vary from day to day, depending on many factors. Learn to listen to your body.

■ *The recipes make too much food, but I don't want to throw it away. What should I do?*

The Wings meals are designed to be refrigerated or frozen and reheated at a later time. You don't have to prepare every single meal within the week; if you have leftovers, feel free to use them and skip meal preparation on a busy day. You may also choose to cut a recipe's yield in half before serving and use the leftover portion for lunch the next day.

■ *My family doesn't need to lose weight. Can they eat this food without losing weight?*
Absolutely! These recipes and menus are designed for the pleasure of the whole family. People who do not struggle with weight will not lose weight inappropriately, but they will experience better health, which is a terrific side effect!

And now, go to page 241 for your menus and recipes!

TODAY'S ASSIGNMENT

EXAMINE YOUR NUTRIENT BALANCE

As you complete your Food Diary this week, try to estimate how many grams of protein you require each day to feel satisfied. (One ounce of animal protein provides about 9 grams of protein.) Does the amount change from day to day? Record the amount(s) in your Food Diary. As you become more conscious of satisfying your protein requirement, keep your other nutrient needs in mind as well. How many vegetables are you eating? You should be enjoying seven or eight servings of vegetables each day (a serving size is about the size of your fist). Record this information too.

LESSON I-2 STUDY GUIDE

1. What are some common reasons for hunger on the Wings Program?

2. How do I determine how much food to eat?

3. I don't want to waste excess food. What should I do?

4. How much protein is required by the "average" man and woman? How do I translate this requirement into portion size?

5. What are some common side effects of the Wings Program and what are the solutions?

6. I lost several pounds this week! Will this rapid weight loss continue?

HEALTH TIP

ANTIAGING ANTIOXIDANTS

I don't mind the natural aging process—but I don't want premature aging. Think antioxidant nutrients!

- Make sure your diet is rich in brightly colored fruits and vegetables, because the natural pigments that give them their colors are a rich source of antioxidants.

- Consider supplementing your diet with other antioxidants like coenzyme Q_{10} (Q-Gel is a good source), Pycnogenol or grapeseed extract, L-carnitine, vitamin E, vitamin C, and a bioflavonoid complex. Each of these supplements is available at your local health food store.

Lesson I-3. Hold Me Accountable, Please!

One of the first tasks you undertook in this program was to write out your personal goals. Your goals probably include such items as "Lose weight," "Eat more healthfully," "Increase energy," or "Feel better about myself." You may have written, "Exercise faithfully" or, "Prepare better meals for me and my family." One thing is certain: you bought this book and started this program because you know you need to make changes. You need to get your life in order.

If you are going to fulfill your goals, you will need to put the Wings principles to use in your life. Don't be afraid to build accountability into your program. Two kinds of accountability are vital: group accountability and self-accountability. We often require the support of the first (group) while we develop the strength to maintain the second (self).

? TODAY'S QUESTION

What is accountability?

_____

_____

_____

_____

_____

The concept of accountability permeates nearly every pursuit in life. We are accountable to parents, spouses, neighbors, teachers, employers, stockholders, government, faith, and even children. We have responsibilities; we are answerable. No matter how old or how important we are, we never escape being held accountable to someone or for something.

Accountability is significant in any health-improvement pursuit because it keeps us on target while we develop new habits and new lifestyle patterns. Studies show that people who are made accountable in their weight-loss program have greatly increased chances of success. Accountability could be one of the main factors in your long-term success.

The Wings Program is not easy to follow. It has been called a hard-core program, and perhaps it is. We are used to ordering pizza or take-out Chinese food, stopping by the local fast-food restaurant, and relying on our favorite food toys. For many people, learning to prepare good, wholesome food instead can be a difficult adjustment to make.

Wings asks you to change lifelong habits, turn your back on the American junk-food culture, and start cooking again. The food plan asks you to spend more time in meal planning and preparation. Purchasing your vegetables from the produce section instead of buying the canned or frozen stuff means more peeling, washing, chopping, spinning, and sautéing. You are being reintroduced to your kitchen!

At first, you may be excited about these changes: you love the new foods in the Wings Program and your family enjoys them too. But more likely, you feel intimidated by the time and commitment required for meal preparation, and your family is fighting these changes because they enjoyed the pizza and take-out foods. Your kids beg for candy, cake, ice cream, and

✎ NOTES

_____

_____

_____

_____

_____

_____

soft drinks. Your husband refuses to eat your new meals, and so on. You may encounter many obstacles on your way to improved health and weight.

You can do it for a week or two. You're determined! But can you do it over the long haul, without much support from your family? Can you do it alone if you have to? Probably not! Let's be realistic. Change is difficult, even in ideal circumstances. There is a great deal of emotional baggage attached to our food selections; we often feel emotionally deprived if we can't have our favorite foods, especially if our kids are begging.

So we need help. We need someone to hold our hand and hold us (firmly) to our commitment. What kind of help do you need if you are going to be successful on this program? Will you be able to hold yourself accountable?

AN ACCOUNTABILITY PARTNER

The role of an accountability partner is simple: to help ensure that you live up to your commitment. Some people even join an accountability group; Wings is often taught in a group setting, and you can inquire at www.flywithwings.com about groups in your area. If joining such a group is not feasible, however, set up your own accountability partnership with your spouse, a trusted friend, or a healthcare professional. Know that you will have to report your progress weekly; this "fearful knowledge" helps keep you on track. A good accountability partner will be kind and supportive—but will not accept excuses! He or she *will* hold you to your commitment, lovingly and faithfully.

I recommend taking the following steps to establish your Wings accountability relationship:

1. Make a list of qualifications your partner must have (examples: unafraid to challenge my excuses, able to understand the program, agrees with my health goals, won't sabotage my program by offering me "treats" or "rewards," and so on).

2. Make a list of people who qualify for this role and might be willing to take on the task.

3. Make a list of exactly what you want your partner to do (examples: have a weekly meeting or talk via telephone, review my Food Diary and point out areas of weakness, brainstorm with me to find solutions to my challenges, and so on).

4. Set up meetings with prospective partners and bring your lists and this book. Once you've chosen your partner, he/she may want a copy of the book in order to go through the material with you.

5. Be prepared to be totally honest with your chosen accountability partner. He/she cannot help you without knowing the whole story.

6. Each week when you talk or get together, review the lesson together, review your goals and how you did with the program or lesson that week, and set up your next goal. Confirm your next meeting. Ask your partner for suggestions on how you can overcome your personal challenges.

An accountability relationship might function as follows: At your meeting, you share with your partner that your goal is to remain faithful to the Wings menus but that you're concerned because your family is uncooperative or your unrelenting time schedule doesn't readily allow the time you need for meal preparation. Together, you find two workable solutions to your challenge. You pledge to use those solutions to solve the problem that week. At your next meeting, you discuss freely how you did. If you blew it, you discuss why it was difficult, and together you review your plan to handle your problem. You may set up another set of goals to be completed in the week to follow, and so on, through the entire program.

SELF-ACCOUNTABILITY

Learning to become accountable to yourself is just as important as having an external accountability partner. After all, your accountability partner may not be with you for the rest of your life—but you will be. Just as children learn how to behave in public with their parents' coaching and then become well behaved even when mom and dad aren't looking over their shoulder, you will soon learn to hold yourself to your commitment. You will then learn to do the Wings Program, without even thinking about it, for the rest of your life. That is when you'll know you have achieved long-term success.

You, Yourself, and Your Food Diary

The most important element in self-accountability on this program is keeping an honest Food Diary. To do that successfully, hold yourself to the following rules:

1. Take your Food Diary everywhere and make entries in it whenever you eat or drink something. Record all water you drink, every breath mint, a sip of wine . . . everything that goes into your mouth!

2. Notice and record any symptoms you may experience so that you're able to identify possible food sensitivities. Remember: listen to your body.

3. Jot down any unusual circumstances that affect your food choices. For example, if an illness makes you unable to eat, write it down. If you attend a wedding and indulge in "forbidden foods," write it down. If you're stricken with uncontrollable cravings, write it down. This information will help you monitor your progress and pinpoint possible areas of weakness.

4. Once weekly, review your Food Diary, asking yourself the following questions: Am I on track with my goals? Am I following the program? What recurring or unusual difficulties am I experiencing, and how can I work my way through them? If you have any special circumstances, strategize with your accountability partner about how to overcome them.

Remember that you are learning new habits and breaking old ones. You are building your health one day, or even one meal, at a time. Give yourself a little grace if you slip—but then start anew. Stay faithful to the eating plan, use your Food Diary to its fullest potential, and you will be successful!

And now, go to page 245 for your menus and recipes!

 TODAY'S ASSIGNMENT

DEVELOP YOUR ACCOUNTABILITY

Get started on your accountability relationship immediately. Follow the steps listed in this lesson, and have your partnership established by the end of the week. Meanwhile, keep up with your Food Diary. Get into the habit of taking it with you and recording everything you eat or drink. Strengthen this good habit throughout the week!

LESSON 1-3 STUDY GUIDE

1. What are two important reasons for accountability?

2. How does keeping a Food Diary make you more accountable and therefore more likely to succeed in your Wings Program?

3. Discuss the benefits of self-accountability.

4. How do you keep an honest Food Diary?

HEALTH TIP

ALLERGY CONTROL

Struggling with allergies? Get control naturally! As you reduce the amount of allergens in your food (an allergen is any substance that triggers an allergic or immune system response), you'll "empty your allergic bucket," so to speak. You can reduce the symptoms of dietary and environmental allergies with products from the health food store:

• Freeze-dried stinging nettles are a great antihistamine.

• Pantothenic acid (1,000–2,000 milligrams) is excellent for stopping an allergic reaction immediately.

• The amino acid L-cysteine thins secreted mucus and promotes healing of the respiratory tract.

• To reduce your allergic potential, take the bioflavonoids quercetin and bromelain thirty minutes prior to each meal.

• Homeopathic remedies such as A. Vogel Allergy Relief are excellent for diminishing the symptoms of airborne allergy reactions.

Lesson I-4. Cheating, Binge Eating, and Other Deal Breakers

People of normal weight cannot imagine the social stigma borne by overweight or obese individuals—even those who only have a few pounds to lose feel the sting of society's scorn. Sadly, some of the most judgmental people are those who have successfully lost weight, those who have never struggled with weight, and those in the medical professions.

As a result, there is probably no segment of the population more ridden with guilt than the overweight. Every time they open their mouths to enjoy a morsel of food, they wonder whether people are watching them and thinking, "Why are they eating when they obviously have so much weight to lose?" They feel guilty when they shop for groceries or clothing. They feel guilty ordering food in a restaurant. They feel guilty if they take up too much space in the car or the airplane, in the church pew or the theater. The fact that people with weight-management problems are often driven by food compulsions that they cannot control does not help to relieve their guilt.

? **TODAY'S QUESTION**

Do you have food compulsions?

_____

_____

_____

_____

Do you have strong food cravings? Do you experience episodes of binge-eating behaviors? Are there any foods to which you feel truly addicted? What food can you simply *not* live without?

Dieters are encouraged to avoid fatty foods, sugary foods—indeed, all the foods that satisfy their emotional and physical hunger. They can usually suppress their longings for a while, in the hopes that they'll lose weight and feel better about themselves. But it is an unusual person who can avoid forbidden treats forever; in fact, you will see that this very process of self-denial sets up uncontrollable cravings.

WHERE DO FOOD CRAVINGS AND COMPULSIONS COME FROM?

If you listen to the "experts," they'll tell you that food cravings invariably stem from emotional deprivation or lack of self-control. Experts and authors often pile on these guilt messages, not realizing that many of our cravings for sugars, fats, or other foods are driven by our internal biochemistry. Sometimes, of course, we do eat for reasons that have nothing to do with biochemistry. But very often, food cravings are a message from your body to you.

Here is a list of some commonly craved foods and the underlying messages that can drive the compulsion to eat them. (*Note:* This list is by no means definitive or prescriptive.)

- Chocolate: magnesium deficiency

- Caffeine: stress, adrenal fatigue, or physical fatigue

- Breads and pastas: zinc deficiency

- Salty foods: stress or adrenal fatigue

- Sugary foods: chromium, zinc, and/or magnesium deficiency, fatigue, or stress

✎ **NOTES**

_____

_____

_____

_____

_____

_____

- Fatty foods: essential fatty acid deficiency
- Spicy foods: boredom or fatigue
- Crunchy foods: stress or repressed anger

Food cravings and compulsions can be related to internal fluctuations in nutrient stores, hormone activity, blood sugar levels, and neurotransmitter levels. As an example, consider the minerals magnesium, zinc, chromium, and vanadium, which are used in sugar metabolism and blood sugar regulation. Deficits in these key minerals (common in the dieting population) lead to problems regulating blood sugar and produce symptoms of hypoglycemia or diabetes—in fact, deficiencies in these nutrients have been causally linked to the onset of diabetes. And when our blood sugar level flags or becomes unstable, we tend to crave the carbohydrates that will boost it.

Zinc deficiency, in particular, often leads to cravings for bread and pasta or other refined carbohydrates, along with distaste for protein foods (especially animal proteins). Other symptoms include impaired wound healing, skin problems, poor nail and hair growth, and white spots on the fingernails; depression to the point of suicidal ideation; anger, aggressiveness, and hostility; and poor digestion.

Hormonal shifts lead to sugar cravings around the onset of menses. Module III covers female hormones in depth and explores their effects on eating behaviors, but for now it is simply important to realize that women commonly crave sweets and chocolate around the time of their period, in response to the normal female cycle.

Binge Eating

Binge eating is more common than you may realize. Interesting research dating back to the end of World War II showed that binge eating might be triggered by periods of severe starvation. Most of us in this country don't typically experience starvation—but dieting is, to the body, very much like forced starvation.

Dieters commonly deprive their bodies of calories and nutrients for long periods of time. The body often reacts to deprivation by slowing its metabolism via hypothyroidism (that is, reduced hormone secretion by the thyroid gland), which, in turn, frequently triggers binge-eating episodes. Researchers believe that binge eating may be the body's way of stimulating thyroid function to restore normal metabolism. Unfortunately, it doesn't work very well. You are better served by *never dieting*, by eating regular,

Chocolate Cravings—and Magnesium?

As some authors have asserted, we may eat chocolate when we feel emotionally deprived. Interestingly, magnesium deficiency also causes numerous mental and/or emotional conditions that feel much like emotional deprivation. Consider the following list of classical magnesium-deficiency symptoms:

- Being easily depressed or discouraged
- Emotional ups and downs
- Easily aroused anger
- Unusual sensitivity to loud noises and sounds
- Anxiety/panic attacks
- Heart palpitations and/or irregular heartbeat
- Constipation (fewer than two easy bowel movements per day)
- Cravings for chocolate and/or other sweets
- Insomnia (waking in the middle of the night and being unable to get back to sleep)
- Fatigue
- Short-term memory loss
- Muscle tremors, twitches, and/or cramping

nutrient-dense meals, and by providing your body with superior nutrition, even when there is a need to lose weight (in other words, by following the Wings Program!).

Food Allergy, Addiction, and Withdrawal

Cravings can also be stimulated by food allergies. For reasons that are not fully understood, the body tries to relieve the discomfort of an allergic reaction by craving the very thing that caused it. If your cravings are stimulated by a food allergy or sensitivity (Lesson I-10), you may require three days of total abstinence from that food to clear the reaction and stop the cravings. Getting through this "withdrawal" period can be difficult for some people, and you may even experience true withdrawal symptoms (such as nervousness, headaches, body aches and pains, heart palpitations, sweating, or fatigue). You should not, however, indulge in the food to relieve your symptoms, or the addiction will never be broken.

SOLUTIONS TO CRAVING AND BINGEING

In Lesson II-2, you will learn more about how important it is to feed the body rather than to try to suppress hunger or other signals. For now, the important point to remember is that when your body is adequately nourished, you will no longer be driven by food cravings or the need to binge eat. By using these simple techniques, you really can solve the problems of craving and bingeing, forever.

Don't Suppress—Satisfy!

Get off to a good start every morning. You should have your first meal of the day within one hour of awakening. Be sure to balance protein, carbohydrates, and fats in that morning meal; if your breakfast is too high in carbohydrates, you will feel the need to "stuff and munch" all day. Use the Wings Breakfast Drink for blood sugar balance and hunger satisfaction.

Make sure you are well nourished in the essential vitamins and minerals. Take a really good multivitamin-mineral supplement that provides adequate amounts of chromium (up to 1,000 micrograms per day), magnesium glycinate (up to 300 milligrams per day), and zinc (up to 30 milligrams per day). If, for example, you are a woman who craves chocolate and/or other sweets around "that time of the month," ensure that your diet is adequate in magnesium throughout the month. As much as 65 percent of Americans may be magnesium deficient, and you are probably in that category.

Can't get ice cream out of your mind? A craving can be very powerful, and it may not be enough for you to say, "I just won't eat it!" Talk to your Wings nutritionist about how to make up for the years of malnutrition that are driving your food cravings or binge eating: you can learn to satisfy these compulsions from within. I often recommend using natural formulas that are designed to ease cravings with herbs and targeted nutrients. (For a consultation, go to the website www.flywithwings.com/pnc.html and click on MyProConnect.)

You cannot grit your teeth and hope to overcome a craving issue by sheer willpower; instead, you must listen to the message and meet your body's needs. Go through the list of food cravings on pages 19–20 to discover your own body's messages. If you crave fatty foods, for example, make sure to eat enough healthful fats like butter, olive oil, macadamia nut oil, flaxseed oil, and so on. One of the best cures for a fat craving is eating half of an avocado slathered with a teaspoon of olive oil, a splash of balsamic vinegar, and a pinch of kosher salt—works nearly every time.

If you are eating because of stress (Lesson III-4), solve the stress problem. If you are eating to increase energy, increase energy naturally by following the Wings Program, taking a good-quality dietary supplement for extra nutritional support, getting plenty of sleep each night, and reducing your workload. Fatigue is an important message, so don't push through it: *rest*.

Eliminate Those Allergens

If you are still eating foods to which you are reactive, you may be craving them as a result of the allergy. Be especially careful to eliminate all wheat, corn, and dairy products, which are the most common triggers of dietary allergy; soy, chocolate, eggs, and citrus are also highly allergenic. Remember that the unpleasant symptoms associated with eliminating allergens will disappear after total abstinence of about three days, so push through it. Be faithful in sticking to your program and you'll soon be free of the addiction.

And now, go to page 250 for your menus and recipes!

 TODAY'S ASSIGNMENT

ADDRESS YOUR FOOD COMPULSIONS

Don't just grit your teeth and suffer. Write a plan of action to deal with cravings and bingeing (see Lesson I-4 Study Guide, on the next page). Contact your Wings nutritionist today for help in resolving your underlying nutrient deficiencies. Start immediately!

Learn to listen to your body, not only your sensory organs. If your mouth is screaming, "Feed me!" listen more carefully to those internal signals. Are you truly hungry for a forbidden food—or could the craving be satisfied another way? Are you actually just tired? Instead of eating sugary foods to increase your energy, rest. Are you eating because you are lonely? (Emotional eating is discussed in Lessons III-4, III-8, and IV-8.)

Whenever you feel the need to eat even though you are not truly hungry, try one or more of the following nonfood techniques to get through the false hunger or cravings:

- Take a nap
- Punch a pillow
- Take a walk

▪ Sip herbal tea

▪ Get a massage

▪ Listen to music (and dance a little)

▪ Call a friend

▪ Read a book

▪ Visit a neighbor

▪ Brush your teeth

▪ Write a letter

▪ Go to work

▪ Kiss your spouse or hug your kids

▪ Rub your feet

LESSON 1-4 STUDY GUIDE

1. What are some of the messages that your body is sending through food cravings?

2. What are the most common food allergens, and how do they stimulate eating behaviors?

3. Identify a common cause of binge-eating episodes, and describe how to resolve it.

4. List two or three dietary supplements that can help reduce food cravings.

5. How does low blood sugar affect eating behaviors and food cravings?

6. Write out your personal plan for eliminating your food cravings and compulsions.

HEALTH TIP

ANXIETY AND PANIC

Are you prone to feelings of anxiety and panic? Try the following tips:

• Make sure your dietary supplements provide adequate amounts of magnesium (up to 500 milligrams per day). For best results, magnesium should be taken in the morning or evening and apart from calcium supplements.

• Several herbs including kava kava and passionflower help reduce anxiety and panic attacks. Valerian root is also excellent, particularly when taken in the evening to promote restful sleep. One of the best herbal products on the market for anxiety is a kava kava–California poppy blend from the Eclectic Institute (www.eclecticherb.com).

• Gamma aminobutyric acid or GABA (an amino acid) taken with the B-complex vitamin inositol has a soothing effect and is particularly helpful for people with mild forms of obsessive-compulsive disorder.

• Avoid caffeine at any time of the day and avoid products containing the herbs ephedra (also called ma huang, and now banned by the U.S. Food and Drug Administration) or guarana. These highly stimulating substances often trigger anxiety attacks.

Lesson I-5. The Real-Food Plan

I learned a real lesson in appetite satisfaction at a church event. I teach a middle-school class on a weeknight, and the kids have dinner as part of the program. Mind you, it isn't a meal I would prepare and serve—it's all packaged, "dead" foods—so I usually eat before the class. One night, too busy to eat ahead of time, I sat down at the table with the kids and stared at their food. "Come on, Carol," I said to myself, "You can eat this. Don't be a food Nazi! It won't hurt you this once."

I loaded my plate with what the kids were having: spaghetti with canned tomato sauce, iceberg lettuce with artificial dressing, canned string beans, and artificially flavored garlic bread. I'd given myself a large portion because I was very hungry, but after cleaning my plate, I was just as hungry as when I started. So I heaped it high again, ate the entire amount—and found that my hunger had still not abated. Suddenly, I realized why Americans eat so much: our bodies are not satisfied because they haven't been *fed*, even on 2,000 calories a day!

❓ TODAY'S QUESTION

What are you eating?

_____

_____

_____

_____

Whenever you mention that you are on a diet, people ask, "What kind of diet is it? Low-fat, high-protein, high-carbohydrate?" The question is never, "What kind of eating program meets your nutritional requirements?" Rather, it is, "What kind of diet do you believe in?"

As mentioned earlier in this book, the current diet culture has become very dogmatic, based on one or another belief system or trend rather than on good nutrition. You will see that a dietary belief system without the solid science and practical clinical experience to back it up is worthless. You'll also see that our diet culture is making us unhealthy—and fatter. If you want to lose weight and keep it off, you must never go on a diet again!

FOOD THEN AND NOW

What did you eat before you began this program? If you followed the American junk-food/fast-food culture, it wasn't good for you. Within the past fifty years, a huge dietary transformation has taken place, changing our foods from natural, whole foods to synthetic, highly processed pseudo-foods. We no longer eat from the earth. We have nearly lost sight of what constitutes "real food." Is it a bottle of Pepsi? A bag of potato chips? A toasted bagel? A can of orange slices? Other than stacking on pounds of unwanted weight, these highly processed foods do nothing for our bodies because they are nutrient bare. They do not satisfy the needs of the body. Some of them actually poison us.

Real food is fresh vegetables—grown in rich soil and prepared fresh from the garden or (worst case) the supermarket—served raw or lightly steamed and flavored with fresh herbs. Real food is fresh fish, chicken, beef, lamb, or other animal meats. Real food is fresh fruit, picked in season from the tree or vine. It

✒ NOTES

_____

_____

_____

_____

_____

_____

is butter and olive oil and raw nuts and seeds. It is fresh water or water infused with fresh herbs or fruits. Real food is vibrant in color, taste, and aroma. It doesn't mislead your palate with the artificial stimulation of processed foods spiked with monosodium glutamate (MSG) and other flavor enhancers. It excites your *real* taste buds—the ones that long for fulfillment.

Real Food Versus "Pseudo-Food"

Food used to be brilliantly colored fruits and vegetables, rich brown grains, milk and butter, lean game meats, and plump fish wrestled from living rivers and oceans. Food used to be plucked from the garden after a summer of planting, fertilizing, raking and weeding. It used to have roots deeply imbedded in soil that nearly pulsated with life forms that enriched the earth. Food used to feed on tender green plants and drink out of pristine streams that sparkled with life from the sun.

Food used to be something we ate to endow strength to our bodies, to heal us when we were sick, to satisfy an appetite at the end of a day filled with purpose and work. We ate to satisfy a need that arose from deep within. We ate when we were hungry, and ate food that satisfied that hunger.

Food *is* different now.

Now, what we are mostly sold is packages, boxes, artificial flavors, coloring agents, and pseudo-foods that strip the body, and leave the brain poverty-stricken. The product is colorful and flavorful, but not from natural goodness. The colors come from a chemist's beaker, from FD&C Blue No. 1, Red No. 40, and Yellow No. 5 or from cochineal (from the female insect *Coccus cacti* of the West Indies). The flavor comes from allyl anthranilate or isopulegol or linalyl benzoate or methyl delta-ionone, while gravies and sauces are thickened with wood fiber and emulsified by dioctyl sodium sulfosuccinate. While some of these agents have been tested for carcinogenic properties, virtually none have been studied to learn their impacts on brain chemistry.

Instead of being eaten when we are physically hungry, food is now consumed to satisfy artificial cravings generated by a brain that isn't working right and whose receptor sites beg for synthetic stimulation from chemicals. We eat but we're never satisfied. We're full but we aren't contented.

From Carol Simontacchi, *The Crazy Makers: How the Food Industry Is Destroying Our Minds and Harming Our Children.* (New York, NY: Jeremy P. Tarcher/Penguin, 2000, page 2)

Food Principles for Healthful Weight Management

1. The body cannot lose weight if it is chronically malnourished. When the nutrients needed to convert food into energy are missing or in short supply, the body cannot complete the conversion process and can only turn food into limited amounts of energy and stored fat.

2. Synthetic or highly processed food is nutrient poor or even toxic to the body. Only natural food can provide the fundamental building blocks of health.

3. When natural food is provided to the body, the body will rebuild its health and will lose its excess weight after homeostasis (self-maintained balance) is restored.

THE WINGS MEAL PLAN

Today, I formally introduce the Wings Program meal plan!

When you think of the word "diet," you simultaneously think "temporary." When you think of dieting, you say to yourself, "Just until I get the weight off . . . I can do this for a little while . . . " But I am not selling a diet. I am not interested in teaching a cute little program that sounds glitzy and unusual. I am interested in promoting lifelong health and vitality. You will notice that I purposely avoid the use of the word "diet" when referring to the Wings plan: I call it a meal plan or an eating plan or a food plan. It isn't a diet!

You saw a sketch of the plan in Lesson I-1, we've waltzed around the edges of the discussion for a few weeks, and you've been experimenting with some new foods in these first few weeks of using the Menus and Recipes section. Now you will learn more specific details about how to eat—and eat well—for the rest of your life.

Remember These Simple Rules

You'll find that people in the Wings Program really enjoy food! We talk about it a lot and share recipes and cooking tips. We eat a wide (and sometimes wild) variety of foods bursting with flavor and nutrition. There is nothing Spartan or diet-like about the Wings meal plan!

Plenty of Protein

Protein is included in each meal and snack. The source can be animal (fish, chicken, turkey, beef, eggs, lamb, veal, and so on) or vegetarian (beans, nuts, seeds, and so on). You are encouraged to purchase fresh organic sources of protein without growth hormone, antibiotics, or other chemicals whenever possible.

Lots of Vegetables

You are encouraged to eat seven or eight servings of raw or lightly cooked fresh vegetables per day. I discourage you from choosing canned or frozen vegetables, because the processing and storage of these foods has already destroyed much of their nutrient content, leaving little but empty calories.

A Few Fruits

Fruits are allowed in small amounts, as in one or two servings of fresh fruit per day. Canned or frozen fruits and juices are not allowed for the same reason that processed vegetables are discouraged (see above). Wings does make two exceptions, however, to those limits: (1) During the summer, when fruit is gloriously abundant and you need cooling foods for the hot weather, you may indulge more freely in fresh seasonal fruit. (2) In the Wings Breakfast Drink, you may use unsweetened frozen fruit and minimal amounts of fruit juice to add carbohydrates to the meal.

No Artificial Anything

Artificial sweeteners and other artificial flavoring or coloring agents are strictly forbidden, as they destroy your health. They also set you up for weight-loss failure: artificial sweeteners have been causally linked to increased overweight and obesity, as well as many neurological problems. (For more information about the impact of artificial sweeteners, MSG, and other chemicals on the human brain and body, read my book *The Crazy Makers: How the Food Industry Is Destroying Our Minds and Harming Our Children* [New York, NY: Jeremy P. Tarcher/Penguin, 2000].)

Cool, Clear Water

The only beverages allowed are pure water and herbal teas. All other beverages are "anti-nutrients" that pull nutrients from the body and cause weight gain and other health problems. Every day, you are encouraged to drink, in ounces of water, half of your total body weight in pounds; for example, if you weigh 150 pounds, you need to drink half of 150, or 75 ounces of water daily. If you find water too plain, squeeze half of a fresh lemon or lime into it.

Training Wheels

This all sounds simple on paper but I know it can be challenging at first, so I strongly urge you to eat nothing but the meals suggested in the Menus and Recipes section for your first sixty days on the Wings Program. The purpose of this is to provide you with a primer or guide (or training wheels) while you learn to avoid common "food traps" and develop new nutritional habits. At the conclusion of those sixty days, you'll have more latitude in your food choices.

Regaining Your Natural Balance

As you learn to enjoy natural foods, your body will slowly regain its nutritional balance and begin to lose excess weight. Ideally, people lose about 10–15 pounds within the first sixty days of the Wings Program, and then their weight loss levels out to about ¹/₂–1 pound per week. At this point, they must begin to address other issues of weight management and meet the total needs of the body. Weight challenges are seldom simply dietary: other issues are almost always present, complicating the weight-loss picture. There is a lot of material to cover in this program— but support and counsel are provided throughout the entire forty-nine weeks. If you wish, we will hold your hand through the whole process!

Personal Portion Control

I do not tell you how much to eat because I simply don't know. Each person's calorie and nutrient requirements are different and may change from day to day or from week to week. I urge you to eat slowly, chew thoroughly, and listen to your body! Stop eating when you feel satisfied, *not* full, even if there is still food on your plate—it is no more wasteful to throw food into the garbage than to eat it if you don't need it. Take smaller portions. Share an entrée with a friend. Make each meal a pleasurable, happy time. Relax while you're eating! You'll find that you are satisfied on far less food than you imagine you need.

How Should You Feel on the Wings Meal Plan?

What should you expect now that you've embarked on this program of health and nutrition?

You should have more energy, especially in the middle of the afternoon and throughout the evening. You should be sleeping well at night and awakening more refreshed in the morning. Food cravings should be reduced, and compulsions to binge eat should be reduced or eliminated. Aches and pains are probably disappearing; headaches may be disappearing or lessening in intensity and frequency. Your fingernails and hair should be growing stronger and faster. Your constipation problem should be solved—if not, make sure you drink enough water, eat enough fiber (or take a fiber supplement), and consume an adequate amount of oils as well as magnesium and other minerals. (Constipation is discussed further in Lesson II-3.)

And now, go to page 253 for your menus and recipes!

 ## TODAY'S ASSIGNMENT

GIVE YOURSELF A FOOD CHECK-UP

Review your Food Diary carefully. Now that you understand the program more clearly, are you following the guidelines? Are you using the Menus and Recipes section? List the areas of your program that need to be tightened up, and get to work on them now. Then, invite friends over for a festive Wings dinner—they won't believe these are weight-loss foods!

It is also time to take your weight and BMI measurements once again, making sure to measure yourself in the same place as before (see inset below to refresh your memory), and record these data in your Progress Chart (Appendix 4a).

Measuring Up

Weigh yourself, and then take five girth measurements: bust at the largest point, waist at two inches above the navel, hips at the largest point, and right and left thigh circumference at the point where your extended fingertips reach with your arms hanging down at your sides. Record these figures, and your calculated BMI value, on your Progress Chart.

LESSON I-5 STUDY GUIDE

1. Why can't you lose weight if you are struggling with chronic malnutrition? What does malnutrition have to do with subsequent weight gain?

2. List the eight main rules of the Wings food plan.

3. What are the only beverages allowed on the Wings Program, and why?

4. What is "ideal weight loss" on this program? How much should you expect to lose each week?

5. Are you following the Wings Program carefully? If so, what benefits have you achieved? What goals are being met?

HEALTH TIP

IMPROVING APPETITE

How is your appetite? Although it may seem strange to include information about appetite improvement in a weight-loss curriculum, a healthy appetite is a sign of a healthy body. To improve your appetite:

• Make sure your diet is adequate in B-complex vitamins and zinc.

• Use digestive enzymes or digestive enhancers from your local health food store.

• Thirty minutes before each meal, drink tea made from ginger root or fennel seed. To brew, mince several slices of fresh ginger or measure 1 heaping teaspoon of fennel seed, put the ingredient into a mug, pour boiling water over it, and let the tea steep for several minutes (once it is brewed, chew or discard the ginger or fennel seed). Enjoy the tea when it has cooled enough to drink.

Lesson I-6. Let's Go Out Tonight!

Eating out has always been a challenge for dieters. Can they stay on their diets if they go to a restaurant or, even worse, to someone else's house for a meal? It is often during these times of change that people give up their diets "temporarily," but then find it difficult to get back on track. And when you diet, you often feel that your eating plan is temporary anyway, so why not "fall off the wagon" just once, because, after all, you aren't going to be eating like this forever . . . except that with the Wings Program, you are. Why not make this a permanent part of your lifestyle when you feel—and look—so wonderful?

? TODAY'S QUESTION

Are you committed to staying on the program?

One of the challenges of the Wings Program is planting within your heart the seeds of permanent lifestyle change, teaching you how to be healthy *forever*. Remember the slogan, "Weight Success for a Lifetime"? This isn't just a clever saying; this is the core of the program! With that in mind, you need to learn how to eat healthfully wherever you go.

Fortunately, it isn't difficult to eat healthful foods,

even on the road or at a friend's house. It just takes a little information (which you'll receive today) and a little planning (I'll help with that, too). You supply the desire and the positive attitude.

Keep in mind that the availability of natural ingredients and foods is usually not the problem. If there is a problem, it is an attitude problem. Most challenges of eating out can be met if approached with an attitude of exploration, creativity, and desire to make it work. You have every opportunity to succeed!

RESTAURANT RULES

Your spouse is taking you out to dinner. Your mother wants you to meet her for lunch. How can you stay on your program during these special events?

Choose Your Eatery Wisely

Don't go to a pasta place, a fast-food restaurant, or an establishment that serves "low-end" food. Don't go to a "greasy spoon." Bagel shops are off-limits, as are coffee shops. They serve highly processed high-carbohydrate foods with little to no protein selection. Instead, choose a restaurant that specializes in fresh vegetables (salads or lightly steamed vegetables) and fresh protein (fish, chicken, beef, lamb, venison, and so on). There are many places like this, and fortunately "gourmet" restaurants are flourishing in our communities.

Take Charge

Ask that the bread be left off the table. Ask for water with a wedge of lime or lemon for added zest. Request that an extra serving of vegetables or a salad be substituted for the mashed potatoes or other starchy side dish. If substitutions are not permitted, ask that the starch be left off the plate altogether, or ask for

✒ NOTES

---

only a tiny portion so you aren't tempted to over-indulge.

Share

Appetizers can be wonderful but if you nibble too much at the beginning you'll eat too much in the overall meal. I frequently order one or two appetizers for the table and then split an entrée with my spouse or friend. Although some restaurants add a sharing charge, it's worth the extra dollars to reduce the temptation to overeat.

Eat Out *and* Take Out

If no one wants to share and your entrée is too large, ask for a take-home box and package half of the meal before you begin to eat. Enjoy it for lunch the next day. (Thanks to my kids, I seldom get the opportunity to enjoy my own leftovers!)

Don't Gobble

When choosing the parts of your meal, order a salad first, then a protein entrée with a vegetable side dish. Feel free to eat as much as you wish but stop eating before you feel full. Remember to eat slowly and chew thoroughly. Did your mother tell you it was wrong to leave food on your plate? Gluttony is wrong: leaving food on your plate isn't.

Experiment with New Flavors and Foods

One of the joys of dining in a restaurant is the pleasure of trying new foods. Go for it! Don't try to make it a low-fat meal, and don't opt for artificially manipulated foods. Just eat real foods in the proportions of the Wings Program.

Shun Goopy Salad Dressings

Ranch dressing, for example, is spiked with MSG. That's why it tastes so good! I ask instead for olive oil and balsamic vinegar to be brought to the table (not every restaurant stocks balsamic, so it's often red-wine vinegar but that's alright), and sometimes for a pinch of kosher salt too.

Ask Yourself the Sweet Question

If your dinner partner wants dessert and you feel you can handle it, just take one or two bites of his/her dessert. You'll find that even if you do want something sweet to conclude your meal, you'll be satisfied with a bite or two. More than that and you won't feel well—trust me! If, however, you are truly addicted to sweets, ask the server not to bring the dessert tray to the table. Do not even take that first bite: avoid dessert altogether, because it may start you down a path that is difficult to reverse.

Sometimes you can satisfy your sweet tooth with a sip of wine or a flavored decaffeinated coffee. An occasional glass of red wine is good for the heart and may be enjoyed without guilt. And although I really don't recommend coffee, even decaf, it can provide the once-a-week treat at the close of a special meal. Don't feel you have to be completely Spartan, but don't jeopardize your program either.

Follow Your Nose

When I walk into a restaurant, I sniff the air. Do I smell rancid fat or other suspicious odors? Let your nose be your guide! Learn to recognize musty or other unpleasant smells, and leave immediately if you notice them.

INVITATION INSTRUCTIONS

It is, admittedly, more difficult to follow the program when you are at someone's home for a dinner party, a cocktail party, or a work party—even at a church supper or at a meeting with food involved. You don't want to be rude or presumptuous by asking special favors at special occasions, especially if your host is someone other than a dear friend. Still, there are many ways to get through these events without totally blowing it nutritionally. Try these suggestions:

- If you are invited to an event where you expect to find snacks or hors d'oeuvres, eat well before you go. If you plan to enjoy a glass of wine or other sugary beverages at the party, focus on proteins before you leave home. Do *not* go to a party hungry!

- Whether it's going to be a full meal or casual refreshments, you can probably find out ahead of time what will be served. If it fits with your program, great! If not, make sure to eat beforehand.

- If drinks are being served, ask your host for a glass of water or sparkling water and make it festive with a slice of lemon or lime. No one will notice that you are not drinking the punch or other alcoholic beverage.

- If your host serves a fresh vegetable platter, enjoy it freely. Load your plate with fresh veggies and a little dressing for flavoring and no one will notice that you are not frequenting the cheese platter, the fresh breads, the chips and dip, or other "party favors" that aren't good for you.

- If you are served a high-carbohydrate dinner (pasta, for example) and you want to eat just enough so that your host is not offended, nibble around the edges. Don't feel you have to polish off something that isn't good for you just because everyone else is indulging.

- When I go to a potluck dinner, I bring foods that I can eat and happily dole them out. (People often look on my plate and follow my lead.) Many of the Wings dishes can easily be transported to a potluck and your friends will enjoy your "diet foods"—so be ready to share your recipes!

- If you are close to your host, you may feel comfortable enough to explain your special needs. If not, saying "it's doctor's orders" can often pave your way. Most of the time, your needs will be cheerfully accommodated.

Don't Be Embarrassed

Above all, don't feel embarrassed or uncomfortable about making your food preferences known. We all have challenges in life; your challenge happens to be dietary. That isn't the worst circumstance in the world. You simply have to plan ahead. Most people are happy to accommodate your requests, so just ask.

FORGIVE YOURSELF

Occasionally, you will eat something that is not in the Wings food plan. That is okay! Give yourself a little grace to indulge once in a while. You are permitted to eat a treat occasionally, so don't feel guilty—and don't feel as though you have blown your whole program. If you go out with family or friends and have a piece of pie or an extra glass of wine, remind yourself, "It was just for tonight. Now I'm back on the program. No harm done." Believe me when I tell you that your body can tolerate little deviations without adding weight, as long as these deviations are infrequent and small and you get immediately back on the program.

And now, go to page 255 for your menus and recipes!

 TODAY'S ASSIGNMENT

ANTICIPATE AND PLAN AHEAD

Make a list of the occasional situations that will tempt you to forsake your meal plan. Brainstorm with your accountability partner about what you can do to make good food selections, even in these challenging situations.

Then, stick to your plan! Plan, plan, plan! Take charge of what goes into your mouth! And don't feel sorry for yourself that you can't indulge in what everyone else is eating. Chances are they are overweight, in poor health, and envious of your vibrant health. You are building your health for the future and that's a great thing!

LESSON I-6 STUDY GUIDE

1. What does it mean to say, "Staying on the program is more a matter of attitude than availability"?

_____

_____

_____

2. What types of restaurants will you select when eating out? Make a list of ten restaurants that serve your new kind of food.

_____

_____

_____

3. What will you say to the server who brings the bread or dessert tray to the table?

_____

_____

_____

4. What proactive steps will you take before attending a party or other social event?

_____

_____

HEALTH TIP

ANTI-INFLAMMATORY SUPPLEMENTS

Achy bones and joints? Fleeting inflammations? As you reduce your consumption of allergenic foods by following the Wings Program, many aches and pains will disappear, because the allergic triggers that stimulate inflammation are being eliminated; for example, you should notice fewer "arthritic symptoms" as you progress further into the program. A number of nutritional supplements can also be helpful against inflammation and related pain:

- Bromelain (pineapple enzyme) is an excellent anti-inflammatory agent. For best utilization, take four to six capsules on an empty stomach.

- Fish body oil, also called salmon oil, is a source of essential fatty acids such as EPA (short for eicosapentaenoic acid). Use up to 10 grams of this oil per day to reduce inflammation.

- Glucosamine sulfate (a naturally occurring amino-sugar combination) is important for the formation of bones, tendons, ligaments, and cartilage, as well as for the synovial fluid that lubricates them. Studies show that joint pain is gradually eased when 1,500 milligrams per day of glucosamine sulfate is taken over a long period of time.

- In addition to being a natural anti-inflammatory, Pycnogenol (grapeseed extract) is a powerful free-radical scavenger. Free radicals, which are highly reactive molecules that damage cell membranes and even DNA, are causally linked to premature aging and many degenerative diseases, including arthritis. Scavenging anti-inflammatories like Pycnogenol can be very helpful in dampening free-radical production, subsequently easing inflammation and pain.

- A new anti-inflammatory product, SierraSil, is a combination of minerals mined from the Sierra Nevada Mountains. Preliminary research and clinical observations indicate that these minerals can reduce the pain of many inflammatory conditions by dampening the trigger to inflammation. For more information, visit the website www.sierrasil.com, or ask at your local health food store.

ADDITIONAL NOTES

Lesson I-7. A Trip through the Supermarket

We often feel that strolling through the supermarket is like strolling through a minefield. Dangerous traps are set everywhere around us. It is no accident that the worst, junkiest foods are displayed most prominently, because these nonfoods provide the biggest profit margins for the supermarket. Don't kid yourself—supermarkets have no interest in building your health; they are interested in making money. So don't let the marketers decide what you buy. Take charge of your mouth!

? TODAY'S QUESTION

Is grocery shopping fun or frustrating?

_____

_____

_____

_____

What is your favorite food to buy in the supermarket? What sections of the supermarket do you (or should you) avoid? How much time does it take you to do the grocery shopping?

GENERAL SHOPPING TIPS

We have become so accustomed to eating altered food that we have lost our ability to choose healthful foods even when we go grocery shopping. Should I purchase potato chips or corn chips? Are diet soft drinks better than regular soft drinks? What kinds of snacks are best? Should I buy the low-fat or the nonfat mayonnaise? Are frozen vegetables better than canned?

Get Fresh

Choose fresh produce instead of canned or frozen. By its very nature, processing food for preservation (whether by canning or freezing) causes nutrient loss. What's more, chemicals are often added in the process. One of your goals in eating on the Wings Program is to make every bite count toward good nutrition and good health. You'll soon learn to love the tastes and aromas of fresh fruits and vegetables and wonder what you ever saw in their canned or frozen counterparts.

Instead of dried herbs, buy fresh herbs—they taste wonderful! You probably won't use them quickly enough to keep them from spoiling, so wash and dry them gently and freeze them in tightly fastened freezer bags. When a recipe calls for fresh herbs, you can simply break off the amount you need.

Go to the Garden

Stroll through the fresh produce section and allow yourself to be tempted by the bright colors and pleasing aromas. Try a new vegetable or fruit every week, even if it isn't specifically listed in your Wings menus. Vegetables are always a healthful choice and can be freely enjoyed without fear of gaining weight or disrupting your program.

Avoid the Aisles of Temptation

Aisles of the supermarket you should avoid include cereal, fruit juice, soft drink, baking, chip and cracker,

✐ NOTES

_____

_____

_____

_____

_____

_____

candy and cookie, bread, sale-rack or sale-end displays, frozen, and alcohol. This leaves only the perimeter, which contains fresh produce, meats, and odds and ends like brown rice and legumes. That's about it. See how quickly you can get your shopping done?

Find Your Inner Gourmet

I enjoy browsing through the gourmet section for delicacies like pesto, roasted peppers, olive tapénades, and the like. I use the pesto in Homemade Hummus (page 241) and my "world famous" Salmon Rice Salad (well, it's famous in my small world; page 247), the peppers and tapénades on salads, and so on. Again, don't be afraid of food! Don't be afraid to try new flavors, as long you avoid artificial ingredients.

Never Shop Hungry

You've heard that before, haven't you? When you're hungry, everything sounds and looks good. You'll make little compromises that will sabotage your program. Always shop on a fully satisfied stomach.

Stick to Your List

One of the hardest habits to break while shopping for groceries is succumbing to the lure of impulse items— or to pressure from family members. Always shop with a grocery list and hold yourself to it. Do not allow your eyes to wander lustfully over the "forbidden" sections. Do not allow your spouse or your kids to wheedle, beg, or coerce you into buying something you shouldn't.

What mother hasn't done her shopping with a child pulling on her leg and wailing, "Please Mommy, can I have this? Can I have that? Please, Mommy, please!" If your kids won't respect your expressed boundaries, don't take them with you. Don't be afraid

---

Cutting Food-Prep and Clean-Up Time

No sense dirtying the kitchen every day; after you bring your treasures home from the market, prepare as many of the vegetables as possible before you put them in the refrigerator. Carrots can be peeled and stored in a plastic bag for several days. Onions can be peeled, washed, chopped, and stored in a sealed plastic bag for a few days. Peppers can be halved, seeded, washed, dried, and stored in a sealed plastic bag for several days. Lettuce can be washed, dried, wrapped in plastic wrap, and stored for days as well.

---

to take charge of your kids. If they don't respect you when you say no, tell them that they will not be permitted to shop with you in the future if they continue to beg. Stand firm in your discipline and explain why. If the food isn't good for you, it isn't good for them either.

REMEMBER REAL FOOD? LISTS TO SHOP BY

I am often asked, "What is real food?" This concept was introduced in Lesson I-5. Use the following lists to help you with your grocery shopping. Remember: real foods are to be enjoyed daily. Nonfoods and pseudo-foods are not allowed on your Wings Program. *Note:* For a treat or for convenience, the program does utilize some canned items such as legumes and tomatoes, as well as dried herbs, baked chips, and certain specialty and gourmet items. Unsweetened frozen fruits are also allowed in the Wings Breakfast Drink.

Real Food

- Fresh fruit
- Fresh vegetables
- Raw or lightly processed oils such as olive oil or cold-pressed oils
- Raw or lightly toasted nuts and seeds
- Brown rice, amaranth, barley, Kamut, millet, spelt, and other ancient grains
- Fresh meats, poultry, and seafood (preferably organic)
- Water
- Herbal teas
- Fresh herbs
- Rice crackers (or other non-gluten crackers)

Nonfood or Pseudo-Food

- Canned fruit
- Canned vegetables (except for legumes, tomatoes, or other "occasional stuff")
- Canned meat (except for tuna fish canned in water—but use sparingly)
- Chips (except for baked chips)
- Crackers (except for non-gluten crackers)
- Candy
- Cookies and pastries (except for your own home-

made natural goodies; see the Menus and Recipes section)

- Soft drinks
- Fruit juices (except for occasional use in the Wings Breakfast Drink or a holiday fruit punch)
- Coffee and tea (except for herbal tea)
- Alcoholic beverages (except for an occasional glass of wine)
- Frozen entrées
- Packaged entrées or entrée helpers
- Broth with added MSG, salt, or sugars
- Any products containing MSG or artificial sweeteners (such as aspartame, Splenda, sucralose, and the like)
- Synthetic fats or fat substitutes (such as margarine, olestra, and the like)
- Any other synthetic or highly processed foods (such as Egg Beaters, artificial creamers, and the like)

SNACK ATTACK

If your children enjoy snacks (and what kids don't?), plan to make healthful snacks instead of buying junk food. If you don't buy junk food, they won't eat it as frequently, and you won't be tempted by it yourself. Learn to alter your snack recipes (or use the delicious snack recipes in this book), and you and your family will become accustomed to healthier nibbling.

Some good snacks include fresh fruit, lightly roasted unsalted nuts, baked potato chips, baked tortilla chips with homemade salsa, nut butters on celery stalks or apple slices, carrot and celery sticks with or without hummus, roasted pumpkin or sunflower seeds, and homemade cookies. Increase the appeal of any of these natural snacks by displaying them attractively on the table or the kitchen counter.

And now, turn to page 255 for your menus and recipes!

 TODAY'S FIRST ASSIGNMENT

TAKE OUT THE TRASH

You're going to hate this one. Review the lists of real foods and nonfoods on page 32 and above. Go through your cabinets and refrigerator and remove all nonfoods. Yes, it is going to be painful, but just do it. Throw it away! Don't give one thought to the expense—think of the joy of building your health! And then replenish those bare shelves with real foods that your entire family can enjoy freely.

Does this sound overly restrictive? Do you have to toss out a lot of food? Remember: it isn't actually food! It is junk that is clogging up your body, making you ill, and making you overweight. Get rid of it. And forget about feeding it to your family, your dog, or your relatives; it isn't good for them either. Just pitch it!

 TODAY'S SECOND ASSIGNMENT

MAKE STOCK WHILE YOU TAKE STOCK

For today's second assignment, try out the recipe for Homemade Turkey Broth (page 240). Using commercially prepared broth, soups, and gravies can load your body with excess sodium that will make you retain water; most also contain MSG, a flavor-enhancing chemical that must be avoided. Making your own stock is simple, inexpensive, and delicious. It does take a little time, so put a pot of broth on to simmer while you are preparing a meal or cleaning out your cabinets. After the stock is finished, store it in containers in the freezer (it will keep for several weeks) and defrost it for use as needed.

LESSON I-7 STUDY GUIDE

1. Describe how the lure of impulse items can sabotage your Wings Program.

   _____

   _____

   _____

2. What are some ways of getting your children involved in your program (instead of begging in the supermarket)?

   _____

   _____

   _____

   _____

3. Why does Wings promote the enjoyment of fresh instead of frozen or canned? What are some benefits of whole, fresh foods?

_____

_____

_____

_____

4. List some of the pleasures you have experienced from following the Wings food plan so far. Has food become an enjoyable part of your life instead of a fearful part of your life?

_____

_____

_____

_____

5. List some common nonfoods. How many of these nonfood items have sullied your kitchen cabinets and refrigerator? What steps have you taken to get rid of them?

_____

_____

_____

_____

HEALTH TIP

BUGS AND BITES

Insect stings are annoying—but most insect sprays are toxic to the body! The following are some tips for keeping insects out of your home and dealing with bites and stings.

- Keep your home clean. Do not leave open food containers in your cabinets or on your countertops. All food should be stored in airtight containers that keep out bugs.

- Keep all garbage out of the house. Empty your kitchen pails frequently and keep the garbage outside in a garbage can.

- Look for herbal insect repellants so you can keep pests at bay without rubbing harmful chemicals such as DEET (a possible carcinogen) on your skin. Excellent natural repellants, such as herbal products made by Quantum and other companies, are available through your local health food store.

- Pantothenic acid at a dose of 500–1,000 mg per day helps inhibit allergic responses.

- When you get bitten or stung, rub an ice cube over the bite for a few minutes to relieve the pain and itch. If the itching resumes later, rub the area again with an ice cube.

- Also for a bite or sting, a poultice of finely minced onion packed over the affected area and closed off with plastic wrap can be helpful.

- Try a homeopathic cream to reduce the swelling and itching of insect bites. An example of this type of cream is Sssting Stop, made by Boericke and Tafel.

ADDITIONAL NOTES

_____

_____

_____

_____

_____

_____

Lesson I-8. Why Diets Don't Work, Part One

The first grim fact to be faced is the high failure rate of all the diet plans on the market today. This is particularly true for diets that seek to temporarily alter how you eat rather than encourage a lifetime commitment to healthful eating and getting the body back into nutritional balance. But Wings is geared toward making permanent lifestyle changes so you can feel good about yourself—and about your program.

The next two lessons present different types of diet protocols, their pros and cons, the nutritional consequences of following them, and their weight-loss effects.

?   **TODAY'S QUESTION**

What diets have you tried, and what happened?

_____

_____

_____

_____

If you are like legions of frustrated dieters, you have probably tried every diet on the planet. You may have lost weight, or not. Studies show that most of the time, people lose about 5 percent of their body fat when they embark on virtually any type of diet, and then weight loss slows or stops. A young and vibrant dieter, however, may even lose weight down to his or her ideal—but does it last?

If you are reading this book, it is likely that you haven't completely succeeded in your weight-loss and health goals by dieting. Let's look at how the body reacts to diets and why you should *never* go on a diet again.

HIGH-PROTEIN DIETS

A high-protein protocol focuses on eating excessive amounts of protein foods, particularly animal proteins (chicken, fish, beef, and so on), and restricts the intake of carbohydrates. Examples of high-protein diets are the Atkins Diet and Protein Power, among others. People on these types of diets will often eat significantly more than 100 grams (g) of protein per day and limit their carbohydrate consumption to less than 100 g per day. Because the protein sources are typically flesh foods, high-protein diets tend also to be high in saturated fats.

Benefits of a High-Protein Diet

Excessive amounts of carbohydrates can cause the body to hold on to water, so embarking on a high-protein diet that limits carbohydrate intake causes an immediate loss of water weight ranging from 5 to 25 pounds in a one- or two-week period. This type of instant gratification is very exciting for dieters (especially those who have tried unsuccessfully to lose weight on a high-carbohydrate plan).

Eliminating highly processed carbohydrates in particular is certainly a "plus" for any dietary strategy. Highly processed carbohydrates include sugary foods, breads, other pastries, and pasta. These types

 NOTES

_____

_____

_____

_____

_____

of foods (to which many Americans are addicted) are harmful to the body and cause weight gain, even if they are low in calories and fats.

A high-protein diet is also very filling. The appetite is satisfied by less food and hunger is diminished because proteins and fats are digested slowly, creating a feeling of satiety for long periods of time. The thought of going on a diet but never being hungry again is enticing to people who struggle with their weight.

Negatives of a High-Protein Diet

A diet based on meat is necessarily high in saturated fats and low in the unsaturated oils that are so beneficial to the brain, immune system, gonads, and other systems of the body. Although consuming some saturated fat is essential to health, an optimum balance between saturated and unsaturated fats is very important, and high-protein diets tip this critical balance to the saturated side. Saturated fats can be pro-inflammatory because they are metabolized into a type of hormone called prostaglandin 2, or PGE2. The prostaglandins are a series of hormones, some of which incite inflammation of the joints, among other effects.

Excessive protein intake, if combined with soft drinks, produces an imbalance between calcium and phosphorus that can lead to osteoporosis. Unless one's digestive system is extremely competent, with a very low pH in the stomach and a high pH in the intestinal tract, digestion of the excessive dietary protein will be impaired. Unfortunately, most people over the age of forty experience diminished digestive health. (Lesson II-5 discusses the importance of recovering and maintaining optimum digestion.)

Undigested proteins in the intestines ferment and produce gas that causes bloating and belching. The products of the food's putrefaction can damage the delicate intestinal lining, causing a condition called "leaky gut syndrome" in which the intestines develop tiny holes or lesions; food particles then leak into the bloodstream, leading to inflammation throughout the body and to the development of food allergies. Ironically, the allergies that are due to poor digestion lead to weight gain!

The body struggles to meet its energy demands on a high-protein diet. Muscle wasting can occur as the body breaks down muscle tissue to convert it into carbohydrates. Deficiencies in most minerals, most of the B-complex vitamins, and other vitamins are inevitable because high-protein diets do not in-clude the quantity or quality of foods to provide those nutrients in adequate amounts. These deficiencies lead to poor health and reduced ability to maintain the initial weight loss.

Animal proteins produce an acidic residue in the body, causing an acidic internal pH (Lesson I-1). Restoring the normal, alkaline pH that is essential to health cannot be achieved on a high-protein diet.

Weight Loss on a High-Protein Diet

The bottom line is that following a high-protein diet causes immediate loss of water weight and then moderate amounts of fat loss for a short period of time, but the long-term success of this type of diet has not been consistently shown. A high-protein plan tends to be more effective for men than for women, possibly because more men struggle with carbohydrate-induced weight gain (beer bellies, for example). Women often struggle with a complex of weight- and food-related issues, none of which are addressed by a high-protein plan.

Given the major issue of nutrient deficiencies, the lack of data supporting long-term positive results, and the probability of inducing major health consequences like heart disease, cancer, arthritis, and osteoporosis, I do not recommend high-protein diets. Wings is not interested in short-term solutions to long-term problems.

HIGH-CARBOHYDRATE DIETS

Many diet books focus on reducing dietary fat and increasing carbohydrates in the form of grains, fruits, and vegetables—essentially, the opposite of the high-protein diet. The better-known high-carbohydrate diets include the Dean Ornish and John McDougall programs, but there are hundreds of permutations on the market today. Unfortunately, they seldom differentiate between healthful and unhealthful carbohydrates. Because these diets restrict protein, fat intake is also limited, sometimes to as little as 10 percent of total calories.

Benefits of a High-Carbohydrate Diet

The most significant accomplishment of a high-carbohydrate diet is increasing the amount of vegetables that the dieters eat—which is great *if* that really happens, rather than increasing consumption of unhealthy carbohydrates like pasta and bread. Vegetables are rich in minerals, vitamins, and fiber, nutrients that confer huge benefits to the body.

High-carbohydrate diets emphasizing vegetables

and whole grains can lower the risk of certain forms of heart disease and cancer by curbing levels of fats in the bloodstream. They can also lower the risk of developing diabetes, as vegetable consumption has been shown to reduce insulin resistance and improve insulin sensitivity; fiber-rich vegetables slow the release of sugars (carbohydrates) into the bloodstream, dampening the insulin response. In addition, this kind of diet can improve the ratio of estrogen to progesterone, which is beneficial for many women (you'll learn in Lesson III-3 about female hormone imbalances that pack on unwanted weight and produce emotional symptoms that lead to carbohydrate cravings).

Negatives of a High-Carbohydrate Diet

Initial weight loss often occurs on a high-carbohydrate plan—but if the diet is too low in calories or protein, much of the weight loss is from loss of muscle tissue rather than body fat. A high-carbohydrate plan also poses a number of nutritional problems. Deficiencies in vitamins and minerals are likely to occur, for example, as nutrients like iron, zinc, and vitamin B_{12} are not abundantly supplied by a predominantly vegetarian diet.

Vegetarian sources of protein do not contain adequate amounts of specific essential amino acids (those that are not made by the body and can only be obtained through food) such as the L-methionine and L-cysteine used in the detoxification pathways of the liver, or the branched-chain amino acids that are used to produce lean muscle tissue. For this reason, high-carbohydrate diets that restrict protein intake or limit protein from animal sources can cause deficiencies in essential amino acids unless the dieter is extremely knowledgeable and disciplined in food selection. You may recall that many essential amino acids like tryptophan, tyrosine, and others are used to build hormones and neurotransmitters such as serotonin and dopamine. An absence or shortfall of these amino acids from the diet means a shortage in the brain and nervous system, which can lead to significant health challenges down the road, including mental and emotional problems.

Because high-carbohydrate (low-protein) diets restrict fat intake, deficiencies in essential fatty acids are also likely, leading again to serious health challenges if the diet is followed for very long. Symptoms of fatty-acid deficiency include poor weight control, lowered immune function, depression, dry skin, poor hair and nail growth, fatigue, and so on.

Weight Loss on a High-Carbohydrate Diet

A little weight (statistics show it's typically no more than 5 percent of body weight) is often lost at the beginning of a high-carbohydrate plan, but this loss only occurs for a short period of time. After a few days or maybe weeks, the body responds to the diet's low calorie count by slowing its metabolic rate. Weight loss then stops, and the reduced weight becomes increasingly difficult to maintain. Rapid weight gain is certain once the high-carbohydrate diet is abandoned—and it is often abandoned rapidly because of hunger. Hunger is inevitable when the body's nutritional and caloric needs are not met; hunger is nearly impossible to defeat for long.

Most high-carbohydrate diets do not differentiate between healthful and unhealthful carbohydrates. Many of their recommended foods are, in fact, guaranteed to cause weight gain! For example, bagels, muffins, pancakes, pasta, and other starchy products made from refined grains are surefire "weight gainers," even when they are low in fat and relatively low in calories. If a high-carbohydrate plan restricted its permissible carbohydrates to fresh vegetables that are low in starch, it might lead to better results.

Wings does not promote a high-carbohydrate diet because of the nutrient deficiencies that ensue and because weight loss on such a plan is either unsuccessful or impermanent.

LOW-FAT DIETS

Low-fat diets include Jenny Craig, Weight Watchers, and similar programs. Virtually everything discussed above about high-carbohydrate diets is also true for a low-fat protocol, because to reduce the amount of dietary fat, one must necessarily reduce protein intake as well, leaving the dieter with a high-carbohydrate plan by elimination.

It should also be noted that when fat intake is reduced arbitrarily, deficiencies in essential fatty acids are inevitable, leading to poor health and poor weight management. Symptoms of fatty-acid deficiency include:

- Eczema-like skin eruptions
- Hair loss
- Liver degeneration
- Behavioral disturbances
- Kidney degeneration
- Excessive water loss through the skin (dry skin) accompanied by thirst

- Gland shrinkage
- Susceptibility to infections
- Failure of wound healing
- Sterility in males
- Miscarriage in females
- Arthritis
- Heart and circulatory problems
- Growth retardation
- Weakness
- Vision and learning impairment
- Lack of motor coordination
- Tingling in the arms and legs
- Premenstrual syndrome (PMS) and other menstrual irregularities
- Depression and other mood disorders

Wings never recommends going on a low-fat diet. Rather, I encourage consumption of the healthful fats naturally found in foods like avocados, olive oil, butter, raw nuts and seeds, and fish. When these are balanced with lots of vegetables, the body is well supplied in the fats you need to build health—and to maintain weight loss. Fat is also satisfying to the appetite. Many hunger problems can quickly be resolved by adding good fats to your repertoire of foods!

And now, go to page 255 for your menus and recipes!

 TODAY'S ASSIGNMENT

REVIEW YOUR DIET HISTORY

Think about any high-protein, high-carbohydrate, or low-fat diet plans you've tried over the past few years. How did you feel on these diets? What weight-loss results did you achieve? How long did your "benefits" last? What other possible consequences followed your dieting? You may have known instinctively that diets don't work; now you know the facts behind your instinct.

LESSON 1-8 STUDY GUIDE

1. What are the basic premises of a high-protein diet? List some common high-protein diet plans.

_____

_____

_____

2. What are some of the nutritional perils of a high-protein diet?

_____

_____

_____

3. What are the natural consequences of following a high-protein diet?

_____

_____

_____

4. What are the basic premises of a high-carbohydrate diet? List some common high-carbohydrate diet plans.

_____

_____

_____

5. What are some of the nutritional perils of following a high-carbohydrate diet?

_____

_____

_____

6. What are some natural consequences of following a high-carbohydrate diet?

_____

_____

_____

_____

7. What are the basic premises of a low-fat diet? List some common low-fat diet plans.

_____

_____

_____

_____

8. What are some of the nutritional perils of following a low-fat diet?

_____

_____

_____

_____

9. What are the natural consequences of following a low-fat diet?

_____

_____

_____

HEALTH TIP

BURNING BLADDER INFECTIONS

If you have ever experienced a bladder infection, you don't need to be told how unpleasant it is. When it begins, you often feel bloated in the abdomen, with a slight burning sensation upon urination; as the infection grows, the burning becomes intense, and you feel an urgent need to urinate even when you can only pass a small amount of fluid. Because of anatomical differences and fluctuations in female hormones, women are more likely than men are to experience bladder infections. Women in the perimenopausal or menopausal phases of life also experience more of these infections than younger women.

If you are susceptible to bladder infections or feel one coming on, consider the following natural options for prevention and treatment:

• Drink lots of water and avoid sugar.

• Use cranberry capsules from the health food store. A couple of capsules taken every hour for a few hours will usually knock out the infection quickly.

• Drink unsweetened cranberry juice followed by a swig of apple juice (to cut the tartness).

• Sit in a basin filled with warm water and a few drops of grapefruit-seed extract for a few minutes several times per day. Grapefruit-seed extract is helpful in killing harmful bacteria. *Caution:* Do not use grapefruit-seed extract if you are allergic to citrus products.

• Do not douche! Douching changes the natural pH of the delicate vaginal tissue and actually increases susceptibility to bladder infections.

• Use cotton underwear instead of nylon or other synthetic fabrics.

• Do not use scented toilet paper or scented feminine-hygiene products.

Lesson I-9. Why Diets Don't Work, Part Two

It seems that anyone can write a weight-loss book: actors, talk-show hosts, or simply people who managed to do it on their own. Virtually every popular magazine for women features a weekly article on how to lose weight. But instead of pulling real science into the discussion and providing the public with honest information, they keep hammering away on the same old nail: Stop eating so much! Exercise more! Buy these products! Listen to this "expert"! As you now know, the solution to the problem isn't that simple. That is the bad news.

The good news is twofold. The first piece, to put it bluntly, is that the weight-loss industry is a fraud and a failure. People writing these books and diet plans should realize that their diets aren't working because they don't account for the incredible complexity of the human body. They fail to address overweight as a holistic issue and ignore the mountains of literature on the complicated reasons why the body hangs on to excess weight inappropriately. So how is that good news? It means that *you* are *not* a failure.

The second piece is that you *can* be successful. Now that you are participating in the Wings Program, you have the opportunity to learn why it has been so difficult to lose weight and maintain your weight loss. Now that you are learning about your body and your health, you'll be able to use that knowledge to lose your excess weight without dieting and without hunger. Good news indeed!

? **TODAY'S QUESTION**

Frustrated yet?

This lesson continues the diet debunking of the last lesson. It is, of course, discouraging to realize that we've been deceived. Reviewing the material on why diets don't work can be extremely frustrating or depressing, especially for people who have put a lot of faith in dieting. Perhaps you followed various diet instructions but didn't lose the weight, and perhaps you blamed yourself for "failing"; now you're beginning to see that maybe you weren't at fault after all.

Over the course of this program, you'll learn about all the other issues of weight gain and loss, like digestive problems, food allergies, hormones . . . Well, the list is extensive, and we have a long way to go. Do not become discouraged at the volume of information you will receive: don't think that the road is too hard or too long. Your good health is a journey, not a destination, and you're making progress. By the time you "graduate" from Wings, you will know and understand more about weight loss than "the professional" does. Best of all, you will be well on your way to weight-loss success—for a lifetime.

LOW-CALORIE DIETS

Review the material from last week about high-carbohydrate, low-fat diet programs, because low-

✐ **NOTES**

calorie diets typically fit into these categories. The Zone diet, however, is a low-calorie program that is balanced among protein, carbohydrates, and fats, so it fits neither the high-protein nor the high-carbohydrate category, and it is certainly not a low-fat program. The Zone diet typically offers less than 1,200 calories per day. For some people, that is an appropriate amount of calories, but for others it is definitely on the low side.

The concept behind the low-calorie protocol is that calories act as a form of currency in the body's "bank." When extra calories are consumed, the body stores them, much like a bank account from which they can be withdrawn when the need arises. The problem with this analogy is that calorie utilization is more complex than banking. When a low-calorie diet is undertaken, the body reduces its metabolic rate. When calorie consumption is later increased (usually because of hunger, or when the diet is "over"), the added calories will then be stored in the body as fat.

Consider, for example, someone who requires about 2,000 calories per day to maintain his/her current weight, neither gaining nor losing. If the individual goes on a diet that reduces caloric intake to 1,500 calories per day, he/she may temporarily lose weight, but the body gradually reduces its metabolic rate to compensate for the reduction in calories. Weight loss then stops when his/her body becomes energy efficient at 1,500 calories per day. If he/she reduces caloric intake even further, metabolism slows even more, so that when he/she subsequently adds calories—which is inevitable—all additional calories above that lowered metabolic level are rapidly stored as body fat.

An additional problem regarding the low-calorie concept that is never discussed in the popular press is that nutrient deficiencies are unavoidable because the dieter simply is not eating enough food to provide the quantity of vitamins, minerals, and other nutrient complexes that his/her body needs. (This problem applies equally to most high-protein, high-carbohydrate, and low-fat programs.) When these nutritional needs are not met, the body's attempt to produce energy from food is diminished; fatigue, hunger, and an array of other physical symptoms set the hapless dieter up for failure.

A Low-Calorie Approach That Does Work

Weight loss simply cannot be maintained for long on a low-calorie plan unless (and it's a *big* "unless") the plan is extremely well balanced among protein, carbohydrates, fats, vitamins, and minerals, and is also nutrient dense with no wasted calories from nutrient-dead food. Under these conditions, the body responds positively by reducing the metabolic rate—and possibly extending the lifespan. However, the caveat is that the low-calorie program must be so well balanced that the body's physical needs are being met and hunger signals are not stirred, so the program can be continued indefinitely. One still runs the risk of dropping the metabolic rate to the point that subsequent weight loss stops. (Other strategies must sometimes be employed to prevent this, which we'll discuss in Lessons III-2 and III-5.)

The Wings Program is a low-calorie plan that is well balanced nutritionally so that the body's needs are being met. Wings focuses on eating only natural foods so that the diet is nutrient dense. Hunger is not an issue because the body is satisfied. Wings also takes into account that most people are dealing with years of nutrient deficiencies, so supplementation is mandatory.

DIET PILLS AND POTIONS

Because losing weight is fraught with failure and disappointment, it is nearly impossible for some people to resist the temptation to chuck the idea of diet management into the garbage and reach for a "magic pill" that will make all the extra weight go away. Even people who are more inclined to use natural products than drugs often resort to the lure of an herb or nutrient that promises immediate weight loss. We will briefly explore some of these options, both natural and unnatural.

This section is not exhaustive; new products appear on the market every month, and we can't possibly explore each one. Most of the new products, however, fall into one or more of the categories below, and these principles will apply to them as well.

Chitosan as a Fat Blocker

Chitosan is a fiber derived from the shells of crustaceans like shrimp and crabs. It magnetically binds to fat and escorts it out of the body before it can be absorbed. One gram (g) of chitosan binds to about 8 g of fat. Theoretically, therefore, chitosan should be the ideal diet pill, especially for those people who subscribe to the idea that fat is the mother of all dietary evils.

Chitosan is not benign, however, and it is not selective about the types of fats that it removes from the body. Essential fatty acids and fat-soluble vitamins are also magnetically attracted to chitosan, so deficiencies of these important nutrients can occur if chitosan is used on a regular basis. Very few human studies of chitosan as a weight-loss product have been conducted, and those that have show that little weight loss is ever achieved by using chitosan. The body simply compensates for the reduced caloric intake and weight loss stops.

Think of taking chitosan as another method of trying a low-fat diet. I recommend only using it for those sporadic occasions when you know you are going to eat a meal high in processed fats and have no other alternative. *Caution:* People who are allergic to seafood should never use chitosan, as allergic reactions could occur. Also, chitosan should never be taken right before or after meals containing healthful fats or fat-soluble vitamins.

Herbal Stimulants

The concept behind the use of herbal-stimulant blends for weight loss is that they increase the activity of a specialized type of fat called brown fat. Brown fat is metabolically active and serves two functions in the body: keeping internal organs warm by increasing core body temperature, and wasting excess calories by converting them into body heat. Brown fat is, therefore, the dieter's friend (this will be discussed in more depth in Lesson III-5).

Herbs like guarana (a powerful source of caffeine) and ephedra or ma huang (now removed from the American marketplace by decree of the U.S. Food and Drug Administration) are typical components of these natural weight-loss products; they stimulate the central nervous system and increase the metabolic rate. Some individuals lose weight by using these types of products, but at a huge cost to their health. Side effects include nervousness, heart palpitations, irregular heartbeat, increased blood pressure, insomnia, panic attacks, and other disorders of the cardiovascular system, adrenal glands, and nervous system. People have died using these "natural highs," and I do not recommend their use. *Caution:* If you have been diagnosed with a cardiovascular problem, adrenal exhaustion, or a nervous condition, do not take any herbal stimulants without the consent of your physician.

Non-stimulant thermogenic agents are being introduced, but none have been adequately tested for efficacy or safety; therefore, I cannot recommend any of them at this time. I strongly caution people not to use thermogenic products unless they have been unable to increase their metabolic rate by any other means, are very well nourished, have not been diagnosed with any of the conditions listed in the caution note above, and do not have a family history of these conditions.

Herbal Laxatives and Diuretics

Another category of natural weight-loss products is made up of herbs that stimulate the elimination system, causing diarrhea or a diuretic effect. As you can easily imagine, this can make the numbers on the scale go down, but it produces absolutely no fat loss whatsoever. Although herbs like *Cascara sagrada,* senna, and others stimulate the bowels and liver, continued use can cause dependence and rebound constipation.

Most people are already marginally dehydrated because they don't drink enough water. Taking herbal diuretics is likely to produce further dehydration, which is dangerous and does nothing to induce fat loss. I don't recommend using these types of products. If constipation is a problem, herbal laxatives may be used from time to time, but the blend should contain no senna and only tiny amounts of *Cascara sagrada* so you do not become dependent upon the laxative. (Constipation is explored in Lesson II-3 and Lesson II-6 discusses body cleansing.)

Chromium

Chromium is an essential mineral that is known to increase the effectiveness of insulin and help balance blood sugar. Some studies (mostly conducted with young, healthy male athletes) seem to show that using chromium may help the body lay down lean muscle tissue; other studies have not borne out this association. Studies of chromium show no weight-loss benefit to women.

The American diet is typically deficient in chromium, so you should ensure that your daily supplement provides a generous supply. I recommend using 400–1,000 micrograms of the GTF form of chromium (GTF stands for glucose tolerance factor). As yet, there is little scientific evidence that simply taking adequate amounts of this important mineral without making other dietary changes significantly affects the body's ability to lose weight, but it will certainly reduce cravings for sugars and chocolate and help normalize blood sugar.

SURGICAL AND PHARMACEUTICAL APPROACHES TO WEIGHT LOSS

Little needs to be said about the possible long-term detrimental effects of using surgery to solve the problem of obesity. Severe malnutrition, malabsorption of nutrients, repetitive vomiting, digestive problems, and cardiovascular problems are among the numerous negative health consequences of such operations. It is easy to understand the lure of surgery, however, considering that gross obesity is one of the most difficult conditions to treat.

Pharmaceutical approaches to weight management are equally harmful, and they seldom cause any more than 5 additional pounds of weight loss over mere dietary restraint. Weight-loss drugs have side effects including lowered mood, angina pectoris (chest pain), faintness, shortness of breath, or water retention in the lower extremities. Some of these drugs pose the risk of even more significant side effects, as follows:

- Dexfenfluramine and fenfluramine: primary pulmonary hypertension, a serious lung disorder

- Anorexigens (drugs that cause reduction of appetite, or anorexia): hypertension

- Phenylpropanolamine: nervousness, insomnia, increased blood pressure, headache, dizziness, rapid and forceful heartbeats, nausea and vomiting, and/or intracranial hemorrhage

- Sibutramine hydrochloride monohydrate: cardiovascular risk factors like rapid heartbeat and hypertension, as well as dry mouth, insomnia, and/or constipation

- Phentermine: sleeplessness, nervousness, and/or euphoria

What's more, abrupt discontinuation of weight-loss drugs can result in extreme fatigue, depression, sleep disorders, irritability, hyperactivity, and personality changes, including a psychosis that is clinically indistinguishable from schizophrenia. There is also a possibility of drug abuse in terms of both psychological dependence and severe social dysfunction. Ionamin (phentermine), for example, is chemically and pharmacologically related to amphetamine and other stimulant drugs that have been extensively abused, and is not effective for long periods of time (more than a few weeks).

Remember that drugs are not benign. Although some medications are needed for medical reasons, a drug should not be considered a magic pill that will make lifestyle changes unnecessary.

NOW HOW DO YOU FEEL?

This very negative view of current weight-loss theory and practice may have been distressing to absorb. It is especially frustrating to realize that we have been duped or misled by people we trusted with our health. Confusion is likely, because much of this information runs directly opposite what you've read in the press or in weight-loss books. But if you feel that you've lost the battle of the bulge, or that you've damaged your health by following some of these diets, cheer up! You are not destined to be unhealthy and overweight forever simply because you have dieted incorrectly: you can lose your extra weight and be healthy at the same time.

Continue to follow your program, knowing that you are in training to be healthy and slim for the rest of your life. Wings is not a temporary fix, to be abandoned when the next fad comes along or as soon as you have reached your weight-loss goal. Wings is a permanent lifestyle change that will allow you to build your health day after day and feel wonderful doing it. Best of all, it is geared toward helping you lose your excess weight—and keep it off forever.

Measuring Up

It's that time again . . . Weigh yourself, and then take five girth measurements: bust at the largest point, waist at two inches above the navel, hips at the largest point, and right and left thigh circumference at the point where your extended fingertips reach with your arms hanging down at your sides. Record these figures, and your calculated BMI value, on your Progress Chart.

And now, go to page 255 for your menus and recipes!

 TODAY'S ASSIGNMENT

RECOMMIT

Why did you buy this book? What were your goals when you began the program? What do you hope to accomplish over the course of this material? Go back over your goals, and re-establish your commitment to achieving each of them.

Ponder your progress. How are you feeling? Have you begun to lose weight? Are you discouraged because your progress is slower than you expected? Are you creating your meals from the Menus and Recipes section?

Recommit yourself to building your health. Abandon the idea that you can achieve good health (and weight goals) by following a program for a few days or weeks; instead, relish the idea that you are going to spend the rest of your life on your health journey.

Remember: if you resume your old way of eating (or dieting), you will regain your weight. Each time you regain your weight, it will become more difficult to lose it and keep it off. Now that you understand why, don't be tempted to fall back into your old patterns. You're doing well! Don't quit!

LESSON I-9 STUDY GUIDE

1. What are the different types of natural pills for weight loss?

2. What are some of the nutritional perils of using these natural remedies?

3. Why is the surgical treatment of obesity not a good idea?

4. What are the names of several common synthetic diet pills?

5. What are some of the perils of using "pill therapy" for weight management?

6. What are some natural consequences of using "uppers" or other prescription or over-the-counter weight-loss remedies?

7. List, again, the fundamental concepts of the Wings Program.

HEALTH TIP

COUGHING

Are you coughing from bronchitis or an upper respiratory infection?

- Make sure no one in your family or work environment is blowing smoke into the air you breathe. Secondhand smoke contributes to the frequency of bronchitis.

- Drink plenty of fluids.

- Take the amino acid L-cysteine to keep mucus thin so it can be easily expelled. *Caution:* L-cysteine is for short-term use only, as it is a chelating agent that pulls minerals from the body.

- Several herbal and/or homeopathic remedies can help soothe the throat, ease coughing, and thin mucus to reduce congestion. Try Bronc-Ease by Nature's Herbs for nighttime relief, or Boericke and Tafel's Cough and Bronchial Syrup (available in daytime and nighttime formulas).

- Avoid mucus-forming foods like sugar, wheat products, or any food to which you are allergic: dairy products, for instance, are notorious for producing mucus.

- Sip a tea of minced onions and garlic (recipe on page 181 throughout the day.

- For a dry cough, try the homeopathic remedy Bryonia.

Lesson I-10. One Man's Food, Another Man's Poison

Allergies—food, environmental, or other allergies—can cause you to gain both water weight and fat weight. Although it can be dauntingly difficult to learn exactly what is causing the problem, the good news is that there are answers. This lesson will help you discover whether an allergy or an intolerance are indeed causing some of your weight mischief, how to determine the allergen (the substance producing the allergic response), and how to rid your body of its effects. This is one of the most important lessons in the entire curriculum! Don't miss a word of it.

? TODAY'S QUESTION

What are your trigger foods?

_____

_____

_____

_____

It isn't commonly known that foods like wheat, corn, and dairy products can easily generate 35 or more pounds of excess weight. This happens through mechanisms that are not readily understood or well researched. The problem is that most Americans consume at least one of these foods every day. What foods do you eat every day? What foods do you phys-ically crave? What are your comfort foods? What foods do you avoid because they bother you? How do you feel in general? Do you have dark circles under your eyes? Stomach pains? Tired?

Dr. Elson Haas, a well-known author, calls allergy-induced excess weight "false fat." In *The False Fat Diet* (New York, NY: Ballantine Books, 2001), he suggests answering the following questions to determine whether your weight problem may be an allergy or intolerance issue:

- Do you have an extra 5–15 pounds or more that you can't shed with normal dieting and exercise?

- Do you sometimes crave specific foods?

- Does your stomach sometimes get bloated after a normal-sized meal?

- Do certain foods seem to affect your mood (up or down)?

- Do you often suffer from heartburn, indigestion, gas, or acid reflux problems?

- Do you tend to eat the same foods almost every day?

- Do you frequently intend to eat only a small amount of a favorite food but end up overeating?

- After eating, do you sometimes develop a stuffy or runny nose, or watery eyes?

- Do your hands, feet, or ankles frequently swell? Are your eyes or face puffy?

- Do you tend to suffer from insomnia, hypoglycemia, chronic joint pain, or skin problems (such as acne or eczema)?

- Do you have asthma, allergies, frequent sinus or ear infections, or frequent headaches?

✒ NOTES

_____

_____

_____

_____

_____

- Do you frequently eat eggs, wheat, soy, milk, or corn syrup?
- If you are a woman, do you suffer from PMS?
- Do you frequently eat foods that don't agree with you, despite your reaction to them?
- Do you feel unusually tired after eating?

If you answered yes to two or more of those questions, Dr. Haas believes that you almost certainly struggle with allergy-induced or intolerance-induced weight gain, and that it will be easier for you to lose the weight once you eliminate the foods that are causing the reactions.

HOW DOES FOOD ALLERGY OR INTOLERANCE CAUSE WEIGHT GAIN?

An allergy is an immune system response to what the body considers to be a foreign invader. An intolerance, on the other hand, may be caused by digestive, enzymatic, or hormonal disruptions. An intolerance does not necessarily stimulate an immune system response but provokes other types of symptoms; its impact on the body can be just as severe. Allergies can attack quickly, often within seconds after the offending substance is touched, eaten, or inhaled. An intolerance, however, can affect the body up to seven days later, making it difficult to connect the reaction with what caused it.

Although many healthcare practitioners do not realize that allergies or intolerances can cause excess weight gain, many others are looking closely at this issue. According to physician Rudy Rivera, M.D., the increased pollution and stress in the world have worn down our defense mechanisms and are leading to increased food intolerance. In *Your Hidden Food Allergies Are Making You Fat,* he writes, "Estimates on the prevalence of food intolerance range from 30 percent to 90 percent of the population suffering from some degree of the condition."

A number of mechanisms make us gain weight when we eat a food to which we are intolerant or allergic. Allergies can reduce the production of the calming neurotransmitter serotonin, stimulating carbohydrate cravings. Food intolerance can cause a surge in the secretion of insulin, making blood sugar control difficult if not impossible. When insulin pulls too much sugar out of your bloodstream, you become lethargic and tired, and you tend to eat more to increase your energy.

According to Dr. Rivera, we often crave the very foods to which we are allergic. He writes, "When the chemical reactions precipitated by the allergic response are pleasurable, the absence of this allergic response results in unpleasant feelings, which can only be remedied by eating the food and creating the allergic reaction again."

Another interesting theory compares food sensitivity to serum sickness: the body produces excessive antibodies to a food antigen, to the point that the individual actually becomes sick from his/her own antibodies. Only when the antigen is reintroduced and binds with the surplus antibodies does the condition improve. Unfortunately, consuming the food also stimulates the production of more antibodies, so the cycle repeats. (For more detailed information on this subject, read *Your Hidden Food Allergies Are Making You Fat,* by Rudy Rivera, M.D., and Roger D. Deutsch, Rocklin, CA: Prima Health, 1998.)

There is also some evidence that allergies can provoke an autoimmune response in which the immune system attacks the body itself: it can attack the thyroid gland, for example, causing hypothyroidism. When thyroid hormone production is low, the body's metabolism slows, making it more difficult to lose weight.

Grain Allergy, Weight Gain, and Me

Although I had been close to my ideal weight for several years, I wanted to drop another 10 pounds nestling around my abdomen and hips. I reduced my calories to the level I felt necessary to lose the weight, but nothing happened; for six months, I was particularly careful about food quantities, and still no weight loss occurred.

I was, at that time, virtually grain-free: I did not eat cereals, breads, or desserts—very much. Once or twice a week, I went out to dinner and enjoyed one or two slices of really good bread, and I'd occasionally share a dessert. The calorie count of these minor indiscretions was relatively insignificant. But when I decided I really needed to lose those 10 pounds, I decided to eliminate *all* grains from my diet, including those one or two slices of bread. Within two weeks, I lost the extra weight and successfully kept it off with no further "dieting" required, as long as I avoided all grain.

I now know from experience that eating just one bowl of cereal will, for me, pack on 5 pounds overnight. This type of weight gain, of course, is not fat but water weight: the water is retained as an allergic response to that particular food. But it looks and feels like fat anyway!

(The role of the thyroid gland in weight management will be discussed in detail in Lesson III-2.)

One of the most dramatic examples I know of weight gain from a food allergy happened to a Wings student who gained 5 pounds overnight from eating one chocolate-chip cookie. Obviously, she didn't gain fat weight from that single cookie; fat is not so easily generated, and that much fat cannot be synthesized from so few calories. Her gain was in the form of excess water that was stored in her tissues—and it took her several days to get rid of it. On the flip side, another woman lost over 65 pounds by simply eliminating the foods to which she was reactive. Her calorie count didn't change; her food choices changed.

IDENTIFYING TRIGGER FOODS

If you tend to crave specific foods or eat certain foods virtually every day, the likelihood of intolerance is high. Some of the foods that most commonly induce an allergic response are eggs, soy, dairy, wheat, corn, peanuts, shellfish, and chocolate. If you still consume these foods, eliminate them totally for a period of six weeks or more and see whether your weight loss is improved (other health challenges may improve as well).

It can be difficult to determine whether you have a food allergy or intolerance, or even to learn what foods cause your body to be reactive. Complicating the issue further, reactions can come and go and can even change form. There are, however, methods for discovering what provokes your body to an allergic response or an intolerance reaction.

Allergy Testing

Some allergies are "fixed," meaning that regardless of how long you avoid exposure to the food or environmental allergen, you will react consistently any time you are exposed to it. On the other hand, "acquired allergies" to certain foods or other substances can appear and disappear for any number of reasons, at different points in our lives. Allergy testing is admittedly imperfect and may even yield inconsistent results from year to year—but it's a start.

Evaluating Your Immune System's Response

Allergic reactions lead to the formation of antibodies that either protect your body or provoke symptoms. Most people only associate allergic reactions with symptoms like sneezing, itchy eyes, diarrhea, constipation, or skin eruptions, not realizing that allergies can afflict any part of the body with any type of symptom, including depression, fatigue, or weight gain.

Allergists often test only for immune responses of the antibodies (immunoglobulins) IgA or IgM, which provide a very incomplete picture of what happens in your body when you are exposed to an allergen.

I recommend that you ask your doctor to prescribe the ELISA/ACT LRA, a combination of the enzyme-linked immunosorbant assay (ELISA), the advanced cell test (ACT), and the lymphocyte response assay (LRA). This blood test detects the delayed or hidden immune responses that trigger the activity of lymphocytes (white blood cells). Many physicians now use this test because it provides a more specific and comprehensive picture of what happens in your immune system when you are exposed to substances to which you are reactive. The ELISA/ACT LRA assesses lymphocyte responses for all delayed immune pathways, including type II (reactive antibody), type III (immune complex), and type IV (cell mediated). It is available by prescription through Perque Laboratories; for more information, ask your doctor to call 1-800-525-7322.

We often associate allergies or intolerances with a skin rash or stomach upset, not with "stubborn fat." But if you are struggling to lose weight—no matter how hard you diet or exercise—I strongly encourage you to explore this issue further. It can mean the difference between weight success and failure!

Pulse Testing

The second measure I recommend checking for potential triggers is the pulse test. Intolerances may be the issue even if a true allergy is not present, as either an allergy or a food intolerance can stimulate weight gain. Intolerances will typically not be picked up by allergy testing, so you may need both the ELISA/ACT LRA and the pulse test to get a clear picture of your body's own reactions. The pulse test is a noninvasive procedure that you can do at home; a pulse-test chart is provided in Appendix 5 to simplify your record keeping.

Performing the Pulse Test

The following directions are extracted from a book written by a physician who used the pulse test in his clinical practice for many years, to the great benefit of his patients. (To study the subject in greater depth, obtain Dr. Arthur F. Coca's book *The Pulse Test*, originally published in 1952 and reprinted by Barricade Books; it is difficult to follow, but the information is excellent.)

1. Stop smoking entirely: smoking will disrupt the accuracy of the test.

2. Count your 1-minute pulse several times per day: just before each meal, three times after each meal at half-hour intervals, just before retiring for the night, and after waking (before rising) in the morning. All counts are to be taken while sitting except for the count upon awakening, which is to be taken lying down. Test your pulse in the neck or wrist, whichever is easiest.

3. Record all foods eaten at each meal.

4. After the first day, conduct single-food tests for two or more whole days, beginning early in the morning and continuing during the waking hours, as follows: Eat a small portion of a single food (for example, a few slices of apple or banana, an egg, or a cup of coffee) every hour. Test every food that you normally eat and other items that you typically put into your mouth like mouthwash, toothpaste, and so on. Count the pulse just before eating and again one hour later. Do not test any food that is known to disagree with you.

Interpreting the Results of the Pulse Test

The first objective of the pulse test is to determine one's lowest pulse rate under normal conditions, that is, nonallergic conditions. The second objective is to find one's "true maximum" pulse rate. According to Dr. Coca, the pulse's normal elevation should never exceed 12 beats per minute. Therefore, if the true low is 60 beats per minute, as an example, the pulse will never normally rise above 60 + 12, or 72 beats per minute. After keeping records for a few days and after testing many foods, an individual will determine his/her normal range of pulse elevation (which should never exceed 12 beats per minute).

These counts are then used to evaluate suspected allergens. Potential allergens should be removed from the diet, causing the pulse to normalize at a lower rate. As allergenic items are eliminated, this "lowest count" will drop, and within a few days a "true low" will emerge from the numbers. If the true low is 60 beats per minute and the normal range of elevation is found to be 8 beats per minute, any food or substance that elevates the pulse above 60 + 8, or 68 beats per minute, indicates an allergy or other sensitivity to that food or substance. Dr. Coca writes that the pulse should never, under any circumstances, rise above 84 beats per minute, and if it does, allergy is strongly indicated.

He provides other guidelines for interpreting the results of pulse testing:

- If your pulse count taken standing is greater than that taken sitting, this is a positive indication of present "allergic tension."

- If at least fourteen pulse counts are being taken each day and if your daily maximal pulse rate is constant (within 1 or 2 beats) for three days in succession, this indicates that all food allergens have been avoided on those days.

- If your daily maximal pulse rate varies more than 2 beats (for example, Monday = 72, Tuesday = 78, Wednesday = 76, Thursday = 61), you are certainly allergic to foods or environmental triggers, provided there is no infection.

- If eating a frequently consumed food causes no acceleration of your pulse (to at least 6 beats above your estimated normal maximum), that food can be tentatively considered nonallergenic for you.

- House dust is, at least usually, a minor allergen; most food allergies cause stronger reactions, which are actually protective against such lesser allergens and reactions.

- Your pulse reaction to an inhaled allergen (particularly house dust) is more likely to be of shorter duration than that to a major food allergen.

- Pulse rates that are not more than 6 beats above the estimated normal daily maximum should not be blamed on a recently eaten food but on an inhalant or a recurrent reaction.

- If your maximum pulse rate does not regularly occur before rising after the night's rest, but at some other time of the day, this usually indicates sensitivity to house dust in mattresses or pillows.

- If you are not susceptible to common colds, you are probably allergic to only a few, if any, commonly eaten foods, though you may be allergic to some inhaled substances such as house dust, which may even cause respiratory symptoms.

Through the pulse test, one of my earliest Wings students learned that she was reactive to garbanzo beans and sesame seeds, two foods she ate regularly in hummus. She was brokenhearted because she loved those foods, but by eliminating them she subsequently lost several pounds that she had not been able to lose through dietary restriction alone. Another student learned she was reactive to corn tortilla chips and bananas, and she lost several pounds just by eliminating these foods. I have found that many individuals who plateau after initially losing weight will resume losing weight when they eliminate their trigger foods—so can you.

And now, go to page 255 for your menus and recipes!

 ### TODAY'S ASSIGNMENT

UNCOVER YOUR ALLERGIES AND INTOLERANCES

Reread this lesson. Do you believe that some of your symptoms could be the result of a hidden food allergy or intolerance? Have you reached a plateau in your weight-loss program and are unable to get those remaining extra pounds to budge? If so, consult your Wings nutritionist (at www.flywithwings.com/pnc. html, click on MyProConnect) or a nutritionally trained physician. Then, read through the Menus and Recipes section and eliminate your apparent trigger foods from the menus. The recipes contain no wheat and very few of the other most common allergens. If you follow the Wings meal plan carefully, it will not be difficult to fine-tune your program to eliminate any other food allergens that affect you.

Ask your doctor to schedule an ELISA/ACT LRA; or, find a holistic physician in your area (see the Resource Guide) who understands the importance of allergy testing and can prescribe it. The books by Dr. Haas and Dr. Rivera are a goldmine of information on allergy-induced weight gain, and also provide good references for your physician. Meanwhile, I encourage you to spend the necessary time to do the pulse test for yourself. Yes, it is complicated, but it is well worth the effort: eliminating all of the foods and non-food substances that trigger allergic or intolerance reactions can make a huge difference in your long-term health and weight loss.

LESSON I-10 STUDY GUIDE

1. What is the difference between allergy and intolerance?

2. How do food allergies or intolerances affect our ability to lose and maintain weight?

3. What are the most common food allergies and intolerances?

4. What are some symptoms of allergy?

5. Explain the "withdrawal factor" in removing allergens from the diet.

6. Write out the protocol for the pulse test.

7. What foods do you eat every day? What foods did you eat regularly before you began the Wings Program? Are any symptoms associated with your consumption of these foods? (Remember that weight gain, or resistance to weight loss, can be your only symptom.)

HEALTH TIP

CANKER SORES AND COLD SORES

Ouch! Canker sores are often a result of food allergies but can also be triggered by other factors. Cold sores are caused by the herpes simplex virus. Try these natural treatments:

- To speed healing, apply some goldenseal extract or tea tree oil directly to the sore twice per day and again at bedtime; you can also use goldenseal tea as a mouthwash several times a day.

- To treat an outbreak of sores in the mouth, use the amino acid L-lysine several times per day (but use this only when needed, not daily).

- To normalize your intestinal flora, take acidophilus and other probiotics (friendly bacteria) on an empty stomach. (Intestinal bacteria will be discussed further in Lesson II-3.)

ADDITIONAL NOTES

_____

_____

_____

_____

_____

_____

_____

_____

_____

_____

_____

_____

_____

_____

_____

_____

_____

_____

Lesson I-11. The Childhood Risk Factor

One of the realities you may have to face is that fat cells originating with weight gain in childhood do not disappear, even if that excess weight is lost later in life. If you gain 10 extra pounds when you are eight years old, your body creates extra fat cells. If you eventually lose those pounds, the fat cells lose their store of fat, but the cells themselves remain, making it easier for you to gain weight at a later time (in adulthood, for example).

It does not mean, thankfully, that you can't lose your unwanted weight; it does mean that if you ever revert to an unhealthful eating pattern, your body will tend to regain the weight because those empty fat cells want to be replenished. You simply have to stay a little more vigilant, work a little harder, compensate a little more, because of a physiological pattern that started when you were young.

? TODAY'S QUESTION

When did you gain your excess weight?

_____

_____

_____

_____

Did you become overweight as a child, during adolescence, or as an adult? Even if it happened in adulthood, you might have been set up for your weight problem by foods you ate as an infant or young child. If you did gain your excess weight in childhood or adolescence, or if your weight issue is a result of childhood eating habits, you should still be able to lose the weight, but you may face different weight-management challenges than if you gained it simply from overeating as an adult.

FIRST FOODS

What childhood dietary indiscretions may have followed you into adulthood and caused you to gain excess weight many years later? To begin to answer this question, we need to look at the history of American food and eating over the past hundred years and into this new century.

At the turn of the twentieth century, Americans were eating well. Because processing and preservation techniques were not what they are today, most people ate their food fresh from the garden or market. For storage, food was canned at home or kept in cool dirt cellars. Organic materials were used as fertilizer for crops. Animals were generally raised on green grass growing out in the field or taken from the wild; they were well fed, and so were the humans who ate them. Nowadays, we mostly eat packaged pseudo-foods, containing additives—from preservatives to chemical flavors and colors, along with huge amounts of sodium and sugar—starting almost from the day we are born.

Breast versus Bottle

In the 1930s, manufacturers started selling and promoting infant formula, and breastfeeding rates plummeted. Babies who are fed formula instead of breast

✒ NOTES

_____

_____

_____

_____

_____

_____

milk from well-nourished mothers are typically fatter and larger than breastfed babies, a trait that tends to continue through childhood. Evidence now shows that infant formulas contribute to the onset of juvenile and adult obesity.

Researchers have also learned that feeding cow's milk products to babies under the age of two increases the risk of developing adult-onset diabetes. We are now seeing a frightening increase in the development of this type of diabetes in young children.

Did Mom Diet?

Here is another startling piece of information: preliminary studies show that when women are exposed to famine conditions during pregnancy, their boy children tend to develop obesity after the age of fifty, regardless of other health or dietary conditions throughout life. This phenomenon of malnutrition in pregnancy may also apply to dieting in pregnancy.

Men, could this be you? Did your mother diet during her pregnancy with you, or use diet pills during that time? Diet pills were commonly prescribed to pregnant women in the 1950s, 60s, and early 70s. Find out whether these or any other condition of prenatal malnutrition may have predisposed you to develop weight problems in the fifth decade of your life.

You Sweet Thing

Americans ate less than 20 pounds of refined sugar per person per year around the early 1900s, but by now that figure has reached well over 200 pounds of sugar and artificial sweeteners. This sugar onslaught begins in infancy when the pancreas and other organs are still developing. The effects of sugar on a child's metabolism are unknown, but it is likely that the child's immature blood sugar regulatory mechanisms are overwhelmed and weakened, leading to obesity and other health conditions.

If you gained weight in childhood by eating too many refined carbohydrates in the form of sweets, soft drinks, and sugared breakfast cereals, you are likely struggling now with Syndrome X, a cluster of symptoms that includes abdominal obesity (Lesson III-10). You will need to pay careful attention to sugars and other refined carbohydrates now, because you have become a carbohydrate-sensitive adult. Your pancreas tends to secrete too much of the hormone insulin, which causes your body to store fat from refined carbohydrates. Syndrome X is a precursor for heart disease, so it is very important to control your blood sugars carefully.

Fortunately, this is easy to do—just stay on the Wings Program! The Wings food plan is designed to reduce your secretion of insulin and help stabilize your blood sugar level by eliminating all refined carbohydrates and emphasizing fresh, unrefined vegetables.

Puberty and Hormone Concerns for Girls

Many girls become overweight in puberty when hormones begin to dramatically influence their physiology, adding weight to hips and buttocks. When the female hormones are "out of whack," girls often crave chocolate or other sweets that pack on the pounds. These issues are not satisfactorily addressed by diet alone. It will be important to stay with your program so you can address the problems of the endocrine system. (The influence of female hormones on weight management is covered in Lesson III-3.)

Often, thyroid function is low, leading to dysregulation of the female hormones. A low thyroid output makes weight management difficult to maintain on any type of program (see Lesson III-2). Help the thyroid so the metabolism burns hotter, and the female hormone issue often resolves as a result.

CAN WE GO BACK AND FIX IT?

We may feel some resentment if we recognize ourselves in this lesson's picture. It seems unfair, doesn't it? We didn't have a choice about our mother's nutritional status, being breastfed or bottle fed, or even the foods we were offered during infancy or childhood. Many of us were raised in homes where we were not allowed to express our own needs, and our parents, not being trained nutritionists, didn't realize they were setting us up for weight-management failure or less-than-ideal health.

But knowing now how these events in our young lives have influenced our weight in adulthood, we can put the issue at rest by dealing with the present. We can forgive the past so we can pursue the future. That is the good news of this lesson: yes, our needs may have deep roots, but they need not determine our health or weight. We *can* and *will* solve the problem!

Steps toward Improved Health

Although many of the following suggestions pertain to everyone, these tips are particularly important for you if your weight gain is due to the influences of childhood. Avoid the following:

▪ Highly processed foods, especially processed fats or rancid fats like bacon, shortening, margarine, and so on. These contain fats called trans-fatty acids, which are extremely toxic to the heart and also lead to Syndrome X and other conditions. Avoid them totally! (You already run a higher risk of developing Syndrome X because of the high sugar content of your early diet, so it is doubly important to avoid any foods that could contribute to this serious condition.)

- Dairy products, except for butter or raw organic dairy products (as long as you aren't allergic to them; drinking a cow's milk infant formula or consuming large amounts of dairy products in early childhood increases your risk of milk allergy). *Note:* Some individuals can tolerate yogurt without a resulting weight gain.

- Sugar in all forms. The pancreatic damage caused by a high-sugar diet in childhood has permanently altered your ability to keep your blood sugar steady and your weight under control. Overweight people (particularly those with Syndrome X) cannot tolerate sugar in any form, including high-fructose corn syrup, honey, white sugar, brown sugar, and such. They also cannot tolerate artificially sweetened foods that may stimulate the same type of pancreatic reaction as to sugar, yet with even more devastating consequences.

It is possible that an adult sweet tooth is a carry-over from feasting on sweets as a child. To bring sugar cravings under control, make sure your diet is adequate in the minerals that help stabilize blood sugar; you may require higher-than-normal amounts of key minerals like chromium, magnesium, and zinc. *Note:* Your Wings nutritionist can recommend a supplement designed to compensate for damage done by the high-sugar diets of processed foods that most Americans have eaten throughout their lives. For a consultation, go to the website www.flywithwings.com/pnc.html and click on MyProConnect.

And now, go to page 255 for your new recipes!

 TODAY'S ASSIGNMENT

LOOK BACK

If possible, ask your mother whether she dieted during her pregnancy with you, whether you were breastfed during infancy, and what your eating habits were like as a young child. Consider whether your current weight problem has to do with an issue from your dietary past. The Wings Program is perfect for resolving these very issues. The emphasis on fresh,

natural produce, adequate amounts of protein, and healthy, natural fats is important to balance blood sugar, reduce insulin resistance, and reduce the risk of developing either diabetes or cardiovascular disease. The emphasis on removing possible allergens like grains and dairy products is important in solving allergy issues stemming from childhood.

LESSON I-11 STUDY GUIDE

1. What are some of the changes in the American food culture over the past hundred years?

2. What do studies show about cow's milk and the development of diabetes and Syndrome X?

3. What has been shown by studies of famine conditions during pregnancy? What does this have to do with dieting?

4. How does sugar consumption during childhood lead to becoming overweight in adulthood?

5. List some important nutritional steps to help correct the consequences of a poor childhood diet.

HEALTH TIP

STOP THAT A-A-A-CHOO!

Coming down with a cold? The key to preventing a full-blown cold is to hit it hard the minute you feel it coming on—don't wait until it is entrenched, because by then it will be hard to stop.

- Take 1,000 milligrams of buffered vitamin C in a little diluted fruit juice every hour until diarrhea occurs, and then reduce your hourly dosage to a level just below that diarrhea threshold.

- Take extra vitamin A (up to 15,000 IU per day, unless pregnancy is possible, in which case no more than 7,500 IU of vitamin A should be taken daily).

- Take a little extra zinc to nourish the immune system.

- Avoid all sugars! Sugar reduces immune system activity and feeds pathogenic bacteria.

- At the first sign of a sore, scratchy throat, use zinc lozenges to boost the immune system and possibly kill bacteria lining the throat.

- A nasal rinse of a little salt, glycerin, and warm water can keep the nasal passages clear. If the nasal discharge is colored, use one drop of grapefruit-seed extract in the rinse as well. *Caution:* Avoid grapefruit-seed extract if you are allergic to citrus.

- Chicken broth is excellent for colds and influenza (Grandma was right!).

- Wash your hands often. Disinfect your toothbrush daily.

- Eucalyptus is excellent for reducing congestion: add five drops of eucalyptus essential oil to a hot bath, or put six drops in a cup of boiling water and inhale the steam.

- Make onion-and-garlic tea (recipe on page 181) to drink or use as a gargle; or, gargle with a tea made from tea tree oil or grapefruit-seed oil.

- Several herbal formulas, available at health food stores, are excellent for immune system support. Keep them on hand to use preventively when you are tired or feel something "coming on." Wellness Formula by Source Naturals, one of the best of these products on the market, is available at most health food stores.

- Homeopathic remedies particularly helpful against cold symptoms are Pulsatilla (for colds with thick, yellow, nonirritating nasal discharge), Kali bichromicum (for colds with nasal congestion and thick, irritating nasal discharge), and Hepar Sulphuris Calcareum (for painful, hoarse, dry cough worsened by cold weather).

ADDITIONAL NOTES

Lesson I-12. Work with Your Set Point

If you were to wander through a museum of paintings from the Middle Ages, you would find that the women admired several hundred years ago would be considered overweight in our century. These women were at least 15–25 pounds heavier than what we now consider to be "ideal."

Somewhere in the middle of the last century, Twiggy burst onto the cultural scene and forever changed the way we think about women. Her shape was certainly not healthy—or attractive, for that matter. Think of Barbie: how realistic is a figure of 36-24-36 for most women? And who said Barbie's is the perfect shape?

Ask yourself this question: what shape is a woman? Is she thin and angular like a runner, or well rounded like a Madonna? Is she muscular? Heavy in the bosom? Does she have generous hips and a rounded face, or does she have a thin face with a body to match?

Women come in all shapes and sizes, don't they? So do men! Our differences should be celebrated, and we should learn to love our differences. We should also learn to enjoy our bodies instead of always trying to change them, especially by dieting, and *especially* if we are trying to reach a goal weight that is not right for our bodies.

? **TODAY'S QUESTION**

What is your ideal weight?

How did you set that number? At what weight did you feel and look your best? Is your current weight goal realistic?

SET POINT THEORY AND IMPLICATIONS

Much has been written about set point, an arbitrary point at which the body stops losing weight and simply maintains its current weight. Unfortunately, our bodies and our brains often disagree. Our natural set point seldom occurs at a point where we think that we look and feel our best. Our bodies seem to take on a mind of their own, and when we're giving weight loss our best shot, all weight loss stops and we plateau. The scales just don't budge.

The scientific basis behind set point is not well understood. A number of theories have been raised about why our bodies stop losing weight when we obviously have so much left to lose, or stop at a point about 10 or 15 pounds above what we consider to be ideal weight. This is where a complex set of factors work together (or in opposition to one another) to cause the body's regulation of fat stores to work inefficiently. Although some biology textbooks explain that the body maintains a predetermined weight through several regulatory systems, scientists do not currently know whether the body establishes a true set point, or what the basis of that set point would be.

In normal-weight adults, the body seems to be regulated in such a way that preserves a specific, appropriate body weight. When individuals have either been

  NOTES

Some Questions to Ask Yourself

- At what weight did you feel the healthiest in your life? At what weight did you look your best? Do these two weights match?

- What is your weight goal? Does it match the weight above?

- What are you willing to sacrifice to be as thin as you would like to be? Your health, marriage, family, vigor? Constant feelings of starvation?

- If your set point is 10 or 15 pounds above what you consider to be ideal, can you learn to be content with your body's perception of ideal?

overfed to induce overweight or starved to induce underweight, their bodies then tend to revert back to their original weight after a "normal" diet is reintroduced. The theory, then, about overweight is that the body has, for some unknown reason, set the "normal weight" at an abnormally high level, a point to which the body will eventually return.

A number of theories have been offered to explain set point, such as the action of a hormone called leptin, reduced thyroid activity, loss of brown fat thermogenesis, and so on, but scientists really do not know why set point happens. It is likely that the body has a type of "cellular scale" that regulates body weight, much like the biological clock that regulates the body's circadian rhythms, or that a complex constellation of factors regulates body weight. Genetics are certainly involved. It is possible that environmental triggers can deregulate the internal scale, or that other conditions contribute to establishing a set point that is seemingly less than optimal.

If the set point theory about weight management is valid, we are left with two choices: accept the set point weight that our bodies have determined to be the right weight for us and forget about weight loss, *or* work diligently to overcome the plateau and keep working on our health. In the absence of good science proving that it cannot be done, I believe that it can be done—and we'll work a little harder.

What Is Most Important: Your Health or Your Weight?

One of the primary goals of Wings is to redirect your

focus from the weight scale to the health of your body. Although we would all like to slink around in a size-eight dress with nary a wrinkle or bulge, most of us will never be that size again. Gravity and age are not kind to the human body! When your body is healthy, it will, for the most part, gradually lose excess weight down to your ideal size—or the size at which your body feels the best.

As you continue through the Wings curriculum, you will see that there are many reasons why you have not yet finished losing your weight. There may still be one or many underlying issues or problems yet unresolved, and so you may not have hit your set point. We will continue to work together on these issues, and we will solve them together.

As we age, we naturally change shape. Women especially tend to become a little heavier in the thighs and buttocks. Men, too, can lose some muscle mass and become heavier around the middle. Part of this aging process is the body's way of protecting us. The thyroid gland tends to slow down gradually as we age, for example, and extra fat serves as insulation to help keep us warm.

Women often gain a few pounds around the perimenopausal period of life because fat produces estrogen that buffers the effects of the ovaries' slowdown. Women who have about 5 extra pounds find that they go through menopause more easily. Women who are too thin are more likely to suffer from degenerative diseases like osteoporosis; they may also find that their sex drive is diminished because fat is used to synthesize the steroid hormones estrogen, testosterone, and progesterone that normalize sex drive.

For these and other reasons, your body may choose to hang on to an extra few pounds. If you have lost about 35 pounds and still have many pounds to go, your body may temporarily halt weight loss until it readjusts its set point, or until you restimulate your metabolic rate. How to do that safely will be discussed in another lesson; right now, concentrate on keeping your diet really clean. Follow the menus diligently and take your supplements so that you are nourishing your body. Don't give your body reason to think that you are starving! You may have reached a plateau for a season, but you will soon start losing weight again.

HOW MUCH BODY FAT DO YOU NEED?

Experts recommend that women have a body mass index (BMI) of about 22 to 25, perhaps even up to 27. Men can have a lower BMI, ranging more toward 18 to 21. That means a woman weighing 150 pounds should have about 35 pounds of body fat. A man weighing 175 pounds should also have about 35 pounds of body fat.

If a woman is overweight at 175 pounds, she will want to drop to about 132 pounds, for a BMI of 25. If a man is overweight at 200 pounds, he will want to drop about 40 pounds, to reach a goal weight of 160 pounds. However, if the woman is very tall and broad shouldered, she may actually be healthier around 160 pounds. Likewise, a man weighing 200 pounds can be very stocky and muscular, and may be within just a few pounds of ideal weight.

As good a measurement as the BMI is, it is not a perfect way of measuring the percentage of body fat, or determining how much weight should be lost.

And now, go to page 256 for your new recipes!

 TODAY'S ASSIGNMENT

REEXAMINE YOUR GOALS

Go over the list of goals that you wrote in Lesson I-1. How are you doing on fulfilling them? Have you started losing weight? Have any of your other symptoms disappeared? Do you have more energy? Is your hair growing faster and thicker? Are your nails stronger? Are you sleeping well at night? Are your bowels functioning properly?

Reevaluate your goals in the light of the information in this lesson. Were your weight goals realistic? If not, adjust them accordingly so you can be successful: don't set yourself up for failure because of unrealistic goals.

LESSON I-12 STUDY GUIDE

1. What are some differences between perceptions of beauty several hundred years ago and today?

2. What is set point, and what are some common theories about how set point is governed?

3. Discuss how age affects weight and body shape.

4. What are some physical consequences of being too thin?

HEALTH TIP

DANDRUFF

Flaky, itchy scalp? Avoid antidandruff shampoos, as they contain toxic chemicals. Fortunately, most dandruff problems disappear when you add natural oil to the diet and reduce your intake of allergenic foods. But if you are still struggling with dandruff, here's how to attack it naturally:

- Take one capsule of kelp per day to nourish the thyroid gland.

- Drink dandelion tea daily for a few weeks.

- Avoid fried foods, dairy products, sugar, flour, chocolate, and nuts.

- After shampooing, rinse your hair with a tea made from chaparral or thyme, or with a vinegar-and-water rinse ($1/2$ cup of vinegar to 1 quart of water—and then rinse it out well!).

MODULE II
Getting the Body Back into Shape

You're starting a new semester, and what an exciting thirteen weeks this will be! Module I covered food issues extensively. This module's theme is completely different but equally important. Weight-loss books or articles seldom cover the concepts of weight loss and health management that we will explore here. I think you will be intrigued and excited as you learn more about how to care lovingly for your body.

This section covers lifestyle issues including digestion, constipation, body cleansing, and exercise; the problem of nonfoods and the problem (or opportunity) of hunger; and special circumstances that can make it more difficult to stay on a good eating program. We will explore scientific findings and clinical experience to discover how these issues influence weight and health. Best of all, you will learn how to overcome unique challenges.

By the conclusion of this module, you will have taken a huge leap forward in improving your whole-body health. You will find that you are healthier than you have been for years (maybe ever!). And instead of relying solely on food management to solve your weight-management problem, you will have learned how to get your whole body working toward your weight-loss goal.

Lesson II-1. Your Personal Energy Crisis

Do not be tempted to skip this material, even if it is uncomfortable at first. This module will challenge you to become physically fit by incorporating a vigorous exercise program into your busy life. If you typically pass over this type of information in the belief that you can't do it or that it doesn't fit with your lifestyle, push through your resistance and *just do it*! You will end up loving the way your body feels.

Now that we are shifting the focus from food, do not revert to your former way of eating. Over the past twelve lessons, you have been building good nutrition habits that will last for a lifetime: do not abandon them now! Continue to follow the menus and recipes in the back of the book. By providing your body with good nutrition every day, you continue to build your whole-body health. Don't ever become discouraged, even if your weight loss begins to plateau. Remember that Wings is not a temporary fix. Forge ahead, knowing that you are learning how to be healthy for the rest of your life!

?   TODAY'S QUESTION

What are you doing really well?

_____

_____

_____

_____

In other words, what part of your health program greatly enhances your weight and health goals?

You have always been told that you gain weight because you eat too much or don't burn enough calories at the gym. But one of the primary reasons most people gain weight is simply that they have left their bodies no choice! Chronic undernutrition, whether caused by years of eating nutrient-dead food or years of dieting, leads to a serious problem of malnutrition that makes it virtually impossible for you to lose weight. Until this problem is corrected, you will not lose weight, no matter how many calories you cut out of your diet.

AN ENERGY PERSPECTIVE

Your body's most basic task is the production of cellular energy. When the cell produces enough energy, it is able to accomplish the functions for which it was genetically designed. When the cells of an organ are able to produce cellular energy and function well (which includes "taking out the garbage" or detoxifying), the organ is able to perform its functions well. When each organ is functioning well, the whole system works well—and you feel good! You have sufficient energy to carry out your responsibilities and (hopefully) enough energy left over to truly enjoy your life.

Enzymes and Energy

Your body spends a great deal of metabolic energy in the production of cellular energy, because converting food into adenosine triphosphate (ATP) is not an easy task. Thousands of biochemical steps are involved in the process: each one requires vitamins, minerals, fats, proteins, and carbohydrates, and is completed by the activation of an enzyme. Enzymes are synthesized

✒ NOTES

_____

_____

_____

_____

_____

_____

from the nutrients in foods, so if these nutrients are missing or in short supply because of poor food quality (for example, from eating processed foods), the conversion of food to energy cannot be completed.

Think of your body as a house under construction. Your contractor needs many different building materials, and if he runs out of money before he can complete his purchases, some part of the building will not be completed. Or, if he runs out of money and cannot hire workers, the building will not be completed, even if all the materials are piled on the site. In your body, foods are the materials and enzymes are the workers that literally make everything happen, so if you have not consumed enough nutrients for the enzymes, some critical function goes undone, or some important structure is never made. The results? Poor health and added unnecessary weight.

Remember that converting food into cellular energy requires hundreds of enzymes—all synthesized from the diet! We cannot lose weight or maintain a healthful weight on a nutrient-dead diet. We simply do not have the raw materials to build the enzymes to make weight loss happen. This is also a fundamental reason that many Americans struggle with chronic fatigue: their bodies simply cannot produce enough cellular energy, and therefore organ energy is depleted. When organs do not receive adequate amounts of energy, the whole body is tired.

What Energy-Building Nutrients Are Lacking in the American Diet?

The key nutrients required to build cellular energy include the whole complex of B vitamins (these act as coenzymes, or part of enzyme molecules), vitamin C, the minerals zinc and magnesium, fatty acids, amino acids, and some carbohydrates. Most Americans are deficient in at least one of the B-complex vitamins, and about 65 percent of Americans are deficient in magnesium. The average American consumes less than 10 milligrams (mg) of zinc per day, but the recommended daily allowance (RDA) for zinc is 15 mg, and some nutritionists believe that even more than that is required for optimum enzyme production.

It is no wonder that we are chronically tired, that we don't have enough energy to exercise, that we don't sleep well at night—and that we can't lose weight. If the building blocks of cellular energy are in short supply, we can't build energy and our food cannot efficiently be converted into energy. Our bodies then have no choice but to store food as fat, even if our diet is relatively low in calories. (And by the way,

undernutrition may be a key reason that "energy-deficiency diseases" like fibromyalgia are becoming increasingly prevalent.)

SOLVING YOUR PERSONAL ENERGY CRISIS

Fortunately, your personal energy problem is not difficult to correct: you must simply eat real food. It is very important that every morsel of food that goes into your mouth contributes to solving your energy crisis rather than making it worse. Unfortunately, dieters are often tempted to shortcut this solution by drinking caffeinated beverages, eating sugary foods, or using other stimulants to feel more energized. How many dieters start the morning with a piece of toast and a cup of coffee? Both are highly energizing and low in calories—but both sabotage the weight-loss process.

Why Is Coffee a Poor Energizer?

Coffee actually robs the body of energy! Caffeine temporarily increases energy by elevating the production of stress hormone (cortisol) and increasing blood pressure and heart rate. The long-term consequence, however, is an exhausted adrenal gland. Additionally, coffee strips the body of nutrients that are critical to energy production, particularly minerals like magnesium, potassium, zinc, and calcium. If you are deficient in any of these nutrients, your body cannot produce enough energy naturally.

So do not be tempted to take the shortcut to energy by starting your day with a cup of coffee. Provide your body with the building blocks of real, natural, vibrant energy by maximizing your intake of healthful foods and supplementing your diet with additional vitamins and minerals.

Begin to address your energy crisis with a good breakfast. I highly recommend using the Wings Breakfast Drink daily; each serving provides a foundation of protein, carbohydrates, and fats to keep energy levels high throughout the morning. Complement the Wings Breakfast Drink with a good-quality multivitamin-mineral supplement (ask your Wings nutritionist for her recommendation: at www.flywithwings.com/pnc.html, click on MyProConnect), and you are off to a great start.

Then at lunch and dinner, when you enjoy a portion of protein and a large colorful salad tossed with olive oil and vinegar, you continue to supply your body with the building blocks of energy. Fresh vegetables are nature's mineral supplement, and fresh fruits are nature's vitamin supplement. Rich in the nutrients that go directly into producing cellular energy, several servings of vegetables should be enjoyed throughout each day.

Be sure to follow the food plan outlined in this book. The menus and recipes were designed specifically to meet the body's energy requirements by emphasizing whole foods. Whole foods contain vitamins, minerals, proteins, fats, and carbohydrates that form the substrate or foundation of energy molecules. Each meal in the food plan contains proteins, fats, and carbohydrates so that blood sugar remains steady. Our goal is to provide your body with whole-food energy every day!

Snacks to Get Your Energy Flowing!

Want a great energizing snack? Stuff almond butter into a celery stalk or spread it on a crispy rice cracker. The wonderful fats in the nut butter are healthful and energizing. Other high-energy snacks are found in the back of the book, and you may "graze" on them throughout the day.

Remember that you can only convert food into cellular energy if your diet provides the nutrients needed to complete this conversion; otherwise, you store the food as fat. It has been found that when dieters reach a plateau, it is often because they need to provide their bodies with extra nutrition to get energy production back in full gear. If you feel this is the case for you, you may wish to double up on your multivitamin-mineral supplement for a short time, as added insurance.

Measuring Up

It's that time again . . . Weigh yourself, and then take five girth measurements: bust at the largest point, waist at two inches above the navel, hips at the largest point, and right and left thigh circumference at the point where your extended fingertips reach with your arms hanging down at your sides. Record these figures, and your calculated BMI value, on your Progress Chart.

And now, go to page 258 for your new recipes!

TODAY'S ASSIGNMENT

REVIEW, REMOVE, AND RELAX

Review the past four weeks of your Food Diary. How many stimulants are you using? Coffee? Sugar? Pastry and pasta? Soft drinks? List some healthful alternatives to these, and make a plan to eliminate the unhealthful stimulants from your diet.

Don't do it "cold turkey." People who suddenly stop consuming highly stimulating and potentially addictive foods and beverages often find themselves "crashing." Because their bodies have adapted to the continuous intake of artificial energy, they may feel particularly fatigued or nearly unable to function, which is so distressing they are then tempted to start using the sugar and caffeine again just to get through the day. Wean yourself off such stimulants one at a time, and substitute a healthful beverage or food that you really enjoy. Allow your body to adapt slowly.

Make sure you are eating at least five servings of fresh vegetables and one serving of fresh fruit daily. Also make sure you have at least 2 tablespoons of olive oil or macadamia nut oil, and a little butter, each day. Fat is very satisfying and energizing. Do not be afraid to enjoy fresh natural fats, because your body needs them.

Write out a supplement plan that includes energizing nutrients (see the Health Tip on page 63), purchase the supplements, and start using them. And throw out your coffeepot! Better yet, use it to brew relaxing or energizing herbal teas.

Pull out your appointment book and review your schedule. Does it include enough down time to allow your body and mind to rest? Remember that fatigue can often be a sign that you are working too hard and not resting enough. If your schedule is too tight, make a plan to eliminate unnecessary appointments and work. Learn to say no! (I have found it extremely important to include a "Sabbath" in my week. On this day, I do not work: I enjoy restful and calming activities instead. It makes a huge difference in my energy levels throughout the week.)

LESSON II-1 STUDY GUIDE

1. What is the body's most basic task?

_____

_____

_____

2. Why does the American diet actually foster fatigue instead of energy?

3. What nutrients are necessary for the production of cellular energy?

4. List some dietary tips for increasing energy.

5. Spend some time in the fresh produce aisle of your supermarket and list every vegetable you find there. How many of these are you enjoying regularly?

6. Design a soup recipe that includes at least ten to fifteen different vegetables and prepare it for your family—and notice how good you feel! You will want to make your soup creation a frequent addition to your menu.

HEALTH TIP

ENERGIZING SUPPLEMENTS

Want more energy? Use supplements!

- Alpha-lipoic or lipoic acid is essential to metabolism and has been found to increase ATP (cellular energy) levels. It also helps regulate blood glucose levels.

- The amino acid L-carnitine acts as a powerful energizer by shuttling fatty acids into the mitochondria (the "furnace" of the cell) to be burned for energy. Without sufficient L-carnitine, fats cannot be burned and instead will remain in the body. Take 1–2 grams per day, just before breakfast or with your Wings Breakfast Drink.

- You must not forget to use coenzyme Q_{10} (CoQ_{10}), which increases the energy-releasing actions on mitochondrial membranes, nourishes the heart, and helps reduce the risk of developing many types of heart and vascular disease. The recommended daily dose is 240–360 milligrams. The Q-Gel form (sold under many brand names) is a good source of CoQ_{10}; take it along with L-carnitine.

- Make sure you get enough B-complex vitamins, particularly if you struggle with chronic stress. On top of those included in my multivitamin, I take an additional 100 milligrams of each of the B-complex vitamins, and I've noticed big differences in my energy and my ability to handle stress.

Lesson II-2. Is It Hunger, or Is It Thirst?

The body does not always communicate its needs very clearly. Often when we feel we are hungry, we are actually thirsty and need to drink water. Both hunger and thirst are regulated by the hypothalamus, an organ in the endocrine system that can be damaged by certain chemicals, including MSG and aspartame. If we are not used to drinking water throughout the day, we may think we're hungry when we are really thirsty. If you still feel hungry when you know you have eaten adequate amounts of food, ask yourself whether you might be thirsty instead—or, simply sip water throughout the day, and avoid the problems associated with inadequate water intake.

?   **TODAY'S QUESTION**

How much water do you drink in a day?

_____

_____

_____

_____

    Review your Food Diary and calculate an accurate answer. Do not include any other beverages in this tally except herbal tea.

    Drinking water as our *only* beverage is not something to which we Americans are accustomed. The average American adult drinks 26 gallons of coffee, 46 gallons of soft drinks, 26 gallons of tea, and more than 26 gallons of alcoholic beverages per year. How much water do we drink? Only 9 gallons of bottled water per person per year. Unfortunately, coffee, tea, fruit juices, alcohol, and soft drinks are not at all equivalent to water in terms of hydrating and cleansing the body.

BAD BEVERAGES

Most beverages can actually be classified as antinutrients because they can strip nutrition out of the body. Beverages other than water simply do not hydrate as efficiently: coffee and other caffeinated drinks, for example, are actually dehydrating. Have you ever noticed that when you drink one or more cups of coffee in the morning, you need to go to the bathroom shortly after? Coffee can act as a laxative or diuretic, both of which flush water out of the body. Coffee likewise increases the excretion of minerals, leading to nutrient deficiencies.

Seductive Soft Drinks

How do carbonated soft drinks damage the body? The carbonation is provided by phosphoric acid, a chemical derivative of phosphorus. Phosphorus, an essential nutrient, is used as a structural component in the bones and other tissue, and the body maintains a specific calcium-to-phosphorus ratio that provides optimum bone-building capabilities. The relatively large amounts of phosphoric acid in soft drinks skew this critical mineral ratio dramatically in the direction of phosphorus, leading to a relative calcium deficiency, no matter how much calcium is consumed. In addition, the acidic sugars in soft drinks disrupt the delicate pH of the blood. Maintaining a correct pH in the tissues is vitally important, so when these sugars

✎   **NOTES**

_____

_____

_____

_____

_____

_____

over-acidify the body, alkalinity must be restored by pulling minerals from the bones—ultimately leading to bone loss.

In a sense, we use coffee and soft drinks as a form of self-medication to stimulate energy, to shore up our flagging, tired bodies that are overworked, under-rested, and undernourished. Drinking these beverages sets up addictive behaviors that are difficult to control. What's more, our ravenous appetite for these anti-nutrients may be setting us up for a frightening epidemic of diseases like osteoporosis and heart disease. In short, coffee and soft drinks may be some of the most dangerous things we put into our mouths.

THE BODY NEEDS WATER

What benefits does water provide?

1. Water cleanses the body's internal environment.

2. Water activates hundreds of thousands of enzymes, stimulating every bodily activity.

3. Water regulates body temperature, cooling the body when it is too hot and making it easier to heat when it is too cool.

4. Water is the fluid conduit (the internal river) that carries nutrients throughout the tissues of the body. The lymphatic and excretory systems provide watery channels to escort toxic materials out of the body.

5. Water is a solvent (dissolving medium) that puts hundreds of chemicals into forms the body can use.

6. Water serves structural functions for all cells and organs; for example, water helps cushion the brain against injury within the hard surface of the skull.

7. Water is the substance that conducts red and white blood cells and hundreds of other substances throughout the circulatory system.

8. The body's electrical system is based upon hydro-electric energy, which is generated by the osmotic flow of water through cell membranes.

Symptoms of "Water Deficiency"

Unless we drink copious amounts of water, many of the processes listed above are curtailed. Symptoms of dehydration include constipation, fatigue, headaches, dry, scaly skin, skin eruptions, sleep disorders, urinary tract infections and disorders, darkly colored urine, sinus and respiratory infections, and so on. A loss of 20 percent of the body's water stores results in death; 10 percent dehydration results in serious ill-ness. Unfortunately, by the time we feel thirsty, we are already 2 or 3 percent dehydrated, and the body's energy production is already diminished.

If you are often bloated with excess water, you certainly need to drink more water! This may seem contradictory, but when you are chronically dehydrated, your body will hold any water it gets, causing bloating and edema (water retention in the tissues). Also, fecal material that is insufficiently hydrated will be compacted in your colon, causing your abdomen to become distended. *Note:* If you suffer from chronic edema that is not resolved by drinking adequate amounts of water, please see your doctor, because edema can also be a symptom of cardiovascular disease.

How to Drink Water

People should drink water throughout the day, not just at mealtimes. How much water do you require? Some doctors believe you should drink 1 ounce for every 2 pounds of body weight. In other words, if you weigh 150 pounds, you should drink 75 ounces of water daily; if you weigh 200 pounds, you should drink 100 ounces of water daily. If that seems like too much water, gradually increase up to that level. Make sure you distribute your water intake throughout the entire day (while you are awake). If you gulp large quantities of water at infrequent intervals, the water often floods the kidneys and you simply urinate much of the water out, which is fine for the kidneys but isn't hydrating for the rest of the body.

I suggest that you drink about $\frac{1}{4}$ or $\frac{1}{2}$ cup of water every thirty minutes or so, whether or not you feel thirsty. As long as you do not drink the water too rapidly or in large quantities at one sitting, you will not find that you have to urinate more frequently. Ideally, though, you should urinate several times per day. Drinking water is very important to the health of your kidneys, and reduced kidney function is a marker for deteriorating health and premature aging.

Keep a water bottle at your workstation at all times. If you live in a warm or dry climate, you may require more water. If you work physically hard enough to break a sweat, increase your water intake proportionately. Preferably, the water should be at room temperature so your body does not have to spend metabolic energy raising the temperature of the water (although that process can burn calories).

Are there any negative side effects from drinking all of this water? None! But the positive side effects include clear skin, increased energy, reduced incidence of headaches and sinus problems, resolution of edema and constipation, and so on. One can only benefit from keeping the body hydrated!

And now, go to page 258 for your new recipes!

TODAY'S ASSIGNMENT

BOTTOM'S UP!

Practice drinking water this week. Buy an athletic bottle or thermos and measure how much water it holds. Calculate the amount of water you should drink daily according to the formula of 1 ounce for every 2 pounds of your body weight. Challenge yourself to drink that amount of water and eliminate all other beverages. For a special treat, you may enjoy a cup or two of herbal tea to take the place of some of the water.

LESSON II-2 STUDY GUIDE

1. What organ regulates hunger and thirst?

2. What two chemicals can dysregulate that organ?

3. What are some of the functions of water in the body?

4. What are some common symptoms of dehydration?

5. How much water should we drink each day? What circumstances could increase that amount?

HEALTH TIP

CALCIUM SUPPLEMENTATION

New research indicates that women—especially dieters—may require more calcium. In a study published recently in the *American Journal of Clinical Nutrition* (2004, Vol. 80:123–130), fifty-seven postmenopausal overweight women took either 200 milligrams (mg) of calcium in a multivitamin or 1,000 mg of supplemental calcium citrate daily for six weeks. Some were dieting and some simply maintained their current weight. The dieting women actually absorbed less calcium than those in the weight-maintenance group; the researchers suggest that dieters need to take supplemental calcium above the current recommendations to prevent the bone-mass reduction associated with dieting.

Lesson II-3. Less Than Two BMs Daily? Help!

You will notice that many people carry a huge amount of excess weight in their abdomens. Often when I see someone who is otherwise thin but carries a protruding belly, I wonder what is lurking in the colon. Is it impacted with pounds of fecal material that impairs the person's health and makes weight loss impossible? This lesson will discuss colon health and why it is important to maintain good bowel habits.

? TODAY'S QUESTION

How frequent are your bowel movements?

_____

_____

_____

_____

What is the consistency? Are they floaters or sinkers? Soft and cleansing, or hard and dry? (Whew! Isn't this embarrassing?)

It has been said, "All disease begins in the colon." Our ancestors used to have several well-formed bowel movements per day, and as a result, enjoyed a lower incidence of colon cancer, diabetes, and many other diseases. Today, however, chronic constipation is an ongoing problem for many Americans. You must start thinking about the health of the lower half of your body and focus on getting it cleaned out!

WHAT DOES THE COLON DO?

After food has been digested and the nutrients have been absorbed into the bloodstream through the inner lining of the small intestine, the leftovers are carried into the large intestine. There they mix with cellular debris that has been deposited into the colon from the bloodstream, and with the yeast and bacteria that normally populate our digestive system. The colon, or large intestine, is an incredibly important part of the body and a very dynamic organ. Its function is twofold: to collect intestinal debris into a solid packet for excretion from the body, and to absorb water from the digestive tract.

Fecal material is very fluid as it moves from the small intestine into the large intestine. As the material passes through the colon, much of the water is absorbed into the bloodstream and the product becomes drier, though it should still contain enough water to make it soft and easily passed. The mixture is then carried by a process of peristalsis (rhythmic, involuntary muscle contractions) to the rectum to be expelled from the body.

Environmental chemicals that have invaded the body through food, air, and the skin are filtered through the liver, kidneys, and lungs, and most of those chemicals are then expelled in the feces along with the byproducts of digestion. As detoxification enzymes are activated in the liver, the byproducts of detoxification are dumped into the colon for removal from the body. Used estrogens are also excreted by the liver into the colon for expulsion in the feces, a process that helps the female body maintain a normal estrogen balance.

✒ NOTES

_____

_____

_____

_____

_____

Bacteria in the Colon

A healthy colon contains more bacteria than there are cells in the entire body. As many as 400 different species of bacteria may live in the colon, and intestinal bacteria can weigh about $3\frac{1}{2}$ pounds (this explains why a violent wave of diarrhea can cause loss of several pounds; some of that lost weight is intestinal bacteria, plus water). The colon's bacterial assortment includes both "friendly" and "unfriendly" or pathogenic (disease-producing) organisms.

Friendly bacteria perform several valuable services for us. They synthesize several B-complex vitamins, which are then absorbed into the bloodstream and used by the body. They help maintain the correct pH of the intestinal tract, which is important for the health and function of the tissue, and they aid in the digestion of several nutrients. They wage war against the pathogenic bacteria, preventing them from proliferating to the point that they could create disease. Friendly bacteria also keep yeasts in check that would otherwise multiply out of control.

Colon Damage

Because the tissues of the large and small intestines are very delicate, they are easily damaged. Some of the most common causes of damage to the intestinal lining include the overuse of antibiotics, the consumption of large amounts of sugar, chlorinated water, or alcoholic beverages, and illness. Chronic use of antibiotics, sugar, or alcohol often disrupts the normal colonization of bacteria in the intestines, which then leads to chronic yeast infections, constipation, and other conditions. (Unfriendly yeast will be discussed in Lesson III-13.) When fecal material is not moved out of the colon frequently and efficiently, toxins (such as the used estrogens and chemicals mentioned above) can be reabsorbed into the body.

CONSTIPATION

There is a huge misunderstanding about the definition of constipation. Many healthcare practitioners do not consider less than one bowel movement per day to be a problem as long as the stool is not hard and dry. Most holistic physicians believe, however, that at least two or three bowel movements per day are absolutely essential if we are to enjoy superior health.

Constipation should be defined as less than two to three easy bowel movements per day, and a stool that is hard and dry instead of large, soft, and well formed. Want to be really healthy? Work toward achieving two or three soft, cleansing bowel movements per day. You will find that every measure of health improves—and you may even often lose weight.

What Causes Constipation?

One or more of the following factors can cause constipation:

- Dehydration (drinking too little water)
- Mineral deficiencies (such as magnesium and potassium)
- Excessive consumption of, or consuming poorly absorbed forms of, iron or calcium
- Hypothyroidism (must be diagnosed and treated by a physician)
- Food allergy or food intolerance (particularly from consuming cheese or other dairy products)
- Antibiotic use or other factors that kill helpful intestinal bacteria
- A diet low in fiber
- Certain types of medications (morphine, codeine, calcium channel blockers, beta-blockers, various sedatives and tranquilizers, calcium carbonate, some antacids)
- Lack of exercise
- Imbalance of the estrogen-progesterone ratio (to estrogen dominance)
- Growth or blockage in the colon (must be diagnosed by a physician and may necessitate surgical removal)
- Constrictions in the colon (must be diagnosed and treated by a physician)

Do any of these conditions apply to you? If so, let's start working on your constipation today.

What Trouble Constipation Can Cause!

Constipation can cause the following conditions:

- Acne
- Appendicitis
- Arthritis
- Bad breath
- Bowel cancer
- Diverticulitis
- Gas
- Headaches
- Hemorrhoids (piles)
- Hernia
- Indigestion
- Insomnia
- Obesity
- Varicose veins

This list should help impress on us how very important it is to take care of our colons!

Colon cancer is one of the most common types of cancer. It is thought that constipation is a leading cause of this deadly disease. As toxic materials sit in the colon for long periods of time, they damage the lining and can increase the risk of cancer development. People in cultures that consume large amounts of fiber rarely get colon cancer. For that matter, they seldom get heart disease, diabetes, and other degenerative diseases!

A Ghastly Illustration

Imagine chewing your food but instead of swallowing it, spitting it into an enamel pan and placing it into an oven set at 98.6°F. Then imagine repeating the process at each meal: pulling out the pan and spitting the chewed contents of your mouth into it. Imagine allowing the pan to sit in the oven for one, two, three days or more. What would be the condition of the contents of the pan within a short period of time? Would you be able to stand the odor in the house?

If you are not moving your bowels on a regular basis, that very food is fermenting (rotting) in your intestinal tract and colon! No wonder we struggle with bad breath, low energy, bad skin, and excess weight. Yuck!

Solving a Constipation Problem

Following are some tips for treating constipation naturally, without resorting to medications:

- Drink eight to ten (or more) glasses of pure water each day, spaced throughout the day as described in Lesson II-2.

- Make sure your diet is adequate in magnesium and potassium. Take up to 500 milligrams (mg) of magnesium per day in supplement form, and 99 mg of potassium per day, or more with a physician's approval. Fresh, green, leafy vegetables are also a good source of these essential minerals.

- Increase the fiber in your diet to 35 grams or more per day. You may need to purchase a good fiber supplement (and take it with copious amounts of water) unless you eat large amounts of fibrous vegetables like garbanzo beans. Purchase a fiber counter and keep track of your daily fiber intake, to make sure.

- Resolve any medical conditions that may cause constipation (see page 68) and ask your physician whether your medications may contribute to constipation.

- Remove all allergens from the diet, particularly dairy and wheat products, both of which are particularly constipating.

- Make sure that exercise is a regular part of your daily routine, especially walking or swimming, which "massage" the lower abdomen.

- Make sure that your dietary supplements do not contain calcium carbonate, iron sulfate, or other forms of minerals that may be constipating.

- If necessary, use herbal laxatives that do not contain senna or large amounts of *Cascara sagrada*.

- If you have used antibiotics for any length of time, eaten large amounts of sugar, consumed soft drinks, alcoholic beverages, or chlorinated water, or have otherwise killed off the friendly bacteria in your digestive system, you should use a good probiotic supplement. Ask at your local health food store for suggestions. Restoring normal bacterial counts will require taking a supplement twice per day (on an empty stomach) for several months or more.

Remember that maintaining the health of your colon is a lifelong project. You will start working on it in today's assignment, but don't forget about it as the weeks pass. Soon, you should "enjoy" two to three easy, soft, cleansing bowel movements per day.

And now, go to page 259 for your new recipes!

 TODAY'S ASSIGNMENT

BE KIND TO YOUR COLON

Pay special attention to your bowel movements this week, making sure to move your bowels at least once per day.

Each bowel movement should be soft and well formed and should not contain any particles of undigested food. They should not be odoriferous; if they smell like sulfur, you may not be digesting your protein to completion. If you notice streaks of blood, or if portions of your bowel movement are black, see your physician immediately to learn the cause of blood in the stool. If the fecal material is long and stringy, you may also wish to consult your physician to make sure that there is no constriction of the bowel that could be preventing the feces from being well formed.

If you have any questions about the quality or quantity of your bowel movements, please check with your physician, who will be able to answer your questions and make sure there is no underlying disease.

As mentioned previously, purchase a fiber counter to keep track of the amount of fiber you consume. If you are not regularly reaching the goal of 35 grams of dietary fiber daily, purchase a good-quality fiber supplement from your health food store and take it each evening before you retire, along with a large glass of water.

And remember: all disease (and all health) begins in the colon. So take care of it!

LESSON 11-3 STUDY GUIDE

1. What could be meant by "All disease begins in the colon"?

_____

_____

2. What are some functions of the colon?

_____

_____

3. What is constipation?

_____

_____

4. What are some causes of constipation?

_____

_____

5. What disease conditions are caused by constipation?

_____

_____

6. How much fiber should one consume?

_____

_____

7. List some techniques for resolving the problem of constipation.

_____

_____

HEALTH TIP

FEVER

A fever is the sign of an active immune system response to an invading pathogen. A fever is therefore a good thing, unless it gets too high. Don't try to bring a fever down unless it climbs above 103°F; allow the fever to do its job. If a fever starts getting too high, you can reduce it by:

- Using an enema of catnip tea twice daily
- Drinking a tea of catnip combined with dandelion
- Taking the herb yarrow

There are several things you can do to support the immune system in cases of fever. They include:

- Enjoy (whew!) a few cups of onion-and-garlic tea (page 181)
- Do an ascorbic acid flush (pages 8–9)
- Take supplementary pantothenic acid, vitamin A, and zinc

For fever's side effects, you should:

- Get plenty of rest
- Drink large quantities of liquids (especially chicken broth, freshly squeezed orange juice, and water) to prevent dehydration and flush out toxins
- Use cool sponge baths on the forehead and face

See a healthcare professional immediately if the following conditions develop:

- Frequent urination, a burning sensation while urinating, or blood in the urine
- Pain concentrated in one area of the abdomen
- Shaking chills or alternating chills and sweats
- Severe headache and vomiting
- Profuse, watery diarrhea lasting more than twenty-four hours
- Swollen glands or rashes

Caution: NEVER give aspirin to a child with a fever.

Lesson II-4. The Problem of Nonfoods

When your great-grandparents went "shopping," they "bought" their food from the garden and pasture. Each morning, they milked the family cow into a galvanized bucket. After the creamy, rich beverage cooled, they poured it into glass bottles and stored it on ice or in a refrigerator. They beat the cream into butter and converted soured milk into cheese. They wrestled their carrots out of the garden soil and washed them off under the pump spigot at the well. The only packaging around their corn was several layers of husks that Bessie munched on as a late-afternoon snack. The shrink-wrap on their beef or halibut fillet was its own skin.

Sadly, the vast majority of what Americans now eat and drink falls into the category of nonfood or pseudo-food: food products that have been altered (for example, low-fat items), that are highly processed, or to which artificial flavoring agents, coloring agents, preservatives, or other man-made chemicals have been added. In other words, we eat huge amounts of synthetic products that cannot be classified as food. Just some of the nonfoods that Americans regularly consume include potato chips, frozen and canned entrées, entrée mixes like Hamburger Helper, dried soup mixes, processed snack and beverage items, and of course, most desserts like ice cream and cookies. Certainly, candy falls into the nonfood category (but we knew that—didn't we?).

? TODAY'S QUESTION

Why are nonfoods harmful to the body?

_____

_____

_____

_____

And how do nonfoods cause side effects like excess weight gain? The answer goes beyond too many calories or too much sugar, and even beyond the lack of nutrients in nonfoods. The thrust of this lesson is how the chemicals routinely added to foods cause a variety of endocrine and other problems for the body.

We've previously discussed how certain nonfood beverages can cause osteoporosis and pH disturbance. Consuming nonfoods strips the body's minerals and disrupts their natural balance, leading to the development of many health problems. For example, when high-sodium packaged entrées are eaten without a counterbalancing amount of potassium, the electrical signals of the nervous system are disrupted. Excessive sodium also causes bloating from water retention. When high-calcium products are eaten without a balancing amount of magnesium, muscle contraction and relaxation is altered, causing hardening of the arteries, kidney stones, and emotional upsets (review the symptoms of magnesium deficiency on page 20).

🖋 NOTES

_____

_____

_____

_____

_____

_____

It may surprise you to learn that nonfoods can lead to weight gain by interfering with female hormones. Xenoestrogens (synthetic estrogens) and phytoestrogens (plant-based estrogens) in our food supply disrupt the normal estrogen-progesterone balance. Plastics leach biologically significant amounts of xenoestrogens into food; this happens, for example, when we microwave something in a plastic container or plastic wrap, or pour hot liquids into plastic containers. Estrogen dominance can pack on 5–35 pounds of extra weight, some in the form of water retention but some as added fat tissue.

When the liver becomes overloaded or is unable to process the glut of chemicals to which it is exposed, the harmful toxins are stored in fat tissue. (You will learn more about the influence of environmental pollutants on weight and health in Lesson III-11.) This long-term storage is another important reason to maintain regular bowel movements and eat lots of fiber to help expel any toxins consumed. The body does not produce enzymes that digest nonfoods, so they clog the body and produce toxicity throughout the tissues. Toxic materials in the body can cause the following health problems:

▪ Increased water retention

▪ Reduced energy production

▪ Disrupted production and activity of enzymes

▪ Disrupted natural hormone levels

▪ Stress on the immune system

REMEMBERING WHAT'S REAL AND WHAT ISN'T

Grandma didn't fill recycling bins with glass, plastic, and paper. She recycled by slopping the hogs, composting, and stoking the woodstove that warmed the family home and heated the family meal.

We have become so accustomed to seeing lists of additives on our food packages that we don't think twice about them anymore. A good rule of thumb to follow is this: If you can't spell it or pronounce it, don't eat it! Perhaps another good rule of thumb should be: If it didn't grow in a garden or walk on the land or swim in the natural waters, don't eat it!

Some of the "stuff" you eat may look like real foods but are, in fact, pseudo-foods that negatively impact your overall health. And they can certainly influence your body's ability to lose and maintain weight. Fostering good health means eating good food and avoiding man-made, synthetic foods as much as possible.

What is real food? Food is a substance naturally produced from the earth that provides the materials needed by the body for health. Food contributes protein, carbohydrates, fats, vitamins, minerals, water, and fiber, all in a form that the body can digest using its own enzymes and other digestive products. Foods include vegetables, fruits, and animal products. That's it!

Food Toys

Being told to avoid nonfoods is hard to take, isn't it? We really love our food toys! We are used to the tastes and aromas blended in a chemist's beaker. We almost don't know how real food looks, tastes, or smells.

Some common nonfoods to avoid:

- Margarine and shortening

- Soft drinks or other canned, processed beverages

- Packaged cereals

- Packaged entrée meals

- Packaged snack foods

- Infant formula (this warning is too late for adults—but make sure you do not feed an artificial formula to your baby)

- Sugary cereals and sugary baked goods

- Candy!

- Fruit juice (unless it is freshly pressed)

AN ENVIRONMENTAL PERSPECTIVE

It is bad enough that nonfoods pollute our bodies; they also pollute the environment. This weekend when you do your weekly grocery shopping, take a careful look around the store. What do you see? "I see food!" you say. Look again. Unless you are standing in the fresh produce aisle or in front of the meat counter, you see packages, cans, and boxes. You see plastic and cardboard and aluminum and glass: you don't see food.

The other day, I was browsing through my local supermarket, loading my shopping cart with a week's supply of groceries. As I walked up and down the aisles, I became fascinated with the assortment of materials on the shelves: brightly colored packages, reds, yellows, blues, greens, cans, boxes, bags—row after row, aisle after aisle, thousands and thousands of packages. Normally while I'm browsing like this, I'm amazed by how few real-food products are sold, but that day my mind was on something different: how much waste is generated by putting pseudo-food into packaging materials and lining it up in the supermarket. How many landfills have to be created before we realize that the best environmental policy is to stock our kitchen cupboards with fresh foods, as close to the garden and pasture as possible?

I remember how we recycled when I was a child. We threw the corn husks to the cows behind the house and dumped the garden waste on the compost pile; what little we couldn't reuse in that fashion, my father burned in a little stove. We never heard of garbage collection in those days.

Imagine how "eating natural" would influence our environment:

1. There would be massive savings of the wood products that are used to produce millions of tons of paper packaging materials.

2. More paper (trees) would be saved if we stopped eating out in fast-food restaurants where meals are served in disposable trays, cups, wrappers, and bags.

3. The production and consumption of plastic products would be reduced significantly, leading to less leaching of xenoestrogens into groundwater, streams, rivers, and our bodies.

4. Think of the energy (water and electricity) used to produce the papers and plastics that wrap our pseudo-foods. What a waste! And think of the chemicals used in paper-manufacturing plants!

5. Newspapers could save the amount of paper used to print grocery ads, and junk mail would be reduced by about half (don't you just remove those four-color flyers from the mailbox and toss them without even reading them?).

6. Instead of driving to the supermarket or fast-food chain, we would forage through our gardens and pantries for dinner, saving gasoline and reducing pollution.

7. Speaking of transportation wastes, think of all the fuel consumed and the pollution generated by trucks hauling our pseudo-foods to the stores and restaurants . . .

Well, if we really started eating natural, the impact on our environment and economy would be staggering.

Ramifications of Getting Real

I love filling my grocery cart with fresh veggies and fruits, dark pink salmon fillets, olive oils, vinegars, and crisp green herbs. I have to admit that I do sneak a few packages into the crevasses between the salad greens and the bok choy, but my packages are usually a few cans of tuna fish (for emergencies), chicken broth (when I don't have time to make my own), and a can or two of olives or tomatoes. I guess I haven't gone totally "green"!

But if we make a conscious effort to buy as few cans, boxes, and wrapped goods as possible, we'll be doing our Earth a huge favor. When we go natural, we're saving our world for our kids and our grandkids. I hate to think that my kids will have to devise a way to deal with the garbage I left behind, or that by the time they are grown and having babies of their own, the world they inherited has become one huge garbage site they'll have to spend billions of dollars trying to fix.

Live consciously and purposefully. What are you doing to preserve the beauty of our world? Think natural. Live natural. *Eat natural.* Your body—and our Earth—will be grateful.

And now, go to page 260 for your new recipes!

TODAY'S ASSIGNMENT

RAISE YOUR REAL-FOOD AWARENESS

In case you could not bring yourself to throw out your nonfoods back in Lesson I-7, here is another opportunity. Those of us who were brought up in the forties and fifties shudder at the "waste" of tossing out what we've purchased, but you need to realize that nonfoods do no good to anyone: your body cannot use them, so even if you eat them, the dollars have already been wasted. Refresh your memory by revisiting the list of nonfoods on pages 32–33. Then, get rid of all packaged and processed nonfood items (and don't forget the nonfood beverages) in your house, car, workplace, gym bag . . . Replace these things with real foods. Think of what you're doing for the health of your body, your family, and the world around you, and feel good!

LESSON II-4 STUDY GUIDE

1. What common food products are categorized in this lesson as nonfoods?

2. What is food?

3. Name several ways that nonfoods harm the body.

4. What are xenoestrogens and phytoestrogens?

5. Discuss some ways that processed foods harm the environment.

HEALTH TIP

SEX AND LIBIDO

A vigorous sex life is the sign of a healthy body—and a healthy relationship. Frigidity can be caused by psychological distress (fear, guilt, depression, conflict with one's mate, or feelings of inferiority). Unresolved past sexual and/or emotional abuse is a common cause.

Here are some tips for naturally promoting female libido and sexual function:

- If intercourse is painful due to insufficient lubrication, use pure body oil (available from your health food store) to provide lubrication.

- Try damiana, called "the women's sexuality herb" because it contains alkaloids that have a testosterone-like effect. Place a dropperful of damiana extract under the tongue an hour or two before sexual activity. You may need to take it for several days before noticing a difference.

- Other herbs to enhance libido include fo-ti, gotu kola, sarsaparilla, and Siberian ginseng.

- Include lots of alfalfa tea in the diet, as well as avocados, olive oil, pumpkin seeds, other seeds and nuts, and sesame oil.

- Consider using DHEA, the precursor to testosterone and estrogen. *Caution:* Do not use DHEA if you have a personal or family history of hormone-driven tumors.

- Make sure your diet contains enough omega-3 fatty acids, zinc, and vitamin C.

- Make sure any possible underlying hypothyroidism is resolved, as hypothyroidism can cause impotence or loss of libido.

And here are some natural tips for men from Dr. James Duke, author of several books, including *The Green Pharmacy* (Emmaus, PA: Rodale Press, 1997):

- Fava beans (8–16 ounces per day) have a reputation as an aphrodisiac.

- Quebracho is considered a male aphrodisiac. *Caution:* Do not use quebracho if you have high blood pressure.

- Ginkgo (60–240 milligrams per day) increases blood flow to the penis.

- Anise may increase male libido.

- Muira puama extract (1–2.5 grams per day) may improve male libido and treat erectile dysfunction.

- Yohimbe increases erections. *Caution:* Be careful with yohimbe, because this herb can also increase anxiety, heart rate, blood pressure, and other symptoms.

Lesson II-5. The Ins and Outs of Digestion

There is no point in eating food if you cannot digest it. Undigested or partially digested food that sits in the colon is rotting and fermenting; it is not being broken down into molecules that the body can use. Nurturing good digestion is a fundamental part of building health that must not be ignored.

? TODAY'S QUESTION

How is your digestion?

Do you ever experience one or more of the following symptoms?

- Bloating, belching, or burping
- Bad breath
- Bad skin
- Constipation, diarrhea, or alternating constipation and diarrhea
- Feeling that your food is "just sitting down there"
- Intestinal gas
- Nausea after eating a meal

These are common symptoms of poor digestion. It is possible, however, to have impaired digestion and not even know it, as it does not always elicit unpleasant symptoms.

A THUMBNAIL SKETCH OF THE DIGESTIVE PROCESS

Digestion actually begins when you anticipate eating. Hunger and the aroma of cooking food alert your liver and pancreas to begin secreting digestive enzymes in preparation for receiving the impending meal.

When the first bite of food reaches your mouth, your salivary glands secrete enzymes that begin digesting the starch and other sugars in the meal. Chewing the food is very important, because as food is broken down into very small pieces, enzymes (both those in the food and those produced by the body) have more access to the bonds holding the food's constituents together. I recommend chewing each bite at least twenty times, or until the food is reduced to a liquid in the mouth. This little step greatly enhances the digestive process.

After food is swallowed, it goes down the esophagus into the pyloric region of the stomach, where it sits for a period of time. Cold foods are warmed to body temperature, the temperature at which digestive enzymes work most efficiently. Digestion of protein and, to a limited extent, fat begins here, in the upper stomach: when the body identifies the presence of proteins or fat, the appropriate enzymes are secreted to begin breaking the food down into its elemental parts.

Hydrochloric acid production reduces the pH of the stomach to about 1.5, creating an extremely acidic environment that kills bacteria, yeast, and other

✦ NOTES

Chewing Liquids and Drinking Solids

The Eclectic physicians of the 1800s counseled patients to "chew their liquids and drink their solids." What does that mean? "Chew liquids" means to swish liquids in the mouth to mix them thoroughly with salivary enzymes before swallowing. "Drink solids" means to chew solid food so thoroughly that it becomes liquid in the mouth. These little steps greatly aid in the process of digestion. Perhaps we buy so many antacids because we simply bite twice and swallow, forcing the body to struggle to break down huge lumps of food through enzyme activity alone. Chewing and mixing thoroughly in the mouth makes the breakdown of food more efficient, improving digestion without the use of drugs.

pathogens, facilitates the action of several protein-digesting enzymes, and serves other functions in the digestive system. As the enzymes do their work, the food particles drop into the lower region of the stomach, where protein digestion is nearly completed. Very little carbohydrate or fat digestion occurs in the stomach.

The partly digested food (now called chyme) then passes into the small intestine, where enzymes on the surface of the intestinal tract complete the digestion of proteins, fats, and carbohydrates. As food particles are digested, they are absorbed into the bloodstream by several different mechanisms; some require energy and others are passive. The absorbent area of the small intestine's inner surface is enormous: if it were spread out flat, it would cover an area about the size of a football field!

Interestingly, each area of the small intestine is responsible for absorbing a different nutrient: some are specific to calcium and magnesium, another is specific to iron, and still another is responsible for the absorption of vitamin C. Imagine, then, what could happen to nutrient absorption if a section of the small intestine were injured or damaged.

After the nutrients have been absorbed into the body, the remainder of the food (fiber and other undigested particles) passes into the large intestine. Much of the water is then absorbed into the body from the colon, leaving a packet of fecal material consisting of fiber, desquamated cells (recycled cellular materials), bacteria, and yeast. Finally, the body eliminates this fecal material in the bowel movement.

WHEN DIGESTION GOES WRONG

Most people struggle with poor digestion at one point

or another because so many things can disrupt the process. Factors that can contribute to poor or incomplete digestion include stress, deficiencies in essential nutrients like the B-complex vitamins or zinc, poor liver function, haste (rushing through a meal so food is not chewed thoroughly, or not allowing the body time to prepare itself for the meal), physical activity directly following a meal, and underproduction of digestive enzymes or hydrochloric acid, among other causes.

Poor digestion can cause constipation, acne, and many other health conditions, so it is fundamentally important to make sure your digestive tract is not only clean but working well. How do you know when your digestive system isn't working properly? Common signs of poor digestion include the following:

- Bloating, belching, burning, and flatulence immediately after a meal
- A sense of fullness that lasts long after eating
- Indigestion, diarrhea, or constipation
- Multiple food allergies or intolerances
- Nausea after taking dietary supplements
- Itching around the rectum
- Weak, peeling, and cracked fingernails
- Dilated blood vessels in the chin, cheeks, and/or nose (in nonalcoholics)
- Acne
- Iron deficiency
- Chronic intestinal parasites or abnormal intestinal flora
- Chronic candida (yeast) infections
- Upper-digestive-tract gassiness
- Undigested food in the stool

Sometimes, however, a person with a digestive problem will experience few or no symptoms.

POOR DIGESTION CAUSES WEIGHT GAIN

As you learned in Lesson I-10, incompletely digested foods (especially proteins) cause food allergies and other inflammatory conditions, which lead to water retention and fat deposition. Foods that rot in the body produce huge amounts of gas that distend the abdomen and stomach. One Wings student, after improving her digestion and releasing huge amounts of gas, lost several inches around her waist and abdomen! (Disgusting, but true.) If the elimination process is inadequate, up to several pounds of fecal material can cake or line the inside of the colon, causing distention of the abdomen and adding unnecessary weight.

When undigested food passes unabsorbed out of the body, the nutrients contained in that food are eliminated as well; the result can be malnutrition, even if adequate amounts of calories and nutrients were eaten in the meal. It is known that long-term malnutrition lowers the activity of the thyroid gland, which then slows metabolism, which in turn hinders weight loss (Lesson III-2). It is not hard to imagine, therefore, how poor digestion leads to a downward spiral of poor health. The goal for this lesson is to reverse that downward spiral.

HOW TO IMPROVE YOUR DIGESTION

It is not enough just to get the body cleaned out occasionally; you must make sure the digestive process is completed satisfactorily after every meal. Here are some simple tips:

- Include substantial amounts of fiber in your diet (up to 35 grams per day).

- Remove all potential allergens from your diet.

- Spend time in meal preparation, anticipating the food's arrival. This allows your body enough time to release digestive juices prior to the meal.

- Before eating, drink a cup of ginger tea to stimulate the flow of digestive juices (see Today's Assignment).

- Use an herbal bitters product twenty minutes prior to each meal to further improve the flow of digestive juices. The Eclectic Institute produces many wonderful herbal digestive products, including tinctures of gentian and other bitters. Their Neutralizing Cordial is one of the best digestive aids on the market!

- You may not be secreting adequate amounts of hydrochloric acid. If you suspect that is the case, ask your doctor for a Heidelberg test of your stomach's acidity, or test it yourself with a "stomach acid challenge"(see inset).

- Drink plenty of pure water *between* meals. Do not, however, drink too much water *with* meals.

- Make mealtime a pleasurable time: do not use the family dinner table to discuss poor academic performance, bad behavior, or other unpleasant topics.

The Stomach Acid Challenge

Perhaps your stomach's production of hydrochloric acid (HCl) is not adequate for your digestive needs? Try the following self-evaluation:

- Take one HCl capsule with a full meal (HCl capsules are available at health food stores).

- If you do not notice any difference, take two HCl capsules at the next full meal.

- If you still do not notice anything, take three at the next full meal, and so on. *Caution:* At no time should you take more than six HCl capsules without consulting your physician.

- If you take too much HCl, your stomach will almost immediately feel acidic, and you can practically taste the excess (it is highly unpleasant); if that occurs, simply eat a little food or take a little bicarbonate of soda to buffer the excess acidity.

- If you notice that you can take one or several HCl capsules with no symptoms of over-acidity, you may find it beneficial to supplement each meal with HCl for a period of time.

- You may find that after taking HCl for a while, you feel the sensation of over-acidity, which means that your body is now producing more stomach acid itself. That's great! Simply cut down your amount of supplemental HCl and let your body take over the job.

- Chew each bite twenty times ("chew your liquids and drink your solids").

- Ask your Wings nutritionist (at www.flywithwings.com/pnc.html, click on MyProConnect) to recommend a digestive-enzyme supplement that you can take twenty minutes after each meal. Supplemental enzymes help relieve the pancreas and liver of the burden of the cardiac stage, or first stage, of digestion. This is when food is broken down into amino acids, simple sugars, and simple fats, thereby releasing the vitamins and minerals for nutritional use. I highly recommend plant-based enzymes from Prevail or Enzymatic Therapy, available at health food stores.

- If you have used antibiotics frequently or for extended periods of time, take a good probiotic supplement containing acidophilus and other helpful organisms to replenish the population of friendly bacteria in your colon. I enjoy and recommend the DDS form of acidophilus, PB8 products from Nutrition Now, and the Natren probiotic product, all available at health food stores; try two capsules upon awakening (on an empty stomach) and again just prior to bedtime.

If you have undergone any type of surgery on the stomach, intestine, or colon, please consult a nutritionally trained physician about the issue of improving digestion. It is likely that the surgery has permanently altered your ability to absorb nutrients, and you may require special assistance or higher doses of supplemental nutrients to compensate for damage to any of these delicate organs.

Measuring Up

It's that time again . . . Weigh yourself, and then take five girth measurements: bust at the largest point, waist at two inches above the navel, hips at the largest point, and right and left thigh circumference at the point where your extended fingertips reach with your arms hanging down at your sides. Record these figures, and your calculated BMI value, on your Progress Chart.

And now, go to page 261 for your new recipes!

TODAY'S ASSIGNMENT

MAKE YOUR TUMMY FEEL BETTER

Implement some good digestive health practices. For starters, reduce mealtime stress by planning pleasurable dinner-table conversation and preparing a fun activity to teach your children (and spouse!) good table manners. Talk with your family about the chewing rule and make a game out of it: be sure to chew each bite at least twenty times before swallowing, and notice how much better your digestion becomes.

Drink a cup of ginger tea before each meal this week. To brew: mince 1 tablespoon of fresh ginger root and place in a mug; pour boiling water over it and let it steep until the tea is cool enough to drink. (Ginger tea is also good for nausea.) Start using your digestive enzyme and bitters products this week as well.

1. Why is good digestion important in the pursuit of a healthful weight?

2. Briefly describe the digestive process.

3. What are some factors that hinder digestion?

4. What are some factors that aid digestion?

5. List some common symptoms of poor digestion.

6. List some ways to improve digestion.

7. What does it mean to "chew your liquids and drink your solids"?

HEALTH TIP

HAY FEVER

Sneezing, sniffing, runny nose? Watery, burning eyes? It's hay-fever season again! The best time to deal with hay fever is before it hits. Start building your immune system and reducing your allergic potential about six months prior to allergy season.

- Increase your vitamin C intake to 75 percent of your bowel tolerance: Take 1 teaspoon of buffered vitamin C crystals in a glass of water every hour until diarrhea occurs. Write down the amount of vitamin C it took to reach the state of diarrhea. Then take 75 percent of that amount daily throughout the hay-fever season.

- Take capsules of echinacea, an herb that builds up the immune system, on an alternating schedule of one week on and one week off throughout the hay-fever season.

- Use a quercetin-bromelain combination thirty minutes prior to each meal to strengthen the mast cells that line the respiratory tract (these sensitive cells, which contain a load of histamine, can rupture easily when exposed to pollen).

- Use a homeopathic anti-allergy preparation throughout the year; one of my favorites is A. Vogel Allergy Relief.

- Use stinging nettles, which is an herbal antihistamine without any side effects, several times a day. The Eclectic Institute of Sandy, Oregon, pioneered research on this herbal remedy and makes an excellent freeze-dried stinging nettles product.

- Take 500–1,000 milligrams (mg) of pantothenic acid to relieve hay-fever symptoms.

- Take a bioflavonoid supplement twice per day along with vitamin C (1,000–2,000 mg per day) as an anti-inflammatory and to strengthen capillaries and mast cells.

ADDITIONAL NOTES

Lesson II-6. The Wings Cleansing Program

In centuries past, because of poor refrigeration and restricted food supplies during the long winter months, people often resorted to eating moldy meat, wilted vegetables, and rancid fats just to stay alive. In Europe and America, the Eclectic physicians encouraged their patients to clean out the body each spring. When the first shoots emerged from the warm spring soil, people gathered whatever fresh food they could find, including greens like crabgrass and dandelion leaves. Physicians of the time found that these "bitters," so rich in natural compounds that stimulate the liver, also cleanse the body, restoring health and vitality. Contemporary healers hold many of these greens in high regard for the same reasons: scientists have shown that dandelion stimulates liver activity, and that other bitters are good for digestion or for stimulating the bowels to eliminate toxic materials. Naturopathic physicians still encourage body cleansing today and often prescribe dandelion or similar bitter greens to help do the job.

? TODAY'S QUESTION

When did you last clean your house?

_____

_____

_____

Do you clean your house from top to bottom every year? Fall or spring cleaning, anyone? Even though you regularly vacuum and dust and try to keep your closets in decent order, you still believe it is necessary to deep clean your house at least once or twice per year. Imagine how it would be if the only cleaning you did was to empty the garbage once or twice a day. Moving your bowels once a day is like taking out the garbage once a day—the rest of the house may still be dirty. So, how about "deep cleaning" your body?

Now that you're following the Wings eating plan, you don't struggle with constipation anymore (hopefully) and you've stopped dumping toxic products into your body. Everyone, however, needs a good internal cleansing at least twice per year. For most people, this process is shrouded in mystery, and for others, it's either a little terrifying or very humorous. But body cleansing needn't be mysterious or even frightening: it is beneficial and can be a pleasant experience. Who knows, once you start the process, you may actually look forward to getting yourself cleaned out, and want to do it often.

GETTING STARTED

This "hard core" internal cleansing program is designed to wash the lymphatic system, lungs, blood, liver, kidneys, and colon, and it works extremely well for most people. The protocol lasts for seven days; afterward, you will resume your normal, healthful Wings food plan, along with a few special additions for a "healing week" (Lesson II-7) to restore the normal pH of the digestive tract and help heal digestive tissue that may have been disrupted during cleansing.

While it is good to clean the colon in particular,

✒ NOTES

_____

_____

_____

_____

_____

_____

cleansing should also happen on an even deeper level. The goal of this cleansing program is to stimulate the cells of several other organs to dump waste products into the bloodstream for transport to the liver and then to the colon for elimination. When doing a cleanse, the bowels must function well so that toxins will be fully eliminated rather than being reabsorbed through the wall of the colon and then back into the bloodstream.

Water is very important! Make sure you drink copious amounts of pure water throughout the cleanse: at least eight to ten glasses per day. This flushes the kidneys of toxic waste materials, hydrates tissues throughout the body so they can more easily dump their waste into the bloodstream, and keeps fecal material soft and pliable so it can be easily excreted. *Note:* The only beverages allowed during the cleansing program are water and your Wings Breakfast Drink.

The protocol is a little intense for some people, especially those who have never done a body cleanse before. Although the process entails several steps, the instructions are not really complicated. Before you embark on this cleansing protocol, you may need to obtain some supplies. Here is a list of what you will need:

- 1–2 canisters Wings Breakfast Drink

- 1 bottle multivitamin-mineral supplement recommended by your healthcare practitioner or your Wings nutritionist

- 1 canister Wings Klean Tea

- 1 canister Wings Healing Tea (this will be used in next week's healing protocol, but it is convenient for you to order the Klean Tea and Healing Tea at the same time)

- Enema bag

- ½ pound organic coffee (not decaffeinated), drip grind

- Ingredients for Module II, Week 6 of the Menus and Recipes section (pages 261–265)

- 1 bottle probiotics (available at your local health food store)

- Stainless-steel or glass pot

- A fine-mesh strainer

- Glass measuring cup with handle and pour spout

- Unsulfured molasses

Cleansing Cautions

- If you are under medical care for any reason or have any reservations, make sure your physician knows that you intend to embark on this cleansing program, and obtain his/her permission prior to starting the process.

- If you are pregnant or breastfeeding, do not do this cleansing program.

CLEANSING WEEK SCHEDULE AND PROTOCOL

The cleansing protocol starts the morning of Day 1 and ends the night of Day 7. Note that you may need to get up a little earlier in the morning for the duration of your cleansing week!

On each day of the cleansing protocol, you will follow these steps:

- Before arising, drink 1 cup of very hot water and lie on your right side for twenty minutes.

- Upon arising, drink 1–1½ heaping tablespoons of a good fiber supplement in a large glass of water. Follow with another glass of water.

- For breakfast, enjoy the Wings Breakfast Drink and take your multivitamin-mineral supplement.

- For lunch and dinner, adhere to the cleansing week menus and recipes that are provided in the back of this book.

- Before bedtime, drink 1–1½ heaping tablespoons of a good fiber supplement in a large glass of water. Follow with another glass of water.

After Day 1, more steps are to be added to your protocol on specific days, as follows:

- On Day 2, brew a batch of Wings Klean Tea according to the directions in the inset on page 82. For the remainder of the cleansing protocol, you will be drinking a dilution of this mixture from one to ten times per day, depending on how your body adjusts to it.

- On Day 3, after your morning water and fiber and before breakfast, drink one serving of Klean Tea, prepared as follows: Pour 2 tablespoons of the Klean Tea you brewed yesterday into a glass of water, and dilute the tea mixture down to the strength you prefer. Then, at each hour throughout the day—until diarrhea occurs—drink one serving of Klean Tea prepared in that same manner. (*Note:* This tea is really bitter, and there is nothing you can do to disguise the bitterness. Sorry!) The goal of this regimen is to drink just enough tea to stimulate several large, cleansing bowel movements per day but not enough to induce diarrhea.

- On Day 4, at each hour throughout the day—until diarrhea occurs—drink one serving of Klean Tea as you did on Day 3.

- On Day 5 and Day 6, continue as on Day 4, but after bowel evacuation, do the coffee enema as described on page 83.

- On Day 7, proceed as on Day 6. After you have evacuated your bowels following the coffee enema and before retiring for the night, do a freshwater enema to refresh the colon; then, complete your internal cleansing with a probiotic enema to recolonize the colon with friendly bacteria, retaining this final enema as long as possible. (Local health food stores generally carry probiotics; good brands include Natren and Nutrition Now PB8, among others.)

How to Brew Wings Klean Tea

Bring 3 quarts of water to a light simmer. Add one canister of Klean Tea herbs and lower the heat so that it just bubbles slightly. Cover with a lid but leave the lid slightly ajar to let steam escape. Don't let the mixture simmer vigorously; let it slowly bubble for twenty minutes, and then remove it from the heat. Put the lid on tightly and let the tea steep for twenty minutes. Strain the tea carefully two or three times to remove the residue of the herbs. Pour the tea into a glass container, cover, and refrigerate. *Note:* This tea will stain virtually any container, so do not use one that you value for its beauty.

Cleansing Foods

During the cleansing period, please follow the corresponding menus provided on pages 261–262 of the Menus and Recipes section. The purpose of avoiding animal products during the cleanse is to give the body a rest from the more difficult task of digesting animal proteins. Meat that is not thoroughly digested putrefies in the intestines and colon, which damages the delicate lining of the digestive tract, causes the proliferation of harmful bacteria, and sends toxins into the bloodstream. A vegetarian diet provides a "clean burn"; that is, vegetarian foods are more easily bro-

ken down and absorbed, giving the digestive tract a chance to cleanse and heal.

The cleansing week menus and recipes are high in fiber to provide more bulk in the stool for better cleansing power. As the different tissues of the body dump toxic materials into the colon for excretion, this waste must be quickly moved out of the body to prevent its reabsorption. The added fiber acts as a kind of broom to sweep the intestinal tract and colon free of debris. The cleansing week meals do contain moderate amounts of protein, although it's probably less protein than you are accustomed to eating. They also contain beneficial oils that are good for energy and for intestinal health.

Most people tolerate the balance of foods in the cleansing week meal plan without difficulty. However, people who are severely hypoglycemic or who require large portions of protein because of heavy physical work may find their blood sugar levels dropping with this dietary change. Make sure you eat enough food and satisfy your protein requirements so you do not slip into hypoglycemia during this week. Listen to your body! Symptoms of hypoglycemia include headache, irritability, difficulty focusing the eyes, anxiety, trembling, and weakness. If these symptoms appear, add about 3 ounces of baked, steamed, or broiled fish to your lunch menu; this small amount of protein should help balance your blood sugar. Also, feel free to have another Wings Breakfast Drink any time during the day if you feel the need for more protein (it provides more than 12 grams of protein per serving).

And remember to take your multivitamin-mineral supplement each day—very important!

Cleansing with—Coffee?

Just talking about a coffee enema brings pallor to many people's faces. We simply aren't used to this employment of one of our favorite beverages!

The coffee is never actually sent into circulation throughout the body. Even coffee-sensitive individuals do not usually experience negative side effects from a coffee enema. The caffeine enters the enterohepatic circulation system through which it moves from the intestine to the liver, where it acts as a strong detoxicant; that is, it causes the liver to unload stored toxins into the colon for elimination from the body. Caffeine's alkaloids stimulate the production of glutathione-S-transferase, an enzyme used in the liver's detoxification pathways to form glutathione, one of the body's prime facilitators of detoxification. The enema also speeds the emptying of the bowel, so the detoxification process proceeds more quickly.

About the Coffee Enema . . .

According to Dr. Sherry Rogers, coffee enemas were part of standard medical practice for many years, as she writes in her book *Wellness Against All Odds* (Syracuse, NY: Prestige Publishing, 1994, 84–89): My first exposure to coffee enemas came from reading about them as an important part of the Gerson program years ago. [The Gerson program is a cancer program.] But frankly it sounded so peculiar, that I readily dismissed them . . . As I read through old medical books from the 1920s, I saw a recurring theme amongst the "natural hygiene" group. Their philosophy was that all disease was merely a question of toxicity. It was the mere inability of the body to dispose of accumulated waste products, before they caused symptoms.

I became seriously impressed, however, with coffee enemas when I watched their effects first-hand when my attorney girlfriend was clearing her leukemia with this program. As her cancer cells were being broken down she would become so toxic that her tongue and liver would visibly swell. She was oftentimes barely able to speak clearly because of such marked tongue swelling. When she did a coffee enema, the tongue swelling, brain fog, and liver swelling were reduced as well as the toxic, sick feeling. She made me promise to write about its effectiveness so that others might benefit . . . .

It's really quite astounding that the old remedies of the 1920s have been forgotten when they could be so useful in these conditions. A coffee enema could save the day for these victims of overwhelming toxicity. As we have found, they are invaluable in numerous conditions, from postoperative healing, severe infections, severe and traumatic injuries, to speeding the recovery time from chemical exposures and cancers.

Caution

If you are under medical treatment for any condition, please consult your physician before doing the coffee enema! People with gallstones should not do coffee enemas. Pregnant or lactating women must not do a coffee enema or any other type of body cleansing.

How to Prepare and Administer the Coffee Enema

The coffee enema is to be done on the fifth, sixth, and seventh days of the cleansing week, once on each of those days, and according to the following instructions. It is preferably done in the morning, after the morning fiber is consumed, but if you work outside the home you may find it more convenient to do the enema in the evening before going to bed.

1. Assemble the following materials: enema bag, stainless-steel or glass pot, glass measuring cup, organic drip-grind coffee, unsulfured molasses (the molasses helps the bowels retain the coffee), a fine-mesh strainer, and pure water (not chlorinated or fluoridated tap water).

2. Bring 1 quart of pure water to a boil in the pot. Add 2 level tablespoons of coffee to the pot, lower the heat, and continue to simmer for five minutes. Turn off the heat and leave the pot on the burner. Add 1 tablespoon of unsulfured molasses to the pot and stir to dissolve it.

3. Cool the coffee to a tepid or comfortable temperature. Never use the coffee when it's hot or steaming! Then strain the coffee carefully to remove the grounds; you may need to strain several times.

4. Pour the coffee into the enema bag.

5. Spread an old towel on the floor. Kneel on the towel with your head down toward the floor, and gently insert the enema bag's nozzle into the rectum (for easier insertion, dab oil or vitamin E on the tip of the nozzle).

6. Release the clamp and let the coffee flow slowly into the rectum and colon. Do not allow the coffee to run into the colon too rapidly, to prevent it from going higher than the sigmoid colon (the bend in the colon). Clamp off the tubing as soon as there is a sensation of fullness; then release and clamp, release and clamp, letting the coffee flow slowly and giving the body time to receive it.

7. Lie on your right side and retain the enema for ten minutes; if an uncomfortable feeling develops, however, do not force yourself to hold it. When finished, clamp the tubing, remove the nozzle, and empty the bowels.

8. Repeat the enema procedure with the remaining part of the coffee, emptying the bowels again when you are finished.

You may hear or feel a squirting in the general area under your right ribcage as the bile duct empties the gallbladder. If you have done several enemas and still have not heard or felt the gallbladder release, you may wish to increase the strength of the coffee (do not exceed 2 tablespoons of coffee per cup), take larger-volume enemas, or take three enemas in succession of 2 cups each or less. If you feel nervous or jittery, reduce the amount of coffee that you add to the water when brewing.

CLEANSING SIDE EFFECTS

It is not uncommon for people to experience side effects during the cleansing week. Typical cleansing side effects include headaches, nausea, skin eruptions, slight fever, cold symptoms (sneezing, coughing, runny nose), gastrointestinal upset, blurry vision, strong emotions, and fatigue. These symptoms are usually a good sign that the cleansing program is working.

But if these symptoms become too intense or you become too uncomfortable, you can slow the cleansing process by cutting back on the amount of Klean Tea and increasing the amount of water you are drinking, until the discomfort has passed. Some people also find that doing the coffee enema can relieve their cleansing symptoms; if you feel it is needed for symptom relief, do not be nervous about doing the coffee enema more frequently than is recommended in this protocol.

HOW LONG TO DO THE CLEANSE

A question commonly asked is, "How do I know if the cleansing process is completed?" The answer varies from person to person, but generally you will just know. For example, your bowel movements will become smaller and less frequent; side effects like headaches or fatigue will disappear; you'll feel more energy; your skin will look brighter and clearer; your breath will be fresher. Some people can achieve good cleansing results in one week; others may want to continue the program for a longer period of time. Alternatively, you may wish to continue doing the coffee enema for a week or so past the cleansing week. Once the cleansing process has been successfully completed, you will move directly into the healing week (Lesson II-7) to attend to the health of the entire digestive tract.

Listen to your body and work with your body. You may also wish to enlist the aid of a healthcare professional familiar with body-cleansing practices. In a book of this nature, it is impossible to personalize the program for you; this is where a healthcare practitioner can be extremely helpful, so don't be afraid to take advantage of any available resources. If you do not feel you have achieved your cleansing goals, do another week of cleansing in about three weeks, or just continue on for a few more days. (At the conclusion of the cleansing period, you should proceed directly to a healing week to give your body a chance to heal and restore the natural pH of the digestive system.)

And now, go to page 261 for your menus and recipes!

TODAY'S ASSIGNMENT

YOU KNOW WHAT TO DO . . .

Spend some time formulating goals for your body-cleansing period. What do you want to achieve? Clearer skin? Better digestion? More energy? Weight loss? Reduced water retention? Write down your goals and post them on your refrigerator door so you don't forget them.

Purchase the necessary products for your cleansing program and decide when to begin. Choose a time period that will not be interrupted by family occasions or by work that will make your cleansing routine difficult for you. For example, if you are attending a family wedding this week, this would not be a good time to embark on a cleanse! Similarly, if you know you'll be working extra hours, traveling, or engaged in hard physical labor, it would be better to postpone your cleansing until you're certain you can complete it successfully.

If you have any questions prior to or in the middle of your cleansing program, do not hesitate to consult a healthcare practitioner who can help advise you in the process. Above all, keep your sense of humor! You're doing a great thing for yourself.

LESSON II-6 STUDY GUIDE

1. What is the purpose of the internal cleansing program?

_____

_____

_____

2. What is the purpose of following the vegetarian diet throughout the cleansing week?

_____

_____

_____

3. What is the purpose of the coffee enema?

_____

_____

_____

 HEALTH TIP

HEADACHES

Headaches are a pain in the . . . head! And their source can be difficult to ascertain. Common causes of headache include hormone imbalance, food or environmental allergies, stress, constipation, consumption of coffee or other stimulants, caffeine withdrawal, sinus infection or pressure, temporomandibular joint (TMJ) syndrome, head trauma, nutritional deficiencies, fever, hypoglycemia, or hypothyroidism. Instead of turning immediately or exclusively to pharmaceutical pain relievers, consider the following dietary and other natural remedies for headache relief:

- Eat several small meals per day, with each meal balanced among proteins, fats, and carbohydrates to stabilize blood sugar.

- As much as possible, eliminate foods that commonly cause headache, including wheat, chocolate, MSG, sulfites (common preservatives), sugar, hot dogs, luncheon meats, dairy products, nuts, citric acid, fermented products (like cheeses, sour cream, vinegar, wine), foods in the nightshade family (tomatoes, potatoes, eggplant), and alcohol.

- Avoid all foods that contain a protein-like substance called tyramine—for example, alcoholic beverages, bananas, cheese, chicken, chocolate, citrus fruits, cold cuts, herring, onions, peanut butter, pork, smoked fish, sour cream, vinegar, wine, and fresh-baked yeast products.

- Eliminate food or environmental allergens. Use the pulse test (pages 47–48) to test every food you commonly eat for allergy or intolerance. Keep an accurate Food Diary and examine it to see whether there is a correlation between consuming specific foods and getting a headache (the headache can develop up to seven days later).

- If you tend to get migraine headaches, try using the herb feverfew daily. Feverfew will not relieve a headache immediately, but taking it over a period of time has a cumulative effect that lessens the frequency and intensity of migraines. *Caution:* Do not use feverfew during pregnancy.

- Other herbs that help relieve headache pain include burdock root, fenugreek, and mint.

- Apply a cold compress to the spot from which the pain is radiating; alternatively, use a heating pad, hot-water bottle, or hot towel to relax the neck and shoulder muscles.

- Make a salve from ginger root, peppermint oil, and wintergreen oil, and rub it on the temples and the back of the neck to relieve tension headaches, or across the sinus area to relieve sinus headaches.

- For a sinus headache, do a nasal rinse using warm water, salt, and glycerin, several times per day if necessary; if the nasal discharge is colored, add one drop of grapefruit-seed extract to the rinse mixture.

- Take a daily fiber supplement and do a weekly cleansing enema.

- Try doing an organic coffee enema (page 83) at the beginning of a headache.

- If the headaches coincide with your menstrual cycle, balance female hormones by using herbs that support and nourish the female system (Lesson III-3).

- See a chiropractor about possible misalignment of the spinal column.

✐ ADDITIONAL NOTES

_____

_____

_____

_____

Lesson II-7. The Wings Healing Week

You have just concluded one of the most interesting weeks of your life (if you had never before embarked on a cleansing program, that is). You may be experiencing some of the effects of dumping waste materials into your bloodstream; some of this waste may still be floating around and causing headaches, cold and flu symptoms, fatigue, or emotional symptoms. Do not worry: these will pass as you "clean out the temple." You are on a good track—even if it doesn't feel like it.

Today's material is to follow directly on the heels of the previous lesson. After you have thoroughly cleansed the inside of your body, you will want to restore the integrity of the digestive tract. However, if you have not finished your cleanse, put the information and procedures in this lesson aside until you are truly finished. There is no need to rush the process.

❓ TODAY'S QUESTION

How does your stomach feel?

_____

_____

_____

By that, I mean how does it feel normally. Do you often feel bloated? Nauseated? Congested? Let's fix that . . .

Intestinal integrity is critical to good health. The in-

testinal tract acts as a type of wall that keeps unwanted materials from being absorbed into the body, and also as a type of gate that allows digested food particles to pass into the body. Concurrently, it allows toxic materials that are destined for excretion to flow from the bloodstream into the colon on their way to the rectum. When this wall or gate is breached and partially undigested materials are allowed to slip into the bloodstream, we develop immune system problems, as you learned in Lesson I-10. When we consistently eat high-acid foods, the pH of the digestive system is disrupted, leading to continued tissue damage.

The purpose of today's lesson is to correct those problems and enhance your digestive health.

INTESTINAL RECOVERY

After the cleansing period has concluded, it is essential to give the intestinal tract and colon an opportunity to heal and restore. This is the time to introduce healing nutrients and herbs. It is also important to re-establish your proper acid/alkaline balance. A high-acid diet (meat, grains, sugar, soft drinks, and such; Lesson I-1) and a stressful lifestyle impose great metabolic stress. To help restore normal pH balance to the diet and the body during this healing week, you will be introduced to several alkalinizing foods (pages 265–266 in the Menus and Recipes section).

The Wings healing week has two major angles. First, the flora residing in your intestinal tract may have been disturbed by the numerous cleansing bowel movements that you experienced last week. And as you may recall, your normal bacterial count may have already been disturbed by unhealthful dietary habits or the use of prescription medications. Antibiotics, for example, kill both friendly and unfriendly bacteria, giving the yeast candida (Lesson

🖋 NOTES

_____

_____

_____

_____

_____

_____

III-13) and other pathogens the opportunity to proliferate. Similarly, frequent consumption of sugar, alcohol, and chlorinated water destroy friendly bacteria and feed yeast. The Wings cleansing protocol concludes with a retention probiotic enema, but that is not adequate to completely replenish your colon and intestinal tract with friendly bacteria. Taking a good probiotic supplement (available at health food stores) should be on your to do list on a regular basis. Beet Kvass (recipe on page 265) can also help maintain the health of your friendly bacteria.

Second, after the cleanse, you need to restore the proper pH of the stomach, small intestine, and colon, and maintain that pH so the tissue in the intestinal tract remains healthy and strong. The Bieler Broth and Barley Juice in this lesson's recipe are very alkalinizing and rich in minerals that help heal the tissue. Barley, one of the oldest seed crops in the world, may provide a tonic to the liver. (For more about Bieler Broth, Beet Kvass, and Barley Juice, please read Sally Fallon's book *Nourishing Traditions* [San Diego, CA: ProMotion Publishing, 1995]. It contains a wealth of information about healing foods and is an excellent reference book.)

If you go through the healing week protocol and still feel that your digestive system doesn't work quite right, please reread the lesson on digestive health (Lesson II-5).

HEALING WEEK SCHEDULE AND PROTOCOL

Here are the steps to follow from Day 1 through Day 7 of the healing week:

- Prior to breakfast, take 1 heaping tablespoon of a good fiber supplement in a large glass of water. Drink 1/2 cup of Beet Kvass (optional). Take two capsules of a probiotic supplement with another glass of water.

- For breakfast, enjoy one portion of the Wings Breakfast Drink, and take your multivitamin-mineral supplement.

- Between meals, drink 1 large cup of Bieler Broth or Vegetable Juice Cocktail.

- Thirty minutes prior to lunch, drink 1 cup of Wings Healing Tea, and take 500–1,000 milligrams (mg) of L-glutamine (this supplement is available at health food stores).

- For lunch, enjoy a normal Wings lunch menu along with 1 cup of Bieler Broth (make sure the meal includes a large salad and at least two other raw or lightly steamed vegetables).

- Thirty minutes prior to dinner, drink 1 cup of Wings Healing Tea, and take 500–1,000 mg of L-glutamine.

- For dinner, enjoy a normal Wings dinner menu along with 1 cup of Bieler Broth (make sure the meal includes a large salad and at least two raw or lightly steamed vegetables).

- After dinner, drink 1 cup of Barley Juice.

- Before retiring for the night, take 1 heaping tablespoon of a good fiber supplement in a large glass of water. Drink 1/2 cup of Beet Kvass (optional). Take two capsules of a probiotic supplement with another glass of water.

What Is the Purpose of the Healing Tea?

The herbs in Wings Healing Tea were carefully chosen for their benefits to the intestinal tract. Chamomile flowers help relax nervous tension that may cause digestive spasms. Peppermint also relaxes the stomach muscles and reduces the production of gas in the digestive system. Slippery elm sooths irritated or inflamed tissues. Mullein helps normalize the pH. Ginger helps stimulate the production and flow of saliva, an important part of the digestive process; ginger also reduces gas production, stimulates the flow of other digestive juices, and relieves nausea.

And unlike the Klean Tea, the Healing Tea is delicious! You will want to enjoy this tea liberally and frequently; its warm, minty flavor makes it a delightful after-dinner beverage.

AFTER THE HEALING WEEK

You may not be sure that you have accomplished all of your cleansing and healing goals during the designated weeks. I recommend doing the Wings cleansing program at least four times a year (for example, once each season). Remember that good digestion is foundational to good health.

If you have chronic digestive problems, follow the healing protocol every day until the digestive difficulty is resolved (or, if you wish, continue it for the rest of your life—you may find that you simply feel better overall). Enjoy Wings Healing Tea as a pleasant dinner beverage every evening. Consider alternating the cleansing and healing weeks for about one month, or until you feel that you have accomplished your goals of total internal cleansing and healing. You may wish to do the coffee enema (Lesson II-6) daily for one month, particularly if you are overcoming some health challenges in addition to weight management.

Now, go to page 265 for your menus and recipes!

TODAY'S ASSIGNMENT

YOU KNOW WHAT TO DO . . . AGAIN

Prepare the special healing week foods on pages 265–266 of the Menus and Recipes section, and refrigerate them until use. Write out your week's schedule, including each element in the healing protocol. Then, start your healing week!

Use your Food Diary to record your feelings and observations this week. During last week's cleanse, you may have experienced many emotional symptoms. Have these abated? If not, you may wish to continue the coffee enema from Lesson II-6 until you feel better. In any case, make sure you drink enough water to help the body flush excess toxins out of your system.

LESSON II-7 STUDY GUIDE

1. What is the purpose of the healing week?

_____

_____

_____

2. What is the purpose of the Bieler Broth? Barley Broth? Beet Kvass? Vegetable Juice Cocktail?

_____

_____

_____

_____

HEALTH TIP

GETTING KIDS TO EAT VEGETABLES

For some reason, some children are highly resistant to eating vegetables—anything green, especially. (It makes no sense to me, but it happens.) Vegetables are very important, especially to growing kids, who need to eat five to seven servings of vegetables (a serving is roughly the size of one's fist) each day for maximum health.

Through the Children's Research Foundation, Juice Plus+ is conducting a national survey on the health and vegetable-eating habits of children. They have found that by introducing kids to vegetables and fruits through a vegetable and fruit supplement, kids are more likely to accept eating real vegetables subsequently. (For more information, visit their website at www.juice plus.com.)

✒ ADDITIONAL NOTES

_____

_____

_____

_____

_____

_____

Lesson II–8. The Importance of Fiber

In the mid-1900s, Dr. Denis Burkitt studied the diet and health of traditional African tribes, and he found that their fiber-rich diet protected them from many "diseases of civilization," including several forms of cancer, heart disease, diabetes, and diseases of the colon and intestinal tract. Many of these traditional people consumed more than 65 grams (g) of fiber per day, a huge amount in comparison to our modern American diet. As a result, they had huge bowel movements daily and enjoyed vibrant health.

? **TODAY'S QUESTION**

How do you keep the inside of your body clean?

_____

_____

_____

_____

How do you feel after your body-cleansing and healing weeks? Any problems? How much weight did you lose? Was it "fat weight" or "toxic-waste weight"—in other words, did you lose inches around your waist or abdomen, or do you simply feel less bloated or stuffed? If you lost more than 5 pounds of toxic-waste weight, what benefits do you think you will experience from getting rid of that harmful material?

Now that you are enjoying renewed health because your body is cleansed, you will wish to keep it that way by scrubbing your intestines each day with plenty of dietary roughage. Eating lots of fiber is sort of like hiring a personal housecleaner to tend to your home while you do other things. As the undigested fiber passes through the intestinal tract, it gathers toxic materials and sweeps them "out the back door."

In our culture, we simply do not consume enough roughage, or fiber. We eat about 5–6 g (or less) of fiber each day, far too little to protect the delicate lining of the intestinal tract, and far too little to keep the colon scrubbed clean of debris. Our ancestors knew the importance of roughage. We will revive that ancient knowledge today and make it part of your modern health system.

WHAT IS DIETARY FIBER?

Dietary fiber is derived from the cell walls and certain other parts of plants. This material cannot be broken down in the human gastrointestinal system because we do not produce the enzymes to digest it. Fiber is classified as a carbohydrate but is a noncaloric carbohydrate: because it is not digested, it contributes no calories or nutrition to the body. It is, however, essential. Several decades ago, many healthcare practitioners ridiculed that idea, simply because they did not understand that although dietary fiber does not contribute to the body's nutritional intake, it nonetheless performs several vital functions.

In general terms, fiber is categorized as either soluble or insoluble. Soluble fibers include pectin, gum, mucilage, and hemicellulose. Pectins are found in fruits and vegetables, and other soluble fibers are obtained from oat bran, barley, and legumes (beans).

✐ **NOTES**

_____

_____

_____

_____

_____

Soluble fibers hold water and form gels, and act as a substrate for fermentation by our helpful colonic bacteria. Insoluble fibers, which consist primarily of cellulose and some hemicelluloses, provide structure to plant cells and are particularly abundant in the bran layers of whole grains. Each of these different types of fiber contributes a different benefit to the body.

DID YOU GET ENOUGH FIBER TODAY?

The average American eats less than 6 g of fiber per day—yet many holistic physicians recommend upward of 35 g per day! Each serving of the Wings Breakfast Drink provides several grams of fiber, but unless you also eat a lot of beans and vegetables with tough outer skins, it is unlikely that you are reaching that daily fiber goal of 35 g. How will you reach it?

First of all, eat several servings of fiber-rich vegetables and fruits every day. Raw nuts and seeds, legumes, dark green and other vegetables, the skins of fruits, and whole grains like brown rice are rich in dietary fiber. It is important to include a variety of these food types in your daily diet because each contains a particular form of fiber with its own beneficial function. Experts recommend, for example, that we eat equal amounts of soluble and insoluble fiber. Make sure to include legumes because beans are rich in soluble fibers. Include one small serving of brown rice per day for insoluble fibers; these are also found in prunes, dates, and figs. Enjoy snacking on raw or home-roasted nuts and seeds.

Second, you may need to supplement these foods with additional fibers found in psyllium seed husks, flaxseeds, and the like. You can obtain such fiber supplements from your local health food store or from your Wings nutritionist (at www.flywithwings.com/pnc.html, click on MyProConnect).

Do not abruptly increase your fiber intake, however. Increase it slowly, and drink copious amounts of water so that your stool remains soft and easily passed. If you are using a fiber supplement, start with 1 heaping teaspoon in a glass of water once per day; after a couple of days, take 1 teaspoon of fiber with water twice per day, and then slowly increase the amount of fiber in each dose until you are taking at least 1–2 heaping tablespoons of fiber per day. Make sure your fiber supplement does not contain sugar or artificial sweeteners, and if possible, does contain live acidophilus cultures with fructo-oligosaccharides (these compounds provide food for the acidophilus and aid in the bacteria's implantation in the intestinal tract).

ADDING FIBER ADDS TO YOUR HEALTH

Dietary fiber has many health benefits. They include the following:

- Stimulates chewing, thereby stimulating saliva flow and gastric juice secretion
- Fills the stomach, providing a sense of satiety or satisfaction
- Increases fecal bulk, decreasing pressure inside the colon
- Increases the transit time of food through the intestinal tract
- Provides a supportive environment for the growth of friendly intestinal bacteria
- Delays the emptying of the stomach, slowing digestion and enhancing nutrient absorption
- Lowers serum cholesterol and normalizes female hormone levels (used estrogens are swept out in the increased fecal material)

The effects of adding fiber to the diet may appear to be subtle. Your bowel movements will be larger and softer: they should float and/or break up into a cloud when you flush the toilet. Bloating and intestinal gas should diminish (if it increases, reduce the amount of fiber until your body has adjusted); your skin should be clearer; you should have more energy. Most important, by consuming more fiber, you are improving your long-term health exponentially. Remember how the high-fiber diet benefited traditional peoples by reducing their risk of cardiovascular disease, cancer (especially colon cancer), and diabetes? You will enjoy those benefits also.

A Cautionary Note about Bowel Disease

If you have been diagnosed with Crohn's disease, irritable bowel syndrome, or another inflammatory disease of the colon and intestinal tract, please speak with your physician about your fiber intake. Make certain that your inflammatory condition is not a consequence of a food allergy or intolerance (wheat and dairy, for example, are common allergens that affect the colon). Many physicians believe that a high-fiber diet is essential for managing bowel disease, but you should consult your physician.

And now, go to page 266 for your menus and recipes!

DIETARY FIBER CONTENT OF COMMON FOODS

Food	Serving	Calories	Fiber
Fruits			
Apple with skin	1 medium	81	3.5 g
Banana	1 medium	105	2.4 g
Cantaloupe	1/4 melon	30	1.0 g
Cherries	10	49	1.2 g
Grapefruit	1/2 medium	38	1.6 g
Orange	1 medium	62	2.6 g
Peach with skin	1	37	1.9 g
Pear with skin	1/2 large	61	3.1 g
Prune	3	60	3.0 g
Raisins	1/4 cup	106	3.1 g
Raspberries	1/2 cup	35	3.1 g
Strawberries	1 cup	45	3.0 g
Vegetables (Raw)			
Bean sprouts	1/2 cup	13	1.5 g
Celery	1/2 cup	10	1.1 g
Cucumber	1/2 cup	8	0.4 g
Lettuce	1 cup	10	0.9 g
Mushrooms	1/2 cup	10	1.5 g
Pepper (green)	1/2 cup	9	0.5 g
Spinach	1 cup	8	1.2 g
Tomato	1 medium	20	1.5 g
Vegetables (Cooked)			
Asparagus	1 cup	30	2.0 g
Beans (green)	1 cup	32	3.2 g
Broccoli	1 cup	40	4.4 g
Brussels sprouts	1 cup	56	4.6 g
Cabbage (red)	1 cup	30	2.8 g
Carrots	1 cup	48	4.6 g
Cauliflower	1 cup	28	2.2 g
Corn	1/2 cup	87	2.9 g
Kale	1 cup	44	2.8 g
Parsnip	1 cup	102	5.4 g
Potato with skin	1 medium	106	2.5 g

Food	Serving	Calories	Fiber
Vegetables (Cooked) continued			
Potato without skin	1 medium	97	1.4 g
Spinach	1 cup	42	4.2 g
Sweet potato	1 medium	160	3.4 g
Zucchini	1 cup	22	3.6 g
Legumes			
Baked beans	1/2 cup	155	8.8 g
Dried peas (cooked)	1/2 cup	115	4.7 g
Kidney beans (cooked)	1/2 cup	110	7.3 g
Lentils (cooked)	1/2 cup	97	3.7 g
Lima beans (cooked)	1/2 cup	64	4.5 g
Navy beans (cooked)	1/2 cup	112	6.0 g
Rice, Bread, and Pasta			
Bran muffins	1 muffin	104	2.5 g
Bread (white)	1 slice	78	0.4 g
Bread (whole wheat)	1 slice	61	1.4 g
Crisp bread, rye	2 crackers	50	2.0 g
Rice, brown (cooked)	1/2 cup	97	1.0 g
Rice, white (cooked)	1/2 cup	82	0.2 g
Spaghetti, regular (cooked)	1/2 cup	155	1.1 g
Spaghetti, whole wheat (cooked)	1/2 cup	155	3.9 g
Breakfast Cereals			
All-Bran	1/2 cup	71	8.5 g
Bran Chex	2/3 cup	91	4.6 g
Corn Bran	2/3 cup	98	5.4 g
Cornflakes	1 1/4 cups	110	0.3 g
Grape Nuts	1/4 cup	101	1.4 g
Oatmeal	3/4 cup	108	1.6 g
Raisin Bran	2/3 cup	115	4.0 g
Shredded Wheat	2/3 cup	102	2.6 g
Nuts			
Almonds	10 nuts	79	1.1 g
Filberts	10 nuts	54	0.8 g
Peanuts	10 nuts	105	1.4 g

TODAY'S ASSIGNMENT

DO THE MATH

Use the chart on page 91 to calculate your daily fiber consumption, and record the numbers in your Food Diary. Set a goal of taking in at least 35 g of fiber per day. If you do not reach that amount, brainstorm with a trusted friend or your accountability partner on how to reach your goal. And then, continue to consume this much fiber every day for the rest of your life!

I have included a wonderful granola recipe (page 266) that is high in fiber—and rich in flavor. If you can tolerate small amounts of oats, you will certainly enjoy this breakfast occasionally. It is also wonderful sprinkled on desserts like apple or berry crisp, or as an occasional treat on top of organic, unsweetened yogurt (for people who can tolerate small amounts of yogurt).

LESSON II-8 STUDY GUIDE

1. What are the two categories of dietary fiber, and where can these fibers be found?

2. How much fiber does the traditional African eat?

3. How much fiber does the average modern American eat?

4. What common diseases can largely be avoided (lowered risk) by consuming fiber?

5. How much fiber should be included in the diet?

6. How should supplementary fiber be added to the diet?

7. List the fiber content of ten fiber-rich foods.

HEALTH TIP

LOWERING CHOLESTEROL

If your cholesterol level is high, how can you reduce it naturally? People who follow the Wings Program nearly always normalize their cholesterol levels within weeks because the food plan is rich in vegetable fibers and encompasses all of these cholesterol-lowering tips:

- Enjoy natural foods including natural fats (olive oil, raw nuts and seeds, avocados, small amounts of butter, and the like).

- Avoid alcohol, sugar, carbonated drinks, coffee, and all highly processed foods.

- Concentrate on eating several large servings of fresh vegetables per day.

- Above all, do not try to reduce your dietary cholesterol by eating unnatural low-fat/nonfat foods: if you do, your liver will simply produce more cholesterol itself, leading to even higher serum cholesterol levels.

For additional cholesterol-lowering benefits:

- Take 1–3 tablespoons of lecithin granules, or 1,200 milligrams (mg) of lecithin capsules, three times daily (make sure the lecithin is fresh; it should not be yellow).

- Take 400–600 micrograms daily of chromium picolinate.

- Take 500–1,000 mg of inositol hexaniacinate, a form of inositol and niacin (part of the vitamin B–complex family), per day.

- Take a supplement called lipotropic factors, which contains choline, inositol, and methionine. These three nutrients prevent accumulation of fatty deposits in the liver and arteries.

- Take up to 2–3 heaping tablespoons of a good fiber supplement per day along with several glasses of water.

- Keep the stool large and cleansing. Work up to two to three such bowel movements per day.

- Get your thyroid gland checked. Hypothyroidism is a common cause of high cholesterol.

ADDITIONAL NOTES

Lesson II-9. Get Up and Get Moving

Today begins a series of lessons on a topic that you may have been expecting: the dreaded "E" word, exercise. We often hate to get out there and get our bodies moving. Many of us would rather sit in front of a computer screen all day, or putter around in the kitchen; if presented with a choice of reading a book or watching a movie on the sofa, or "busting our buns" at the gym, we'll pick the sofa. But we cannot be healthy if our muscles deteriorate from lack of use—and this atrophy begins on the day that we lounge around on the couch! Throughout the rest of this curriculum, I will continue to challenge you to get your body into good shape with exercise.

？ TODAY'S QUESTION

If you could play any sport, what would it be?

_____

_____

_____

_____

When you were a child, what types of sports or other physical activities did you enjoy? Which ones do you enjoy now? If you can't think of any that you actually enjoy, then what physical activity do you find to be the most agreeable (or the least unpleasant)? With whom might you enjoy exercising?

EXERCISE REALLY MATTERS— FOR ALL OF US

The rapidly growing research literature on the benefits of exercise shows that physical movement benefits virtually every part of the body. So, what are some compelling reasons to get up off that chair and get moving? For one, exercise lowers the production of stress hormones. For another, it improves the functioning of your immune system and your digestive system. Exercise builds the strength of the heart muscle, causing it to pump more efficiently, and improves the health of the entire cardiovascular system, putting you at a lowered risk of heart disease. Aerobic exercise, in particular, pumps more air into the lungs, oxygenating the entire body and thereby increasing cellular energy. In other words, exercise is good for your entire body.

The benefits of physical activity also extend to the brain. Some of the "mental" reasons we should exercise are as follows:

- Enhanced mood
- Improved memory
- Increased blood flow in the brain
- Delayed or slowed progression of Alzheimer's disease
- Reduced brain damage after injury

EXERCISE AND WEIGHT MANAGEMENT

A major benefit of exercise, of course, is the loss of extra weight. Exercise is good for the waistline. Studies have demonstrated the following:

✎ NOTES

_____

_____

_____

_____

_____

_____

- Exercise has beneficial effects on body composition, especially when combined with a low-calorie diet.

- Exercise leads to increased expenditures of energy.

- Exercise leads to inhibited food intake (better dietary compliance).

- Long-term weight maintenance is associated with highly restrained eating, regular physical activity, and better mental health.

- Individuals who exercise and diet tend to lose more weight than people who simply diet.

- One can expect to lose 2 percent to 3 percent of body weight through increased exercise alone.

There is no question that exercise helps with weight maintenance. Exercise increases the number of calories burned, uses stored body fat as fuel, and builds lean muscle tissue that increases the metabolic rate of the body. What's more, people who exercise tend to eat better. But much of this you already know.

COMMIT TO EXERCISE

Keep in mind that the Wings Program asks you to make a substantial commitment to physical fitness. For many people, this part of the program does not come easily.

Physical fitness requires time, energy expenditure, and possibly even financial commitment. It involves some level of inconvenience. It requires you to break a lifelong habit of inactivity and create healthful new habits. You can be certain that, unless you really enjoy the process, you will encounter obstacles that are not easily overcome. *Everything* will suddenly seem more important than pulling on those work-out clothes and tying those shoes. The weather won't be perfect, the kids will need something, you'll feel a little tired, a

Measuring Up

It's that time again . . . Weigh yourself, and then take five girth measurements: bust at the largest point, waist at two inches above the navel, hips at the largest point, and right and left thigh circumference at the point where your extended fingertips reach with your arms hanging down at your sides. Record these figures, and your calculated BMI value, on your Progress Chart.

work assignment will need finishing, tomorrow would be a better day, and on and on . . .

Today's lesson is preparatory: examine your lifestyle and your preferences carefully, because in the next lesson you will actually get started on your own fitness routine. Don't close the book now! I will try to make this process as easy—and as fun—as possible, and who knows? Maybe your exercise routine will become one of your favorite times of the day!

And now, go to page 267 for your new recipes!

TODAY'S ASSIGNMENT

EXERCISE SELF-EVALUATION

Review the material in this lesson. Determine your personal level of commitment to building your health, and ponder how you are going to build your exercise program. The next few lessons will provide valuable information on how to incorporate exercise into your lifestyle, how to exercise so you get its full benefits (in terms of both effectiveness and safety), and how to make it fun for the whole family.

If you have not been exercising regularly, why not? What is your biggest hindrance? Is it an issue of time, disinterest, boredom, physical impairment? Take some time to consider this. Be honest. Self-evaluation at this stage of the game will determine whether or not you are successful in your exercise program, and whether or not you will achieve another level of health for the rest of your life.

After you've answered the questions above, consider the following: How committed are you to building your health? If you do not enjoy exercise, are you willing to put aside your personal preference to work exercise into your schedule? If you have previously avoided exercise, are you eager to explore physical fitness? If you aren't actually eager, are you at least willing to start (slowly, perhaps) incorporating exercise into your lifestyle?

Take some time to answer these questions as well. Again, be honest. If the willingness is there, what sacrifices or adjustments are you prepared to make? What can you do to make fitness a family project? How can you get your children involved in exercise or sports so they are also physically fit?

If you are already an exercise buff, consider how you might improve on your efforts and their results. What are your fitness goals? Have you achieved them? Let's make exercise work for you, and let's make it a fun part of your whole-body health program!

LESSON II-9 STUDY GUIDE

1. List some mental benefits of exercise.

2. List some physical benefits of exercise.

3. What are some obstacles in your life that make a consistent exercise program a challenge?

4. What role does exercise play in weight management?

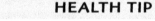

HEALTH TIP

INDIGESTION AND HEARTBURN

Burping, bloating, and belching are common signs of digestive upset. Instead of turning to over-the-counter digestive aids, try settling the problem naturally as follows:

- To facilitate digestion, take your herbal bitters and digestive enzyme products with each meal, particularly large meals. I highly recommend using 1 teaspoon of Eclectic Institute Neutralizing Cordial in a small glass of water after each meal, or when indigestion occurs.

- Ginger tea is an excellent remedy for any type of upset stomach. Catnip, chamomile, fennel, fenugreek, and peppermint are also excellent for indigestion.

- *Aloe vera* gel or juice is good for heartburn. Take 2 tablespoons in a little water when the need arises.

- For intestinal gas or heartburn, take one or two charcoal capsules (available at health food stores).

- Always chew food thoroughly, eat when you are relaxed, and do not drink large quantities of water when eating.

- Indigestion can be a symptom of allergy. If specific foods cause indigestion, avoid them.

You can also determine whether your stomach produces appropriate amounts of hydrochloric acid (HCl) with the following test:

- Take 1 tablespoon of apple-cider vinegar (or one capsule of HCl) with your meal. If your indigestion goes away or seems better, you may require more stomach acid than your body is presently producing. Try taking supplementary HCl with any meal that contains protein, starting with one capsule and working up to five capsules if necessary. However, if at any time your symptoms feel worse or you feel a sensation of burning or acidity in your stomach, reduce the amount of HCl you are taking until you are comfortable.

- If the apple-cider vinegar or the supplementary HCl makes your symptoms worse, your stomach has too much acid. You will need to alkalinize it by drinking a glass of raw cabbage juice just prior to each meal or by taking one capsule of calcium carbonate when your stomach bothers you.

Lesson II-10. Your Personal Exercise Plan

It almost seems like the Western world is divided into two groups of people: buff people and not-so-buff people. On TV commercials, we see the lean, mean bodies of men and women who obviously spend "way too much time" in the gym and have the bulging muscles to prove it. Then we walk down the street and see the rest of us, with lumps and bumps in the wrong places, jiggling body parts that should be firm, huffing and puffing up one flight of stairs.

This dichotomy is not *entirely* our fault. We have been led to believe that unless we commit our entire lives to working out at the gym, there isn't any point. Or, we have been told that a few minutes per day a couple times per week will get us into good shape. We have, unfortunately, been given the wrong information, as both of those statements are untrue.

So I am going to set the record straight by giving you the ungilded truth about physical fitness from a weight-loss perspective. Here it is: If exercise is to be used as a weight-loss tool, we're going to have to really get out there and sweat! We don't have to spend our lives in the gym, but we are going to have to make a serious commitment to personal fitness.

? TODAY'S QUESTION

Are you ready to get up and go?

Pull on those shorts and shoes and get started! Oh yes . . . stop complaining. This is going to be great!

Most of us know that regular workouts benefit the body, but most of us have not been sufficiently challenged to make it happen. Small amounts of exercise alone, or exercise without dieting (or without reducing calories down to a "reasonable level"), will not generally cause weight loss. How much exercise is needed to lose weight? How can we achieve a weight-loss benefit by combining good nutrition (covered in Module I) and physical fitness or exercise? These are some of the questions we will begin to address in this lesson.

YOUR WHOLE BODY LOVES EXERCISE— AND LOTS OF IT!

Any form of exercise benefits the mind (remember the connection between exercise and alertness, enhanced mood, and the like) and the rest of the body. Exercise improves digestion, the immune system, and so on.

Exercise in small amounts is good—but will not produce weight loss. This is not to say a not-so-intense form of exercise is worthless: you learned in the last lesson that even minor amounts of exercise are good for the body. In all honesty, however, walking for a few minutes per day or a few days per week will not help you shed any pounds.

Many people become frustrated and confused to find that when they start walking or swimming a few times per week, they lose no weight at all; in fact, some people have found that light exercise actually

✎ NOTES

causes weight gain. How depressing! No wonder they become discouraged and give up.

The reason that small amounts of exercise do not cause weight loss is that your body is able to adjust, up and down, its caloric intake and energy output. If you begin a low-intensity workout program, your body compensates for the heightened demands by increasing your appetite (so slightly you won't notice it). The increase in appetite is very small—the equivalent of half an apple or less—but that may be just enough to keep those extra pounds afloat.

It is also possible to gain weight by adding muscle tissue without losing a compensatory amount of fat. Worse, we may find that if we are living in a state of chronic fatigue, even low-level exercise can produce a stress response that triggers a cortisol response—which, in turn, adds extra inches to the waistline. (Stress-induced weight gain is discussed in Lesson III-4.)

A Little Bit Will Not Do It

If you are not in a crisis stress state during which you are chronically tired, then low-to-moderate amounts of exercise may reduce stress and produce other physiological benefits. But it is very hard to produce significant weight loss by exercising only an average of three to four times per week, for thirty minutes per session, according to exercise expert Dr. Edmond Burke.

One pound of fat equals 3,500 calories. Theoretically, you need to burn 3,500 calories to burn 1 pound of fat. Exercise, however, does not just burn fat: it also burns carbohydrates and protein. Plus, as Dr. Burke believes, it may actually take upwards of 7,000 calories (of exercise) to burn 1 pound of body fat. This is assuming that the body's calorie intake does not increase to compensate for the added energy requirements.

Ten Exercise Myths

(Adapted from *Nutrition Action Healthletter*, January/February 2000)

1. Strength training will make women too muscular.

   No! Studies show that strength training in women produces greater bone density, muscle mass, muscle strength, and balance.

2. Light weights on your arms or legs can boost your exercise benefit.

   No! Weights on the arms and legs only slow you down; they don't increase the exercise benefit.

3. With the right exercise, you can get rid of trouble spots.

   No! Spot reducing is a myth.

4. Exercise burns lots of calories.

   No! Walking or running a mile burns about 100 calories but sitting still for the same time burns about 50 or 60 calories; but the more you exercise, the more fit you get!

5. If you don't lose weight, there's no point in exercising.

   No! Although most people start exercising to lose weight, there are dozens of other compelling health reasons to exercise.

6. Weight gain is inevitable as you age.

   No! Our basal metabolic rate does tend to decrease as we age, but exercising more and eating slightly less can

accommodate this. And muscle tissue can be rebuilt by resistance training.

7. You can't be fit and fat.

   No! Fitness doesn't necessarily correlate with fatness, as was shown by a study of 25,000 men at the Cooper Clinic in Dallas, Texas. Overweight people can also become fit!

8. No pain, no gain.

   No! Moderate-intensity exercise (done a little longer) is just as effective as high-intensity exercise (done for a shorter period of time).

9. If you can't exercise regularly, why bother?

   No! It takes ten to twelve weeks of regular exercise to become "fit" or to improve performance on a treadmill. But every session of exercise will provide some benefit to the body.

10. If you didn't exercise when you were younger, it could be dangerous to start when you're older.

    No! You are never too old to start exercising, and older people can also lay down lean muscle tissue as they engage in resistance training. But anyone with multiple risk factors for heart disease should check with a physician before beginning, and get into the program at a slower rate.

To achieve weight-loss benefits from an exercise program, you must work up to a fairly strenuous routine of burning roughly 2,500 calories per week through exercise alone; that means burning 2,500 calories above what is normally used during your day-to-day activities and by metabolism. How much exercise does it take to burn those 2,500 weekly calories? You will need to exercise five or more hours per week, at moderate-to-high intensity levels, to have a significant impact on your body weight.

Moderate- to high-intensity exercise can be defined as getting the heartbeat up to 60 to 80 percent of the maximum heart rate for your age (to determine your maximum heart rate, subtract your age from 220). Dr. Burke believes that seven hours of moderate-to-intense exercise per week is more realistic as a weight-loss strategy. That is, for most people, a lot of exercise—and that should become your goal!

THE WINGS EXERCISE PROGRAM

Here, in a nutshell, is the Wings exercise protocol:

- Weeks 1–2: Do five half-hour periods per week of an activity that you enjoy.

- Weeks 3–4: Do five exercise periods per week, recording your "comfortable intensity" (length and duration) in your Exercise Diary (Appendix 2); become aware of your fitness level.

- Weeks 5–6: Do five exercise periods per week; at each session, increase the intensity (length and duration) above that recorded in the previous week.

- Weeks 7–8: Do five exercise periods per week at your increased length and intensity (aerobic); add two sessions weekly of resistance training to improve muscle tone.

- Weeks 9–10: Continue the five aerobic exercise periods per week along with the two weekly sessions of resistance training; step up the intensity of your workouts for both.

- Weeks 11–12: Continue the five aerobic exercise periods per week, and increase the intensity of your resistance training sessions. If you started with one set of repetitions on each exercise, increase to two sets of repetitions, or to the point of muscle fatigue.

- Weeks 13–14: Continue the five aerobic exercise periods and the two sessions of resistance training per week. Add the element of resistance to your

aerobics training: for example, if you're using a treadmill for walking, add incline; if you're walking outdoors, choose a route with hills and valleys, while maintaining the same speed.

- Weeks 15–16: You should now be doing five periods of aerobic exercise per week, at up to one hour each, with resistance or elevations (as above). You should also be doing at least two sessions of resistance training per week, up to the point of muscle fatigue, for each group of large muscles.

- From then on . . . Continue this level of workout indefinitely. As the workout becomes more comfortable, continue to increase the intensity or duration, up to one-and-a-half-hour sessions, five days per week, or more.

Caution

If you have been diagnosed with a cardiovascular condition or any other condition that requires medical treatment, you must seek the counsel of your physician before embarking on a strenuous exercise program! Your safety is of paramount importance!

Two Kinds of Exercise

Aerobic exercise (requiring oxygen) elevates the heart rate and deepens breathing, pulling more oxygen into the lungs and into the muscle tissue. Forms of aerobic exercise include walking, jogging, bike riding, rowing, and so on. Anaerobic exercise (not requiring oxygen) is resistance exercise, which increases muscle strength and endurance. A good example of anaerobic exercise is weight lifting or working out on the resistance machines at a gym.

Aerobic exercise burns calories, improves the strength, endurance, and efficiency of the heart muscle, relieves depression, increases the metabolic rate, and more. Anaerobic exercise builds lean muscle tissue that, in turn, increases the metabolic rate of the body due to the increased metabolism of muscle tissue as opposed to fat tissue. Anaerobic exercise also increases stamina, making it possible for you to remain physically active for longer periods of time, thereby burning more calories.

Aerobic and anaerobic exercises are equally important. A well-balanced exercise program combines them, and this combination produces the best results for weight loss as well as overall personal fitness.

Making a Plan Is Winning Half of the Battle

Most people cannot begin an exercise program at the optimal level of moderate-to-high intensity; they need to begin where they are. If you have been fairly sedentary for a while, start by exercising at a mild-to-moderate pace three to five times per week. Increase your level of exercise so you can work out safely and effectively. I strongly encourage you to work with a personal trainer who can help you customize a personal program.

Included at the end of this lesson are charts that will help you put your own exercise program together. Spend some time with these charts so you are familiar with the information before you start designing your program. Don't get too fancy with it. If you are just beginning to exercise, start by walking several times per week, and then add on to your program as described above in the Wings exercise protocol.

Having read this lesson, you now understand how to keep working your way up into higher and higher levels of fitness. You should work up to doing one and a half hours of aerobics training four to five times per week, along with resistance training for one and a half hours twice weekly up to maximum muscle capacity. If you can develop the discipline to reach and maintain this exercise goal, your fitness level will be superior!

The objective, however, is not only to increase your fitness: it is to develop the lifelong habit of building health, of making sure that exercise is a part of the lifestyle you have chosen. As Dr. Burke says, you'll know you have "gotten there" when you consider your workouts to be just as important as eating healthful meals and getting a good night's sleep. Throughout the entire Wings Program and thereafter for the rest of your healthy life, you must continue to exercise regularly and vigorously. Challenge yourself to new levels of endurance and intensity.

Remember to have fun with it! One of the most important aspects of a workout program is pleasure. Life is not simply an endurance contest. Choose a form of exercise that suits your personality and your lifestyle: walking, running, swimming, hiking, dancing, bicycling, aerobics, something else entirely—whatever works for you, enjoy it! And don't forget the value of accountability: having someone "hold your hand" and keep you steadfast in your resolve can be an important contribution to your success. Make sure to record your activity in your Exercise Diary every day (Appendix 2).

And now, go to page 268 for your new recipes!

Examples of Moderate Amounts of Activity

- Washing and waxing a car for 45–60 minutes
- Washing windows or floors for 45–60 minutes
- Playing volleyball for 45 minutes
- Playing touch football for 30–45 minutes
- Gardening for 30–45 minutes
- Wheeling self in wheelchair for 30–40 minutes
- Walking 1 3/4 miles in 35 minutes (20 minutes/mile)
- Basketball (shooting baskets) for 30 minutes
- Bicycling 5 miles in 30 minutes
- Dancing fast (social) for 30 minutes
- Pushing a stroller 1 1/2 miles in 30 minutes
- Raking leaves for 30 minutes
- Walking 2 miles in 30 minutes (15 minutes/mile)
- Water aerobics for 30 minutes
- Swimming laps for 20 minutes

- Wheelchair basketball for 20 minutes
- Basketball (playing a game) for 15–20 minutes
- Bicycling 4 miles in 15 minutes
- Jumping rope for 15 minutes
- Running 1 1/2 miles in 15 minutes (10 minutes/mile)
- Shoveling snow for 15 minutes
- Stair walking for 15 minutes

*A moderate amount of physical activity is roughly equivalent to physical activity that uses approximately 150 calories of energy per day, or 1,000 calories per week.

**Some activities can be performed at various intensities; the suggested durations correspond to expected intensity effort.

(Adapted from *Clinical Guidelines on the Identification, Evaluation, and Treatment of Overweight and Obesity in Adults: The Evidence Report.* Bethesda, MD: National Institutes of Health, 2000, 78.)

ACTIVITIES THAT EXPEND 150 KILOCALORIES*

*For an average 70-kilogram (154-pound) adult

Intensity	Activity	Approximate Duration
Moderate	Volleyball, noncompetitive	43 min
Moderate	Walking at a moderate pace (3 mph)	37 min
Moderate	Walking at a brisk pace (4 mph)	32 min
Moderate	Table tennis	32 min
Moderate	Raking leaves	32 min
Moderate	Social dancing	29 min
Moderate	Lawn mowing (powered push mower)	29 min
Hard	Jogging (5 mph)	18 min
Hard	Field hockey	16 min
Very hard	Running (6 mph)	13 min

AVERAGE CALORIC NEEDS FOR VARIOUS ACTIVITIES (Thirty Minutes)

Activity	Female (121 pounds)	Male (161 pounds)
Sleeping	28	38
Sitting	29	39
Eating	33	44
Standing, at ease	34	45
Standing, light activity	58	78
Driving a car	72	96
Playing volleyball	83	110
Slow walking, on level	84	112
Playing ping-pong	93	124
Slow pleasure swimming	104	139
Calisthenics	120	160
Pleasure bicycling, on level	120	160
Golfing	130	188
Gardening and weeding	141	188
Fast walking, on level	159	212
Walking downstairs	160	213
Playing tennis	166	221
Playing basketball	169	225
Fast swimming	213	286
Mountain climbing	241	321
Running, long distance	361	481
Walking upstairs	416	555
Sprinting	516	748

TODAY'S ASSIGNMENT

DESIGN YOUR PERSONAL EXERCISE PROGRAM

For this assignment, enlist the aid of this book and, ideally, a personal trainer. Design an individualized program for yourself that extends at least fourteen weeks, and that builds in intensity and endurance each week, until you have reached your fitness goal. Record both your program and your success in your Exercise Diary (Appendix 2). And then . . . do this for the rest of your life!

LESSON II-10 STUDY GUIDE

1. List some benefits of exercise.

2. How much exercise does one need to do to achieve a weight-loss benefit?

3. List some common exercise myths, and the truth behind each myth.

4. What are the two categories of exercise? What types of activities fit into each category?

5. What types of activities burn more than 100 calories per hour?

🌿 HEALTH TIP

INFLAMMATION CONTROL

Fleeting inflammations are a common sign of allergy. There is much you can do to lower your inflammatory response naturally. Consider the following:

- Avoid all foods that commonly cause inflammation (Lesson III-14).

- Avoid all processed foods, sugar, white-flour products, and soft drinks.

- Do the pulse test (pages 47–48; see also Appendix 5) on every food that you commonly consume, and eliminate those foods that appear to pose an intolerance or allergy problem.

- Bromelain and quercetin are excellent anti-inflammatory agents. Take them on an empty stomach for best results.

- Fish oil (up to 10 grams per day) is another excellent anti-inflammatory agent.

- Eat a diet composed of 75 percent raw foods; in other words, eat two large salads each day, accompanied by other vegetables, and make vegetables the mainstay of your diet.

- Drink plenty of herbal teas and freshly squeezed juices: alfalfa is a good source of healing minerals, and echinacea, red clover, and yucca are excellent for reducing inflammation.

✒ ADDITIONAL NOTES

Lesson II-11. Hunger Is a Good Thing

Yes, you read it correctly. Hunger is (can be!) a good thing, a sign that everything is working right, but that the body's nutritional needs have not been met. Learning the lessons of hunger—how to stimulate a healthy hunger in the absence of clear and appropriate hunger signals, how to satisfy the hunger needs of the body, how to interpret the body's hunger signals, and how to make hunger work for you instead of against—is an important part of being healthy (and thin).

? TODAY'S QUESTION

How often do you get hungry?

_____

_____

_____

_____

Does anything other than the need for food stimulate your hunger? How do you resolve your hunger?

Hunger, both false and true, gets us into a lot of trouble nutritionally—and weight-wise. We feel hungry, so we eat. But often, the pangs that rumble around in our midsections are erroneous signals that we mistake for true hunger. Our bodies send messages that they want specific foods (or nonfoods) that actually have little or nothing to do with legitimate physical needs; or, we misinterpret the messages. Our hunger can even be psychological instead of physical, but we eat food instead of caring for our inner person.

WHAT IS HUNGER?

According to the *American Heritage Dictionary*, hunger is "personal states of wanting to eat and drink materials perceived as foods and beverages . . . " This definition, obviously, is a gross oversimplification, as the body has constructed a very complicated system of hunger regulation and eating behaviors. Babies may be the only true depletion-driven eaters; after childhood, the body interacts with physical depletion signals (such as an empty tummy) to stimulate both hunger and eating through what is called the incentive-based hunger system.

Hunger and satiety are governed by the brain, and hormones throughout the body are involved. Appetite is certainly controlled, at least partially, by the senses of sight and smell. The sight of appetizing foods and the smell of tantalizing aromas wafting through the nasal passages send messages to the digestive system to prepare to receive the meal. Our mouths water and we feel hungry for that food.

The presence of food in the stomach and small intestines then triggers receptor sites to send messages to the brain about the amount of food, its nutrient composition, and the rate of nutrient digestion. Key peptides (proteins) secreted in the gastrointestinal tract also signal the brain, affecting appetite. Somatostatin and cholecystokinin, for example, send satiety signals via sensory nerve fibers. Bombesin sends messages to inhibit hunger or to inhibit further eating, and stimulates the release of cholecystokinin, which enhances feelings of satiety even more.

The brain neurotransmitters beta-endorphin and

✒ NOTES

_____

_____

_____

_____

_____

_____

neuropeptide Y (both opioids) and galanin stimulate food intake; the calming neurotransmitter serotonin and corticotropin-releasing factor (CRF) diminish appetite. Depending on the insulin cycle (insulin is secreted on command when sugars or carbohydrates are ingested, and pulled back as blood sugar levels diminish), insulin either increases or decreases hunger. The hypothalamus, an endocrine organ, is responsible for much of the secretion and regulation of these neuropeptides (hormones and neurotransmitters). Even the amount of body fat you have may also help regulate appetite and hunger.

Complicated, isn't it? Most of this internal activity is out of our control: it is regulated by numerous "states of being" and by delicate negative feedback loops that alternately ramp up and dampen hunger response and eating behaviors. We do not even have to think about it. Hunger signals, therefore, are simply part of normal homeostasis, or biological balance. If these messenger systems are working efficiently and correctly and we are eating a nutrient-dense diet, the following occurs: we feel hungry when nutrient and blood sugar levels drop; we feel satisfied (although not necessarily full) at the conclusion of eating an appropriate amount of food or, more accurately, the needed nutrients; and we remain satisfied until the food has been digested, blood sugar levels have normalized, and the hypothalamus again signals the need to obtain food.

It is supposed to work like that, anyway, but these normal bodily circumstances can be disrupted by various factors, including chemical additives, physical or emotional stress, allergy, food addictions, and chronic malnutrition or undernutrition. Although physiological hunger signals can relay real, important information about critical shortages in the body's nutrient levels, false messages can stimulate inappropriate eating behaviors.

We have a rudimentary understanding, for example, that some food additives trigger false hunger. MSG and aspartame, both classified as excitotoxins (chemicals that artificially and powerfully stimulate brain cells, particularly in the hypothalamus), increase cravings for carbohydrates and for foods containing these synthetic chemicals. Little research is being done on the other biochemical effects of taste enhancers, preservatives, and other chemicals in processed food, but we are beginning to see that synthetic foods can be powerfully addictive. We are drawn to eat them even when we are not hungry in the biological sense.

A purely biological definition of hunger is obviously incomplete, because we also feel a type of hunger (and satiety) that is induced by social and psychological influences. Much of the diet world focuses on suppressing hunger. But hunger is not our enemy: hunger is an important messenger. It is very important to understand our personal hunger signals and what causes us to eat. Let's not "shoot the messenger." Let's listen to the message—and respond appropriately.

WHY DO YOU EAT?

Consider the following questions:

- Do you abstain from eating until you feel hunger, or do you eat to prevent feelings of hunger?

- Do you eat out of habit? For social reasons?

- Do certain activities stimulate a feeling of hunger (such as for hot dogs at a ball game, or for coffee and cake at a business meeting)?

- Do cravings for certain foods make you think you're hungry?

- Do foods you are allergic to make you feel hungry?

- Are you meeting the nutritional needs of your body on a regular basis?

Many of us find ourselves rummaging through the refrigerator an hour or so after dinner each evening. Is it habit, or are we still unsatisfied? One possible reason for feeling hungry at the end of a meal is that we have not eaten to fulfill the body's nutrient requirements; in other words, our bodies are still deficient in one or more nutrients, even after consuming a sufficient number of calories.

You should feel physically satisfied on relatively small amounts of food, as long as the food is high in nutrient content and the physiological needs of your body are being met. Are you eating enough protein, carbohydrates, fats, water, and fiber? Are you getting more than the recommended daily allowance (RDA) in micronutrients? If you still feel hungry after eating what you know is a nutritionally adequate meal, discuss your hunger with your Wings nutritionist (at www.flywithwings.com/pnc.html, click on MyProConnect). She may refer you to a nutritionally trained physician.

Another good question to ask yourself is, "What am I hungry for?" If you listen carefully, you will hear your body's response. Sometimes you will "sense" or "know" that your blood sugar is low and you need protein, or you need energizing fats. You may crave chicken salad, or guacamole, or other familiar foods that meet your immediate need.

Sometimes your body needs rest instead of food, so it is asking for stimulating "foods" to increase body energy; for example, you may crave dessert when you are very tired. Sometimes you are simply feeding a habit, not a hunger; for example, you are accustomed to snacking on chips while watching TV in the evening, so when you turn on the TV you "feel hungry" for chips. Rethink that! Are you truly hungry, or are you indulging a habit?

HEALTHY HUNGER—OR A LACK THEREOF

Remember that true hunger is a good thing, a signal that your body's needs are not being met or that other issues need to be addressed. Do not think that struggling through hunger pangs will make you more likely to lose weight: it will actually impair your ability to lose weight and maintain your weight loss. Don't ignore those pangs, but don't automatically indulge them, either. Discover their source so that you can deal with them, nutritionally or otherwise.

Keeping in mind that hunger is one sign of a healthy body, we should also be concerned if we seldom or never feel hungry no matter how long it has been since we have eaten. There can be several reasons for a failed hunger system. Many prescription medications such as pain relievers, sedatives, and antidepressants are well known for reducing or eliminating appetite, making it difficult to eat at appropriate times. Other medications can cause nausea, constipation, or other stomach upsets, and no one enjoys eating when feeling unwell.

The liver is responsible for much of the process of digestion: it secretes enzymes and digestive juices into the intestinal tract, detoxifies the body, and stimulates waste removal. If the liver is not functioning efficiently, the body's digestive capabilities are compromised, resulting in a lowered appetite. If the body cannot physically handle food, it doesn't "want" it and shuts off the appetite in order to control food intake.

Very obese people often lose their sense of hunger for reasons that are not understood. These people have often dieted frequently and severely, and their reduced appetite may be one of the ways their bodies are seeking to restore homeostasis. It may also be that their bodies are in strict "conservation mode" and refuse food because of their drastically lowered metabolism.

And now, go to page 269 for your new recipes!

TODAY'S ASSIGNMENT

CULTIVATE A HEALTHY HUNGER RESPONSE

Pay special attention to your hunger signals this week. If you find yourself feeling hungry when you know you shouldn't be, use the information you learned in this lesson to determine the real origin of the feeling, and then address it by meeting your body's needs. If you suspect that you get hungry out of habit, establish new habits to satisfy those false hunger signals.

If you seldom or never feel hungry, concentrate on improving your digestion so that you can again feel hungry at appropriate times and for appropriate reasons. Reread Lesson II-5 and follow its digestive tips. Drink a cup of ginger tea several times per day. Make sure your diet is adequate in the B-complex vitamins and the mineral zinc (you may need to increase your supplementation of these nutrients to achieve this goal). If you are taking a prescription medication, ask your pharmacist whether appetite suppression or stimulation is a potential side effect. Do the detective work—and solve the "crime"!

LESSON II-11 STUDY GUIDE

1. What is the purpose of the hunger sensation?

2. What triggers true hunger? What can trigger false hunger?

3. What are some common reasons that we feel hungry when we should feel satiated?

4. What are some reasons we may not ever feel hungry?

_____

_____

_____

5. How can we appropriately stimulate a healthy hunger?

_____

_____

_____

HEALTH TIP

FLU PREVENTION

Got the flu? Did you wake up achy, headachy, and feverish? The best solution for a full-blown case of the flu is prevention. Prevention! Prevention! Prevention! During the cold and flu season, wash your hands frequently, and avoid all sugar and other processed foods; remember that sugar disables the immune system for up to four hours.

- At the first sign of flu, take a homeopathic flu formula. Two of the best known are Oscillococcinum from Boiron and Flu Solution from Dolisos; dissolve a capful of the pellets under your tongue every fifteen minutes or until all symptoms disappear. Another classic flu remedy is Source Naturals Wellness Formula; take one tablet (or two capsules) every hour until you feel well, then reduce the dose to three or four tablets per day for a week or so.

- Do an ascorbic acid flush (page 8–9), then reduce your daily intake of vitamin C to 75 percent of the amount needed to stimulate the flush reaction. If you do this at the first sign of flu, you can often prevent it from taking hold.

- Drink teas of echinacea, ginger, and/or yarrow throughout the flu season, and drink more if you feel a bout of flu coming on.

- Drink onion-and-garlic tea (recipe on page 181) throughout the day, or try taking several garlic capsules daily (Kyolic is one of several good brands).

- Increase your daily intake of vitamin A up to 15,000 international units (IU), unless you are pregnant. *Caution:* Do not exceed 7,500 IU of vitamin A per day if you are pregnant or may become pregnant.

- Take 15–30 milligrams of zinc per day with meals. If your throat is sore, suck on zinc lozenges throughout the day.

- Try a homeopathic cough syrup (one of the best is Boericke and Tafel Cough and Bronchial Syrup) to relieve bronchial congestion and allow you to sleep at night.

- Consume plenty of liquids, particularly hot chicken broth (good as both prevention and remedy), freshly squeezed fruit juices, herbal teas, and water.

- Get lots and lots of rest, and sleep as much as possible. There is no substitute for a good night's sleep.

ADDITIONAL NOTES

_____

_____

_____

_____

_____

_____

_____

Lesson II-12. The Fidget Factor and Other Freebies

Calories are not inherently bad; they are a measurement of energy, and they are an essential part of the diet. Foods are burned in the mitochondria of the cell to produce heat and energy. There are many ways to burn additional calories other than exercising to near exhaustion—although you might have to do that too!

❓ TODAY'S QUESTION

What are some easy ways to burn calories?

_____

_____

_____

_____

What activity could you do to burn an additional 10 calories per hour? 100 calories per hour?

Today's lesson is a collection of simple truths—and a bit of fun thrown into the weight-management mix. Did you know that you can help control your weight simply by doing little things that help burn calories? Some of these little things require little to no effort on your part, and some are really fun. This will be one of the most creative lessons in the entire book. The goal here is to get you to become more active, even in little ways. And do not be content with the suggestions in this book alone: I encourage you to get creative and think of new, unusual ways to burn calories and get those energy juices flowing!

What modern conveniences could you forego to make yourself more active? Consider these ideas: Chop your vegetables yourself, the old-fashioned way. Sing instead of listening to the radio. Take the stairs instead of the elevator. (It's my personal policy, when staying in a hotel, to take the stairs instead of the elevator if my room is on the fourth floor or lower.) Whenever you drive somewhere, park as far from the door as possible and walk. Carry your groceries instead of wheeling them in the shopping cart. Keep the temperature of your house cooler than is comfortable, forcing your body to burn more calories to produce more heat and keep itself warm.

Let me explain the "fidget factor." When you're fidgeting, you're keeping some part of your body moving at all times. As it turns out, studies show that you can burn up to 10 calories per hour just by continually jiggling your leg! (It will, however, drive your spouse and coworkers crazy.)

Life is full of these freebies. Every half hour of a romantic encounter, for example, burns about 150 calories. Do lots of hugging and kissing—and enjoy regular periods of lovemaking with your spouse!

Thinking burns calories. Increase your mental activity by reading a book or by doing something else to make you think and concentrate. Taking a class is another way to keep your mind active. What do you want to learn? Painting? Sculpture? A foreign language? Cake decorating? (No, not *that* one!) Public speaking? Whatever gets you excited, learn about it, or teach it.

Housecleaning burns calories. And don't make it too easy for yourself: clean the kitchen floor on your hands and knees; wash the windows manually; scrub

🖋 NOTES

_____

_____

_____

_____

_____

the pots and pans instead of putting them into the dishwasher; hang the clothes out on the clothesline instead of tossing them into the dryer. If you get your kids involved, they'll learn to be good cleaners, and they'll keep physically fit in the process. Don't handicap your children by giving them an easy life (so says Socrates!).

Spend time with your kids in active conversation, play, or jobs. Go catch frogs. Build a healthful, fun social life with friends and family. Instead of inviting friends over for a big dinner, invite them to go bowling with you, or bike riding, or swimming. Are there any elderly or disabled people in your neighborhood? Mow their lawns, shovel their sidewalks, rake their leaves, clean their homes, and take them shopping. In other words, get richly involved in life—it burns calories!

Do you need other freebie-activity ideas?

- Go hiking
- Take a flower-arranging class
- Take a cooking class
- Wash the dog
- Clean out the garage
- Lead a study group
- Write a book
- Learn how to water-ski
- Go clam digging
- Teach your kids how to rollerblade
- Take up yard work or gardening
- Plant and tend a row of raspberries
- Plant an herb garden on your deck
- Plant some fruit trees
- Do massage therapy on your spouse
- Learn how to sew
- Wash the car
- Clean under your bathroom cabinets
- Start a book club
- Explore all the bike paths in your community
- Learn how to parasail (it's marvelous!)
- Teach your kids how to swim
- Pick strawberries

A Chortle a Day Keeps the Doctor Away?

Laughing Clubs International was formed in Bombay, India, to teach people how to laugh. After warm-up exercises, their meetings consist simply of laughing practice, both aloud and silent. Laughing is perhaps the most fun freebie of all. And laughter burns calories! According to one expert, 100 laughs is equivalent to ten minutes on a rowing machine. (Tip: putting your hands up in the sky helps laughing to come easier.)

Although today's focus is activity, remember to get plenty of rest as well. If you are not getting enough rest, your body slows its metabolism to conserve energy. Get a good seven to eight hours of sleep each night. Get mental rest too: take one day off each week to do nothing but spiritual and fun activities. And quit your night job! For reasons not clearly understood, people gain weight just by going on the late shift. According to one review article evaluating thirty-one security guards and sixty-two nurses and nurse aids in New York, evening workers gained an average of 8 pounds after they were hired, while those who worked the day shift lost an average of 1 pound.

And now, go to page 269 for your new recipes!

 TODAY'S ASSIGNMENT

THE PURSUIT OF HAPPY ACTIVITY

Make a list of three freebies you will practice this week. Use the suggestions in this section or come up with your own. Start a laughing club—you'll be the hit of your block!

LESSON 11-12 STUDY GUIDE

1. What is the fidget factor, and how does it help burn calories?

_____

_____

_____

2. List five "minor" activities that increase your activity level.

_____

_____

_____

_____

3. What influence does working at night have on weight management?

_____

_____

_____

HEALTH TIP

GET A GOOD NIGHT'S SLEEP

A night without sleep is a long, dark night—and bad for your health!

- If the problem is a breathing disorder called sleep apnea, allergies can be a common cause, especially wheat or dairy allergy; as these are eliminated, apnea often disappears or lessens. Weight loss can also reduce or eliminate sleep apnea.

- Make sure not to drink or eat any stimulating foods in the daytime. A morning cup of coffee, for example, can cause insomnia twelve hours later for someone who is sensitive to caffeine. Avoid all caffeine, alcohol, and tobacco. (Check your medications, as they often contain caffeine.)

- Do not consume tyramine-containing foods (bacon, cheese, chocolate, eggplant, ham, potatoes, sauerkraut, sugar, sausage, spinach, tomatoes, and wine) close to bedtime. Tyramine increases the release of norepinephrine, a brain stimulant.

- Take a good calcium supplement (calcium citrate malate) in the morning with breakfast, and take magnesium glycinate or a magnesium amino acid chelate in the evening with dinner. (If you prefer, you can switch the order to take the magnesium with breakfast and calcium with dinner.)

- Taking supplemental melatonin can be helpful, especially for people who do shift work (Lesson II-13), travel across time zones, or do not produce enough melatonin naturally.

- Certain herbal teas can be very helpful for calming the brain at night. Try California poppy, hops, kava kava, passionflower, skullcap, or valerian.

ADDITIONAL NOTES

_____

_____

_____

_____

_____

_____

_____

_____

_____

_____

Lesson II-13. Special Circumstances for Certain People

Most of us wrestle our schedules to the ground every single day. We go to work, take care of the house, do the grocery shopping, wash the clothes, and go to religious services. We chauffeur our kids to their after-school sports activities. They have to be reminded to get up on time, eat breakfast, take vitamins, brush teeth, change underwear, pack a lunch, be nice to their siblings, go to sleep on time, and the like. And beyond the usual craziness of daily life, many of us work odd hours or travel a great deal or drive a truck for a living. There are so many special circumstances that make following any type of a health program difficult.

? TODAY'S QUESTION

What makes your life difficult?

_____

_____

_____

_____

What life circumstances make health and weight management difficult for you? Do your work hours change frequently? Do you travel a great deal? Can you change any of these circumstances?

Developing new habits is never easy for anyone, but developing new lifestyle habits becomes even more challenging for people who lead "irregular" lives. Not everyone gets up at 6:30 A.M., eats a quiet breakfast, heads off to work at 8:00 A.M., arrives back home at 5:30 P.M., enjoys a quiet dinner with the family, and drops off to sleep at 10:00 P.M., like clockwork. In fact, very few of us lead that type of orderly life.

You may need to be more creative in the resolution of your personal health and weight issues. Today's lesson presents some ideas for solving problems posed by several special circumstances that make it particularly difficult to lose weight.

NIGHT WORKERS

As noted in the previous lesson, a few medical sources have made reference to the fact that many people gain weight when they start working nights instead of days. Some night workers only gain a few pounds, and some gain a substantial amount of weight, but both men and women seem to experience this phenomenon. So far, the research is inadequate to indicate why night-shift-related weight gain occurs.

Part of the problem may be hormonal changes that affect the body's metabolism. Melatonin, for example, is a hormone that regulates circadian rhythms and helps us fall asleep at night. Melatonin is produced in response to the time of day and total darkness; it is subsequently converted into serotonin, one of the brain's calming neurotransmitters. If you cannot produce adequate amounts of melatonin because you aren't sleeping in a dark room at night, you may also become deficient in serotonin, and this deficiency often leads to cravings for carbohydrates (the junky kind).

Melatonin deficiency may also lead to other types of hormonal imbalances or physiological problems that aren't clearly understood. Your body is thrown

✐ NOTES

_____

_____

_____

_____

_____

_____

into hormonal confusion particularly if you change back and forth from working days to working nights, as is the situation for most shift workers. Companies know that working the night shift is physically exhausting, so they often change people's schedules back and forth in an attempt to make it easier, but this may actually make it harder for the body to adjust. And in fact, it never really adjusts completely.

Chronic fatigue frequently accompanies working the late shift, and eating more calories may be the body's way of increasing energy, which may also contribute to shift-work weight gain. Think about how tired you feel when you are awake when you should be sleeping. Plus, if your shift is quiet and you sit for long periods of time, you may find yourself eating to relieve the boredom. Maintain a caloric intake that is appropriate according to your weight goals, and make sure you do not eat out of boredom.

Have you ever noticed that if you eat a heavy meal late at night, it just seems to "sit there"? Medical literature suggests that the digestive system needs to rest at night. Normally, the body receives and digests food during the day; during the night, it rests and "cleans up"; when you awaken in the morning and drink a glass of water or eat breakfast, you eliminate the waste materials, and then the process begins again.

Breaking down foods and absorbing nutrients at night when the body should be resting "confuses" the digestive system, so you will need to optimize your digestion by using digestive aids like the bitters and enzymes your nutritionist recommends (at www.fly withwings.com/pnc.html, click on MyProConnect). Drink a cup of ginger tea twenty minutes prior to each meal, eat small, frequent meals instead of large meals, try to maintain a regular eating schedule even when your schedule changes frequently, and do *not* eat junk food. In other words, make every calorie count for good nutrition (aren't you doing that anyway?).

Ideally, you should stay on the same eating schedule regardless of whether you are working days or nights: an early morning meal, a midday meal, and a meal around dinnertime. Have a small snack in the late evening, if necessary. If that schedule simply does not work, I suggest that you figure out one that does and stick with it, to allow your body to adapt to it. Don't change your eating schedule back and forth when your work schedule changes. If you simply must eat at night, have small, frequent meals every four hours, and do not indulge the temptation to eat between meals.

Be sure to get enough rest. Remember this axiom:

Ten minutes of sleep prior to 10:00 P.M. is equivalent to one hour of sleep after 10:00 P.M. You may not always be able to sleep for long periods or at the same time each day, but you can use natural sleep aids (like melatonin or relaxing herbs) to help you sleep more deeply. Keep your room pitch-black when you sleep to increase your production of melatonin. Before going to sleep, use relaxing herbs like kava kava, California poppy, valerian root, and chamomile to help your mind rest.

LONG-DISTANCE DRIVERS AND TRAVELERS

It is nearly impossible to eat healthful foods on U.S. highways. The quality of truck-stop restaurant food is absolutely appalling, nearly as appalling as airplane food. I travel a great deal, and I am always disgusted by the lack of healthful food options in most airports, in *all* airplanes, and in nearly all restaurants lining the highways. Frankly, I think there is no excuse for it. (Well, I got *that* out of my system! Do you hear the traveler's angst in my voice?)

I have learned to plan ahead. If you are driving, pack a cooler with fresh salads. Keep salad dressing cold in a separate container within the cooler. Purchase tuna fish to accompany the salad, or order a chicken breast at a restaurant to complete the meal. If you are flying, the quality and quantity of food available *en route* may be a little better—but only a little. It is still preferable to pack your own meal. I often prepare a tuna salad garnished with Greek olives, hummus, or other "yummies," and I take nut bars, dried fruits and nuts, or vegetable packets. Many of the recipes in the back of this book are perfectly portable; just keep them iced or otherwise safe to eat after you have been traveling for a few hours.

Pack a portable mixer for your Wings Breakfast Drink. You can order fresh-squeezed orange juice or purchase bottles of fruit juice to mix with the drink each morning. Remember to keep the Breakfast Drink cold, because it contains oils that can easily become rancid if exposed to warm temperatures. I like to mix almond milk with my Breakfast Drink; I take a fresh container with me, and after opening I keep it on ice or in the small refrigerator that is often in a hotel room, so I can enjoy it for several days.

Keep bottled water with you at all times and drink it throughout the day. Do not be tempted to indulge in coffee or soft drinks if you get tired. Rest frequently and stay hydrated with fresh water. Take herbs and drink plenty of water to resolve any constipation.

Take portable exercise equipment along so you can exercise on the road; or, stay in a hotel that provides a workout room. Pack your walking shoes and take a walking tour of your destination.

PEOPLE LIVING AWAY FROM HOME

If you are dismayed by the poor quality of airplane or truck-stop food, you'll be equally appalled at what colleges or nursing homes feed their residents—terrible! If you want to stay healthy, you simply must take charge of your own meals. Fortunately, there are easy ways to accomplish this.

Purchase a small blender to whip up your Wings Breakfast Drink in the morning. If necessary, purchase a small refrigerator to store fresh fruit, the Breakfast Drink, almond milk, and other small food items. Stock your personal refrigerator with fresh vegetables; broccoli and cauliflower florets, carrot sticks, and celery stalks are good snack foods. Keep olive oil and balsamic vinegar in your refrigerator for salad dressing.

One of the best gadgets for dormitory meals is a Crock-Pot. I love mine and use it frequently. Because I work outside of the home six days per week and yet want my family to enjoy the benefits of freshly prepared meals, I often take the Crock-Pot with me, fill it with the recipe ingredients, and let the dish simmer while I work (the delicious aroma wafting through the office drives my customers crazy). At the end of the day, I pack the Crock-Pot carefully in a box so it doesn't tip over in my car on the long drive home, and our "home-cooked" dinner is ready when I walk through the door. You can do the same in a college dorm. Many of the Wings recipes can be adapted to Crock-Pot use—you will love it!

If you must eat in the cafeteria, speak to the cook and ask for salads with each meal. Ask for freshly prepared proteins like grilled fish or chicken. Make your needs known to the people who prepare the meals, and if they cannot fully accommodate your needs, select carefully from what is available. Don't just indulge in what you know you shouldn't eat simply because it is the easiest thing to do.

Keep bottled water with you at all times and avoid soft drinks and coffee. And above all, avoid the dessert table! Take charge of your health!

PEOPLE WHO HATE TO COOK

I know that not everyone enjoys cooking as I do. But with a little creativity and determination, everyone can learn to prepare simple, healthful meals. And who knows? Perhaps you will even learn to enjoy the creative process . . .

Using the Wings Breakfast Drink each morning takes care of breakfast. Each weekend, spend a couple of hours in the kitchen doing advance meal preparation for the week ahead. Prepare your fresh vegetables and store them in sealed ziplock bags in the refrigerator so you can put together a quick salad for lunch by tossing a handful of each vegetable in a sealable bowl. Pack some olive oil and balsamic vinegar dressing in a separate container. Complete the meal with a can of tuna fish or a grilled chicken breast.

If you choose to purchase some meals away from home, select the restaurant or store carefully. Supermarkets often feature rotisserie chicken, grilled salmon, or other fresh entrées. Under no circumstances should you purchase frozen or freeze-dried entrées: they are nutritionally deficient and high in sodium, which causes water retention and mental symptoms, and otherwise erode your health. Make sure each meal contains a good, fresh source of protein, carbohydrates, and fats.

Commit to cooking at least two home-cooked meals each week. Teach your kids or spouse to cook. Reward your kids with a prize for each meal they prepare. Just because you don't enjoy cooking doesn't mean that the rest of the family can't!

Make one home-cooked meal a pivotal part of the week. Make it festive. Put a cloth on the table. Light candles. Use your best serving dishes. Make one meal a really terrific one for the whole family and let the entire family share in the preparation of the meal. You might even start to enjoy it after all!

"I GET NO SUPPORT!"

Many men and women are in relationships that do not support their health goals. This can be difficult to overcome, especially if the unsupportive spouse is dominant in the relationship, or if the food-preparing spouse won't make the types of meals that are needed. There are, however, choices to be made. Answer the following questions:

- What are my goals?

- Have I clearly articulated my goals and needs to my spouse (or other nonsupportive person)?

- How can I fulfill these goals without his or her support?

- Am I willing to forego the support and approval of my family to achieve my goals? Am I willing even to risk ridicule or annoying comments and pursue my goals until I have accomplished them?

- Are my sense of self-worth and my personal happiness important to me? Am I willing to work for them alone if necessary? What can I do to make sure my sense of self-worth is nurtured if I never get the support I want?

- Can I do it by myself, with the help and support of my Wings support network?

- What support do I need from my Wings instructor or accountability partner to make it easier for me? Have I expressed that need to my instructor and/or partner? Are they willing to work with and for me?

After you have answered these questions, put together your personal plan to handle the situation. Remember that your needs are just as important as those of your unsupportive spouse or other family member. After you construct your plan, do it. It may take constant reinforcement, you may need to keep expressing your needs and controlling your boundaries, but you can overcome this obstacle. ("Loving saboteurs" are discussed more fully in Lesson IV-9.)

Measuring Up

It's that time again . . . Weigh yourself, and then take five girth measurements: bust at the largest point, waist at two inches above the navel, hips at the largest point, and right and left thigh circumference at the point where your extended fingertips reach with your arms hanging down at your sides. Record these figures, and your calculated BMI value, on your Progress Chart.

And now, go to page 271 for your new recipes!

TODAY'S ASSIGNMENT

MAKE LIFE A LITTLE EASIER FOR YOURSELF

Spend some quiet time reflecting on your life. What is making it difficult for you to succeed? What can you do to solve the problem? Are you in control of your life, or is your life in control of you? Are you willing to make sacrifices for the sake of achieving your health goals? Can you bring your family beside you in your journey? It is up to you to make it happen.

Remember: you are never left without options.

Life isn't always very tidy—but who says we need an easy life anyway? The reward and pleasure of life is not in the achievement of our goals but in the struggle it takes to get there. Learn to enjoy the process as much as the accomplishment!

LESSON II-13 STUDY GUIDE

1. What are some special circumstances that make losing weight or optimizing health more difficult?

_____

_____

_____

2. What are some strategies for overcoming these difficulties?

_____

_____

_____

HEALTH TIP

TAKE A REAL BREAK

We lead such busy lives that we often do not spend time caring for our mental and emotional health. The Scriptures teach the importance of a Sabbath: a day that is devoted to spiritual pursuits and precludes any type of work. In this modern age, many of us have drifted away from taking one day a week for complete rest, but we shouldn't have. Mental and spiritual rest is just as important as physical rest.

Plan to include one "Sabbath" day in your week. Do no work on that day, other than light meal preparation. Spend time with your loved ones. Pursue spiritual activities: go to religious services, pray, and meditate. Read enjoyable books. Sprawl on the family-room floor with your kids and play a board game, or let them read to you.

Better yet, plan a twenty-four-hour "noise fast" each month. During your noise fast, allow no sounds at all: no radio, no TV, no talking, no music, no telephones, no computer . . . Get the idea? Have your family do it with you. You will find that mental and spiritual rest is the healthiest thing of all. And I promise that you will *love* your days of noise fasting.

MODULE III
Hidden Issues of Weight Management

People frequently send me articles or websites on weight loss. With skepticism, I check out the information, which is almost always based on a single theory of weight loss, be it caloric intake, exercise, or some physical problem. Recently, I've been receiving "news bulletins" about other influences on weight management like stress, depression, and the like, and I say to myself, "We've already looked at this. We've already discovered this." It isn't news, even though it is just now appearing in the mainstream press. And still, the media and the "weight-loss experts" aren't looking at the big picture—which is why, as a nation and as individuals, we are getting bigger.

That is why I am so excited about the Wings Program. This curriculum puts it all together, in one place. It looks at every part of the body, as well as the heart and the mind. It looks at weight management and health management holistically. That is the beauty and the success of Wings! And you will love this new section of the curriculum: it delves into areas never before covered in weight-loss material, and it is organized so you can make sense of it—for your own good health. Best of all, it provides solutions to very difficult problems,

It is the conclusion of the medical literature that the conditions covered in this module contribute to the problem of weight management by causing weight gain through various mechanisms. An interesting writer/doctor believes, however, that it is the other way around: that as we lay down more fat tissue, these physical problems then develop. In other words, instead of hypothyroidism causing weight deposition, excess weight causes a problem with the thyroid gland; instead of female hormones exacerbating a weight problem, excess fat causes a hormonal imbalance. (For more information, read *The Butterfly and Life Span Nutrition* by Majid Ali, M.D., Institute of Preventive Medicine: 1-201-586-4111.)

So which comes first, the health problem or the weight problem? No one knows for sure. And does it even matter? It may be mere semantics. If being overweight does indeed cause these health problems, then that only makes losing the weight more difficult. It simply means that we must work on the weight and the medical problems as a unit, not as separate issues. If the added weight causes these health problems, it then becomes even more critical to deal with the weight to maximize overall health and vitality! We can't answer the "chicken or the egg" question, but we can dig into these issues and look for solutions.

Lesson III-1. A Quick Review and Another Cleanse

It is always easy to "slip a little." We have concentrated our efforts on exercise and other issues of the body for the past few weeks. That does not mean, however, that food is secondary. Remember the rule of education? Repeat! Repeat! Repeat! So we'll repeat some of the food issues to make sure they stick. And as we delve into the intense issues in this section, you will need to keep your focus on feeding your wonderful body.

 TODAY'S QUESTION

What is your new favorite comfort food?

_____

_____

Perhaps you used to eat chocolate or ice cream for comfort, but you've learned to enjoy many new foods during these past few months as you've become reacquainted with your kitchen! What is your favorite new food toy, and why do you like it so much?

It has been a few weeks since we discussed food issues. Are you staying true to the Wings food plan, or slipping a little? At this point, it is easy to add a little bread here, a little ice cream there, an occasional soft drink or slice of pizza—and before you know it, you're not complying with your program, and then your weight loss comes to a halt. Worse, the weight starts creeping back again. You may be baffled as to why you are stuck at this plateau, not realizing that those "little vices" are impeding your progress.

Well, it is time to shorten your suspenders, tighten your belt, and hike up your trousers! Get back into the program fully so you can enjoy vibrant, glowing health. This lesson reviews some of those critical food issues so the information remains fresh in your mind.

REMEMBER THE ALLERGY/ INTOLERANCE LESSON

One of the most important parts of Module I was the lesson on food allergies and intolerances. It will be helpful to review that material at this point in your program. Resolving a food allergy or intolerance issue solves many difficult weight-loss cases: it may be the answer to the puzzling question "Why have I reached a plateau in my weight loss?"

As you may remember, a food allergy is an immune system reaction to a food allergen. A food intolerance does not provoke an immune system reaction but affects the body in other ways; a common example is lactose intolerance, caused by a deficiency in lactase, the enzyme that digests dairy products. (Remember that environmental allergens can be a significant problem as well.) Both allergies and intolerances can stimulate a wide variety of reactions, in virtually any part of the body.

Allergies or intolerances cause weight gain by several mechanisms. Our bodies tend to sequester

✒ **NOTES**

_____

_____

_____

_____

_____

_____

_____

extra water when we eat foods to which we are reactive; when we stop eating those foods, we rapidly lose that water weight. Allergenic foods can impair the function of the thyroid gland, causing hypothyroidism and lowered metabolism. Food allergies can also produce intense cravings, leading us to overeat the very foods that are causing the mischief in the first place. This information frequently causes a great deal of consternation, because we tend to react to the very foods that we eat frequently and/or to the foods we most enjoy.

Your Personal Food Triggers

Wings students have found they are allergic to garlic, bananas, corn, nuts, apples, lettuce—the list is virtually endless! Many allergenic foods are so healthful that we would never suspect them. The most common food allergens are wheat, corn, and dairy.

People often comment, "I eliminated wheat from my diet and it didn't make any difference." They may not associate their symptoms with grain allergy because they only eliminate wheat while continuing to eat other foods that contain gluten, the grain protein that causes so many problems. Gluten is found in every grain except rice, millet, and some ancient grains like kamut and teff. Simply "going off" wheat is insufficient; that is why Wings students are counseled to remove all grains from the diet, except for rice or the ancient grains named above. Keep in mind also that it can take up to a year to completely rid the body of stored gluten, so a few weeks of eliminating grains may be too short a time to experience the benefits.

Testing Yourself

The topic of allergies and intolerances remains controversial among medical practitioners. How many people actually have food and environmental allergies? Are they a significant issue for most people? How do these allergies present themselves? These are just some of the questions in hot debate. The controversy will probably continue to rage for many years, but this is really of no concern to us, because the real question is highly personal: "Do I experience negative consequences from eating certain foods?" Keep in mind that the only symptom you may notice is weight gain or an inability to lose weight.

In *The False Fat Diet* (New York, NY: Ballantine Books, 2001), Dr. Elson Haas notes that allergies cause

weight gain by a variety of mechanisms, including fluid retention, hormone release (causing fluid retention), intestinal permeability, disrupted cell chemistry (causing fluid retention), leaky capillaries, and gas production. If you are unable to lose weight on any type of program, or if your weight loss plateaus before you have achieved your weight-loss goal, you should suspect that allergies or intolerances may be a problem, and I highly recommend that you read *The False Fat Diet*. According to Dr. Haas, many medical conditions have their primary roots in food sensitivity. The diverse and extensive list includes arthritis, asthma, candidiasis, cardiovascular disease, chronic ear infections, chronic fatigue, and chronic pain, among others.

Can your challenges be solved by eliminating foods to which you are reactive? The best approach may be to try it out. If you have not yet purchased *The Pulse Test* by Dr. Arthur F. Coca (mentioned previously in Lesson I-10), you may want to do so now. Although the book is a little difficult to read, it contains interesting and valuable information on food allergies and how to identify and monitor your own allergies by using the pulse test. Dr. Coca's method is unconventional but effective, if done properly. (A pulse-test chart is included in Appendix 5 of this book to help you with the test, which can be a little complicated.)

Review Lesson I-10. Completely eliminate all foods that cause a pulse reaction. At first, the sensation may not be pleasant: you may find that you crave the foods to which you are reactive, and you may go through a period of withdrawal complete with headaches, fatigue, depression, or other upsets. Generally, however, you will only feel uncomfortable for about three days. You may then feel better than you have felt for many years! And you may (probably) lose weight.

The best way to deal with an allergy or intolerance is to avoid the food totally for a period of at least three months. At that point, you can reintroduce it into your diet to see if the allergy has been eliminated by the abstinence, but be ready to remove the food completely if a reaction is provoked. *Caution:* People who are severely reactive to a particular food must *never* reintroduce that food into their diet *at all* without consulting their physician for guidance. After having abstained from a food, a heightened reactivity to it can be life threatening.

If the foods you react to have been a major part of your diet on the Wings meal plan, you may not know what to eat. Don't worry—you can learn to enjoy many other foods and still stay on your program. Some people find that virtually everything they eat is producing a reaction; if that is the case for you, I strongly urge you to seek the counsel of a nutritionist. He/she can work with you on getting superior nutrition despite being limited to a narrow variety of foods, and on healing your body to reduce your allergic potential. (To contact your Wings nutritionist, go to www.flywithwings.com/pnc.html and click on MyProConnect.)

It is important to develop your own support network to help you sort through your allergy and/or intolerance issues and to keep you on track. Tracing the roots of your reactions can be extremely challenging and I suggest you work with someone who is trained in this field; your support network may include, for example, a caring physician, nurse practitioner, personal trainer, or nutritionist. Don't try to do it alone, as it may be too difficult; you may not be able to navigate your way through the maze of symptoms, reactions, and other information your body is sending you, get lost, and feel like giving up. You will benefit greatly from working with a professional who can bring clarity to this confusing realm.

CLEANSING AND HEALING—AGAIN

Did you follow the body-cleansing and healing protocols outlined in Module II? Do you feel that you achieved a good cleanse? The regimen is powerfully effective, and most people feel better after they complete the cleansing and healing weeks. In fact, it is important to continue working on body cleansing throughout the year. We are all exposed to thousands of chemicals in our food and ambient environment, and our livers have to deal with all of that under less-than-ideal circumstances. Most of us experience some type of reaction to these chemicals; some people stop losing weight or even gain weight because of chemical exposure.

Dr. Paula Baillie-Hamilton, author of *The Detox Diet* (London, UK: Penguin Books, 2002), believes that environmental toxins poison our weight-control mechanisms. She writes eloquently that "our metabolism appears to be affected by a massive range of synthetic chemicals…with the 'fattening' effect intended for animals in all probability working on us too." She continues:

Different synthetic chemicals achieve this in one or more ways in humans and other mammals. First they appear to damage the appetite 'switch,'

so that more food is eaten than is generally needed. Another way is by reducing the amount of food the body needs by damaging the ability to burn off food and so making the food that is eaten go further. But possibly the most important way is by seemingly preventing the body from burning up existing fat stores.

So in effect, many synthetic chemicals appear to possess the potential to poison critical parts of our weight-control system, effectively putting it out of action. What's worse, unless properly tackled, the effect could be cumulative or even synergistic, dooming us to become fatter and fatter as long as we keep exposing our bodies to these chemicals. (*The Detox Diet*, page 26.)

Dr. Baillie-Hamilton's book sheds light on why we often cannot lose weight, no matter how well we eat. It also points out why body-cleansing on a regular basis may be one of the most important parts of a health-management program.

For the first two weeks of Module III, repeat the body-cleansing and healing protocols you learned in Module II, and incorporate an emotional cleanse if you wish. The importance of emotional and spiritual health is discussed more fully in Module IV, but I mention it here because it dovetails so beautifully with the physical cleanse. Most of us go through life never considering that harmful emotions like unresolved anger and fear lie buried in our body tissues, causing as many health problems as stored physical toxins.

In the words of one well-known writer, "See to it that no bitter root grows up to cause trouble and defile many." (Hebrews 12:14) Bitterness, fear, and other negative emotions are poisons that harm the bitter person and all those around him/her. There is so much in this world, and in our personal lives, about which we can be angry. I have personally found that of all my health challenges, anger and the inability to forgive are the hardest to confront.

Considering emotional and spiritual issues can bring a deeper dimension to the body-cleansing week. Readers of any faith, as well as those who do not subscribe to a spiritual belief system, can create an emotional cleansing program that encompasses their own beliefs. If you desire, incorporate any of the following ideas into your personal program to restore your heart and mind as well as your body:

- Take fifteen to thirty minutes for silent meditation after your morning cleansing routine.

▓ Ask yourself such questions as: Am I harboring hidden anger, fear, guilt, or shame? What are the sources of my negative emotions? Am I still grieving over past losses?

▓ Think about the wrongs, committed by others or by yourself, that you have not forgiven.

▓ Think about your many blessings and feel gratitude for the goodness in your life.

As we undergo physical cleansing, strong emotions and even unresolved issues from the past often flood our consciousness. I encourage you to record your thoughts and impressions in a journal for contemplation, review, and resolve.

 ### TODAY'S ASSIGNMENT

MAKE THIS A POWERFUL WEEK

First, review the past month in your Food Diary. Are you sticking with the Wings meal plan? Where are you slipping? Make a plan to get yourself back on track so you can fulfill your health and weight goals.

Then, do the one-week body cleanse, this time incorporating any emotional or spiritual elements of your choice along with the physical cleansing protocol (Lesson II-6). Plan ahead to set aside the final day of your cleanse for a silent retreat: Retire to a location in your home or community where you can be totally silent and removed from the stress of everyday life. Do not speak. Do not listen to music or other sounds or noises. Do not interact with other people; spend this day completely alone and quiet. Allow the quiet to bring new thoughts to your mind so that you can deal with any unresolved issues in your emotional and/or spiritual life. Be purposely thankful, allowing thankfulness to permeate your mind as you are silent.

Follow your cleansing week with a healing week (Lesson II-7), and then proceed to Lesson III-2.

LESSON III-1 STUDY GUIDE

1. List some of the foods commonly associated with food allergies.

2. How do food allergies cause a problem with weight management?

3. Why is internal body cleansing an important part of your health program?

4. List some of the problems caused by environmental pollutants, and how they can influence weight management.

5. List some possible elements of an emotional/spiritual cleansing protocol.

 ### HEALTH TIP

IRRITABLE BOWEL SYNDROME

Irritable bowel syndrome (IBS) is the most common digestive disorder seen by physicians. Its symptoms may include constipation and/or diarrhea, or alternating constipation and diarrhea, pain in the abdomen, mucus in the stools, nausea, flatulence, bloating, and food intolerance. These symptoms can be very severe, to the point that the sufferer may dread eating. Malnutrition due to malabsorption is also common in people who suffer from IBS. Thankfully, much can be done nutritionally to set things right.

- First, identify and avoid your "allergic foods." The most common food triggers are wheat, corn, and especially dairy, so eliminate all dairy products and wheat. Perform the pulse test on every commonly consumed food and eliminate your trigger foods (Lesson I-10).

- Take psyllium fiber to help regulate bowel movements (Lesson II-8).

- Take a good probiotic (acidophilus) to improve the flora in the gut (Lesson III-13).

- Take several capsules per day (on an empty stomach) of a free-form amino acid supplement and include extra L-glutamine, which is used specifically to heal the intestinal tissue.

- Take N-acetylglucosamine (NAG), which is available at health food stores; this compound helps protect the intestinal lining from enzymes and other potentially damaging chemicals.

- Take herbs like burdock root, red clover, and milk thistle to support the liver and bloodstream.

- Licorice root is very healing to the intestinal tract.

Note: Do not use licorice root if your blood pressure is elevated.

- Alfalfa helps rebuild intestinal flora.

- *Aloe vera* gel or juice is healing to the digestive tract. *Note:* Don't take too much, as it can produce diarrhea and cramping of the intestinal muscles.

- Peppermint relieves gas in the intestines. Use the enteric-coated form so it is released directly into the intestines rather than the stomach.

- Avoid all stimulating foods like hot spices, caffeine, fried foods, junk foods, and processed foods. Avoid alcohol and tobacco.

- To relieve gas and bloating, use charcoal tablets, as many as five tablets per episode of distress. *Note:* Do not use charcoal daily, however, because it can absorb other nutrients.

- Chew food thoroughly, at least twenty times per mouthful.

- Eat while relaxed.

If your IBS continues, consult your healthcare practitioner, as this disorder is linked to higher incidence of colon cancer and diverticulitis. Vitamins and minerals are lost in diarrhea, and IBS increases malabsorption of nutrients, so you may need to increase your supplements.

ADDITIONAL NOTES

Lesson III-2. The Little Giant Who Fell Asleep

Dieting has become a way of life, and many of us have dieted frequently over the past few decades. It is frightening to realize how many people go on short-term, extreme low-calorie diets that limit the variety of foods they consume, causing chronic malnutrition. After temporarily losing weight, these dieters rapidly regain it as soon as they resume a fairly normal eating pattern, often putting on even more pounds than they lost. Their rapid weight gain is partly due to an accumulation of excess water, but it is also because previous low-calorie diets have made their bodies more efficient in the use of calories and have reduced the activity of their thyroid gland, which makes it even more difficult to lose weight. They go on another crash diet, which further reduces thyroid function . . . and the vicious cycle spirals downhill rapidly.

This is a prime reason that I say you must never go on a diet again—it will ruin your health and make it virtually impossible to keep the weight off! It is so important that I must say it again: *Don't diet! Dieting ruins your health!* Dieting causes hypothyroidism, which negatively impacts your entire body. Dieting creates chronic malnutrition that erodes your health.

? TODAY'S QUESTION

Is your thyroid interfering with your weight loss?

How many of the following symptoms apply to you?

☐ Weight gain

☐ Sensitivity to cold weather (demonstrated by cold hands and feet)

☐ Elevated cholesterol

☐ Elevated triglycerides

☐ Edema, or fluid retention (particularly in the face)

☐ Loss of libido, or sex drive

☐ Prolonged and heavy menstrual bleeding, with short menstrual cycle

☐ Dry, rough skin

☐ Hair loss or thin or coarse hair

☐ Thin, brittle nails with transverse (horizontal) grooves

☐ Depression

☐ Weakness

☐ Fatigue

☐ Loss of short-term memory

☐ Muscle weakness and joint stiffness

☐ Muscle and joint pain

☐ High blood pressure

☐ Shortness of breath

NOTES

❏ Constipation

❏ Goiter

❏ Abnormal apron of fat

❏ Lethargy

❏ Decreased sweating

❏ Thick tongue

❏ Intolerance to temperature changes

❏ Hoarse and/or slow speech

❏ Anxiety

Depending on what estimate you read, upwards of 5 percent to 35 percent of individuals may struggle with a thyroid problem that makes weight management—and overall health management—more difficult. Are you in that group? The list above shows the standard symptoms of hypothyroidism. If you have a number of them, you may have a thyroid problem; each of these symptoms, however, can signal problems in the body other than a thyroid issue. So read the rest of this lesson first, as it may provide valuable additional information, and then seek the counsel of your physician for an accurate diagnosis and treatment.

THE LITTLE GIANT OF THE ENDOCRINE SYSTEM

The "little giant" of this lesson is, of course, the thyroid gland, a "master organ" that functions under direct orders from the pituitary gland. Despite its diminutive physical size (it weighs less than 1 gram), the thyroid regulates virtually every metabolic process and wields an enormous influence over the entire body, including other organs in the endocrine system.

The endocrine system is the hormonal communication network of the body: the adrenal glands, thyroid gland, ovaries/testes, hypothalamus, pancreas, pineal gland, parathyroid gland, pituitary gland, and thymus. Each endocrine organ secretes hormones into the bloodstream. These hormones lock onto receptor sites on cells all over the body, where they stimulate and regulate numerous physiological functions. Some of the many actions of hormones include the following:

▪ Regulating the composition and volume of extracellular fluid (fluid outside cell membranes)

▪ Regulating metabolism and energy balance

▪ Regulating contraction of muscles

▪ Maintaining homeostasis (biological state of balance) during physical and emotional stress

▪ Regulating activities of the immune system

▪ Playing a role in growth and development

▪ Regulating reproduction

As you can see by this list, the endocrine system plays a fundamental role in weight and health management.

Tasks of the Little Giant

The thyroid is a small butterfly-shaped gland that nestles in front of the esophagus, below the Adam's apple and just above the breastbone. It has a tremendous effect on the body through the hormones it produces or oversees, controlling the rate at which the body utilizes oxygen, the rate and efficiency of various organ functions, and the speed with which the body utilizes food.

Thyroid hormones determine "how hot the fire burns in the cell" and the speed of activity within cells. They also regulate the metabolism of proteins, fats, carbohydrates, vitamins, and minerals, the secretion and breakdown rate of virtually all other hormones, and the response of their target tissue to those hormones. No tissue or organ system escapes the beneficial effects of adequate thyroid hormone levels, or the adverse effects of either excess or insufficient thyroid hormone levels.

The primary product of the thyroid gland is thyroxin or T4, which is synthesized from the amino acid tyrosine and the mineral iodine. The most bioactive thyroid hormone is T3, which is produced in the thyroid by enzyme conversion of the relatively inactive T4. The activity of the thyroid itself is regulated by thyroid-stimulating hormone (TSH) produced in the pituitary gland, which in turn is controlled by thyroid-releasing hormone (TRH) produced in the hypothalamus. This delicate control system is called a negative feedback loop. Other conditions that can trigger this loop to increase the secretion of thyroid hormone include cold temperatures, hypoglycemia (low blood sugar), high altitude, and pregnancy.

When metabolic activity is reduced because of low thyroid production or activity, the body retains excess amounts of water, salt, and protein. Cholesterol levels increase. Hypothyroidism also contributes to mental and emotional disorders, female (and presumably male) hormone imbalance, and disordered blood sugar regulation (diabetes or hypoglycemia).

The Thyroid Gland and Weight Management

Low thyroid function contributes to female hormone problems (the role of estrogen and progesterone in weight management is explored in Lesson III-3) and lowers the production of glucagon, which is the hormone that stimulates the burning of stored calories. Low energy levels also lead us to eat high-energy foods, like highly processed carbohydrates. By eating sugars and salts to feel more energetic, the body "self-medicates" against fatigue that isn't relieved by a good night's sleep.

However, the most fundamental reason for weight gain due to hypothyroidism is reduced metabolic rate. Because the thyroid controls the rate of metabolism (the rate at which calories are burned), low thyroid causes the body's calorie burning to slow down. The body becomes more and more efficient, burning fewer and fewer calories, and the slowed metabolism causes everything to decelerate by virtue of fatigue. The metabolic rate can be reduced by as much as 40 percent—a staggering figure! It means that although you may physically try to maintain your normal activity levels in the face of this chronic fatigue, you still burn fewer calories than you should be when you are active, and even when you are at rest.

Because thyroid hormone stimulates digestion, hypothyroidism impairs digestion and contributes to chronic constipation. It also leads to edema and bloating due to retained excess water, salt, and protein, causing the body to feel puffy and heavy. When hypothyroidism is treated successfully, immediate weight loss from water loss can follow. It is easy to see why maintaining the health of the thyroid is so important.

CAUSES OF HYPOTHYROIDISM

Many practitioners believe that we are seeing an epidemic of problems leading to both hypothyroidism and hyperthyroidism. Pregnancy can contribute to thyroiditis, an inflammation of the thyroid gland. Many other factors may contribute to these problems, including accumulation of toxic metals (especially mercury), diets deficient in fats or other essential nutrients, low-calorie diets, high-fat diets, excessive consumption of soy products or of plants from the *Brassica* genus (cabbage, Brussels sprouts, and the like), exposure to radiation, food and environmental allergies, environmental toxins (like polychlorinated biphenyls, or PCBs, and organophosphates), use of hormone replacement therapy (HRT), stress, and so on.

That is an extensive list, isn't it? It appears that most individuals are at risk of developing hypothy-roidism. Many of these contributing factors are out of our control (exposure to environmental toxins and toxic metals, for example); others we have created ourselves. It is scary to realize that dieting itself can cause hypothyroidism—making it more and more difficult to lose and maintain a healthful weight. Diets that are too low in calories or too low in fat directly contribute to lowered metabolism through lowered thyroid function.

DIAGNOSING HYPOTHYROIDISM

If you checked off more than a few of the symptoms in the list at the beginning of this lesson, you will want to read further.

Accurate diagnosis of thyroid problems is a three-pronged process, starting with recognizing the symptoms of hypothyroidism. An author writing in one peer-reviewed journal noted that the blood work typically used to diagnose hypothyroidism may be inadequate, and recommended that physicians also use clinical symptoms in their evaluation process (John L. Bakke, M.D., "Rethinking Thyroid Guidelines," *Cortlandt Forum* 1991, Vol. 79:46–20). Physicians generally use a blood test that measures the levels of T4, T3, TSH, or TRH to diagnose thyroid problems. Although this information is valuable in diagnosis, it is not, in itself, adequate. Many doctors now realize that blood tests may not present the whole picture in terms of thyroid function, and that they may not accurately diagnose what is termed "subclinical hypothyroidism."

The first prong in the diagnosis of hypothyroidism is the symptom profile. How many symptoms of hypothyroidism do you experience? The second prong is medical blood work to measure thyroid hormones in the bloodstream, a test that can only be done by your physician. The third prong is basal metabolic temperature. Dr. Broda Barnes pioneered the work on the correlation between basal temperature and thyroid function, and many doctors now use his work in their clinical practice.

Metabolic rate is reflected in body temperature. Normal body temperature is 98.6°F, which is very important to maintain, as enzymes function optimally at that temperature; when body temperature is lower than normal, enzyme activity is reduced. Low body temperature is a prime symptom of lowered metabolic function, and is a fairly significant problem. Remember that calories are a measurement of the amount of energy required to raise the temperature of a certain quantity of water; when you can't raise your body temperature, you simply aren't burning as many calories. Although it may seem to be a simple or trivial piece of information, a low body temperature is a very important signal that something is amiss—and it needs to be addressed, particularly in light of a continuing weight challenge.

Over the years, I have asked hundreds of people, most of whom struggle with weight issues, to check their own body temperature. The vast majority of these people, especially women, do not have a normal body temperature, with temperatures at least 2–3°F lower than normal. It is difficult for them to lose weight while their body temperature remains low.

Other conditions can affect body temperature, such as low progesterone levels (Lesson III-3) or loss of brown fat thermogenesis (Lesson III-5). We know, however, that low thyroid function often causes these problems with female hormones or brown fat activity, so dealing with the thyroid must be the first priority in getting all the other organs and hormones back to functioning properly.

In summary, remember the three-pronged approach, and make an appointment with your physician. Take

Time to Take Your Temperature

Following are instructions for the basal temperature test:

- Before retiring for the night, place a shaken-down thermometer beside the bed. Make sure you do not have an infection, and women should take their temperature when they are not ovulating; both conditions temporarily increase body temperature and will throw off the test results.

- In the morning, before you sit up, take your axillary (armpit) resting temperature. Place the thermometer in the base of the armpit, lower the arm against it, hold it there for five minutes, and then read the temperature. If the reading is below 97.6°F, you should discuss the test with your physician and possibly seek treatment for low thyroid function. If you find that your oral temperature is less than 98.6°F, you likewise need to seek the counsel of your physician.

- Body temperature, however, is normally a little lower in the late evening and early morning. You may get a clearer indication of your basal temperature by measuring it several times per day, at times when it should be the highest, or normal: for example, at 10:00 A.M., noon, 3:00 P.M., and 6:00 P.M.

a list of your possible deficiency symptoms, along with a chart of your body temperature for at least five days, so your physician can get a clear understanding of your concerns. He/she will then use this information, along with blood work, to make a diagnosis.

CARE AND FEEDING OF THE THYROID GLAND

Only your physician can treat hypothyroidism—but only *you* can feed your thyroid. The first step in nurturing a healthy thyroid is to feed it. Chronic dieting is associated with hypothyroidism; conversely, we can feed our thyroids to promote optimum thyroid health. Medications are sometimes necessary and helpful, but in the face of chronic malnutrition, your thyroid still won't work right. Follow these dietary tips for nourishing your thyroid gland:

- Make sure your diet is high enough in beneficial oils like olive oil, butter, and the fats naturally occurring in unprocessed, whole foods. Remember that low-fat diets can cause hypothyroidism. Include at least 1–3 tablespoons of natural oil in the diet each day.

- Make sure your carbohydrates and proteins are balanced appropriately (the Wings menus do this). Diets that are too high in either carbohydrates or proteins will slow down the thyroid gland. Balance is the key to good health.

- Drink plenty of water to keep your body hydrated. Remember that water is essential to enzyme function, including thyroid enzymes.

- Make sure to consistently eat the right number of calories for your metabolic rate (easier said than done!). You should eat slowly and stop just before you become full. You may wish to eat several small meals per day instead of three larger meals.

- Do I have to repeat that *all* foods that you eat should be energizing foods, that is, live foods? Eat lots of salads, lots of other vegetables, lots of olive oil and other healthful fats, good sources of protein, real fruit! These whole, live foods energize your flagging thyroid gland and help with weight loss.

- Make sure to eat some seafood each week to provide your body with iodine. Other sources of iodine include sea vegetables like kelp. *Caution:* Do not ingest large amounts of iodine, because excessive iodine can lower thyroid function just as too little iodine can. Be especially careful of thyroid-support supplements that contain large amounts of

Hyperthyroidism

Hyperthyroidism is also a problem: many people suffer from an overactive rather than an underactive thyroid gland. One of the predominant physical features of hyperthyroidism is a noticeable protrusion of the eyes. Other symptoms include increased heart rate, weight loss (in spite of increased appetite), diarrhea, feeling "wired," insomnia, excessive perspiration, weakness, sensitivity to heat, and excessive energy. As with hypothyroidism, treating hyperthyroidism is not a do-it-yourself project. See a physician if you suspect this disorder!

iodine, sea vegetables, or desiccated thyroid products: you may be overdoing it.

- You may wish to use herbs that nourish the thyroid gland: horsetail, oat straw, and alfalfa, among others.

- The amino acid tyrosine can be beneficial, especially when taken with a good multivitamin-mineral supplement. I recommend starting with 200 milligrams (mg) of tyrosine per day, taken in the morning on an empty stomach; then you may slowly increase to 500 mg, in divided doses. *Caution:* Be careful with tyrosine, as is so powerful that it could stimulate excessive production of thyroid hormone, kicking you into hyperthyroidism, a potentially life-threatening condition. Consult your doctor before you use tyrosine to make sure it is safe for you.

Thyroid Therapy with a Washcloth

This treatment, called water therapy or hydrotherapy, is sometimes used by naturopathic physicians. To help stimulate the production of body heat (which is an important part of the thyroid's job), dip a washcloth in ice-cold water, wring it out, and apply it to the front of your neck, leaving it there until the cloth warms up. Do this several times per day. Try alternating hot and cold compresses on this area to further increase thyroid gland function.

Along with targeted nutrition, moderate amounts of exercise are beneficial in stimulating metabolism. Make sure you participate regularly in a form of moderate exercise—preferably one you enjoy (Lessons II-

9 and II-10). Remember that too much exercise can increase stress hormone production, which can lower thyroid hormone function: don't overdo it!

And now, go to page 272 for your new recipes!

 ## TODAY'S ASSIGNMENT

THINK ABOUT YOUR THYROID

Review this lesson's material carefully. What lifestyle, medical, or environmental issues in your life are hindering the health of your thyroid gland, and how can you change them? Does your diet support a healthy thyroid? What dietary changes need to be made this week?

Take the basal temperature test for five days (several times per day) and record your temperature. Is it in the normal range?

If, based on your symptom profile and your body temperature, you believe you may have a thyroid condition, make an appointment with your physician. Take the information you have gathered (your symptom list and five-day body temperature record) with you to the appointment and request a diagnosis. If hypothyroidism is indeed your problem, your doctor will then counsel you on the best way to treat it.

Whether or not you have a thyroid condition, follow the recommendations in the lesson for providing good nutrition to your thyroid gland. Get plenty of rest and moderate amounts of exercise. Know that supporting your thyroid gland is critically important, and that when your thyroid functions well, it will aid you in your quest for a healthy body and a healthful weight.

LESSON III-2 STUDY GUIDE

1. List some of the functions of the thyroid gland.

_____

_____

_____

2. How does the thyroid gland contribute to a healthy (or an unhealthy) weight?

_____

_____

_____

3. How does dieting affect thyroid function?

4. What is the function of the endocrine system?

5. What is the three-pronged approach to diagnosing hypothyroidism?

6. List some of the dietary and lifestyle approaches to nourishing the thyroid.

7. What are some symptoms of hypothyroidism?

8. What are some symptoms of hyperthyroidism?

 HEALTH TIP

MOTION SICKNESS

Motion sickness can be totally debilitating to a traveler! Symptoms include cold sweats, dizziness, excessive salivation, yawning, fatigue, pallor, severe emotional and physical distress, sleepiness, weakness—and of course, nausea and vomiting. Natural remedies are excellent for motion sickness; prevention, however, is the key. Once motion sickness starts, it is difficult to bring it under control naturally.

If you are prone to motion sickness, start your preventive treatment before the motion begins:

- Ginger is an excellent preventive (and treatment) for nausea and upset stomach. Take two ginger capsules every three hours or more, drink ginger tea, or use ginger ale (the real stuff, not the usual artificial soft drink).

- Peppermint is soothing to the stomach. Drink peppermint tea, or take oil of peppermint with you and place drops on the tongue or rub them into the temples.

- Avoid spicy, greasy, fatty junk foods: they contribute to stomach upset.

- Avoid alcohol and odors and aromas that can trigger nausea. Avoid smoke and exhaust.

- Stay cool. Keep an ice pack handy and put it on your forehead or the back of your neck. Stand in the wind, if possible, letting the coolness blow directly in your face.

- Limit visual input. Close your eyes, if possible. Keep the mind relaxed. Breathe deeply.

- Homeopathic remedies are often helpful if these other suggestions do not work.

- Drugstores also carry an acupuncture gadget that is used to prevent motion sickness and can be quite helpful, especially when used in conjunction with ginger and the suggestions listed above.

Lesson III-3. Female, Fat, and Frustrated

Note to male readers: This lesson concerns female hormones and weight management. Although the information does not pertain to you personally, I encourage you to read it. Your understanding can help those wonderful women in your life who struggle with weight or other hormonal problems—and they'll love you for your "sensitive nature." Whether or not you read the entire lesson, don't forget to check out the Health Tip, as it is not for women only.

The title of this lesson really resonates with women. "That's me!" they exclaim. The vast majority of women struggle with hormone issues, starting in puberty and extending until well after the last menstrual cycle several decades later. The fact that hormones can cause weight challenges, however, is fairly new information for many of us. It is much easier for medical professionals, authors, and other weight-loss experts to "blame the victim" than to look deeply into the endocrine system.

The guilt that women feel about excess weight is enormous, so when someone says, "You really must stop eating so much _____ (insert the name of your favorite food here) to lose your weight," you believe it. You think, "I really am not perfect with my diet, so it must be my fault." Guilt-based messages are not fair. The reality is that putting on excess weight can be a consequence of hormonal imbalances—and in fact, that is exactly what is often seen in women. Not only can hormonal imbalances drive unhealthful eating behaviors, but they can also make the female body more prone to being overweight.

? TODAY'S QUESTION

Women, when did you gain your weight?

_____

_____

_____

_____

At puberty? Around childbirth? After taking birth control pills or hormone replacement therapy? When menopause hit? If your weight challenge began around a time of hormonal change (puberty, childbirth, and so on), and if your excess weight is centered in your buttocks and hips, it is likely more of a hormonal issue than a food issue. This is particularly true for weight that creeps on during the perimenopausal period of life, from age thirty-five and up.

Women tend to gain weight later in life for a number of reasons, as you will learn in this lesson. Discovering that your weight problem may be hormonal (not dietary) can free you from the guilt you have carried for so many years. I hope to relieve you of your guilt forever! I hope that you will be able to put your weight problem in perspective and understand that, really and truly, "My fat is not my fault!"

THE FEMALE CYCLE

The innate purpose of the menstrual cycle, of course, is reproduction. Two hormones govern the activities of the female reproductive system: estrogen and progesterone. These hormones are equally important but serve different functions. A normal cycle lasts about

✒ NOTES

_____

_____

_____

_____

_____

twenty- eight days, starting on the first day of menstruation itself, when bleeding begins. Estrogen is dominant during the first fourteen days of the menstrual cycle; when the cycle begins, estrogen levels begin to increase, peaking about day seven, and then waning until day fourteen. During the second fourteen days of the cycle, progesterone is dominant.

Estrogen is required for normal female maturation, and its physiological actions include the following:

- Stimulates the maturation of the vagina, uterus, and uterine tubes at puberty, as well as the development of secondary sex characteristics such as body shape and female image

- Stimulates normal growth and development of the structures within the breasts

- Responsible for the pubertal accelerated-growth phase and maturation of the long bones

- Alters the distribution of body fat to produce female body contours, such as around the hips and breasts

- Stimulates development of pigmentation in the skin, primarily in the nipples, areolae, and genital region

- Plays a role in the development of the endometrial lining of the uterus

- Helps regulate the normal menstrual cycle

- Helps maintain the normal structure of the skin and blood vessels in women

- Decreases the rate of bone resorption (that is, the leaching of minerals back into the bloodstream, or bone breakdown)

- Reduces the motility of the bowel

- Stimulates enzymes leading to uterine growth, and alters the production and activity of many other enzymes in the body

- Assists with normal hormone regulation by increasing the liver's ability to bind and transport female and thyroid hormones for excretion from the body

- Enhances the coagulability of blood (the blood's ability to form clots)

- Helps balance the ratio between HDL (high-density lipoprotein) and LDL (low-density lipoprotein) cholesterol

- Responsible for estrus (mating) behavior in animals, and influences libido in humans

- Pulls fluids into the extracellular space (the space between cell membranes), producing edema or bloating

- Causes retention of sodium and water by the kidneys (thereby causing fluid retention)

- Enhances the activity of LPL, an enzyme that actually increases fat deposition

It is clear from this long list that estrogen is very, very powerful. And did you notice that some of these functions directly affect weight management? But consider that a primary purpose of estrogen is to bring the female body to ovulation and possible pregnancy, which would be one reason that estrogen enhances sex drive, increases the deposition of fat tissue (fat is needed for energy if pregnancy occurs), increases the retention of water (more water is needed for pregnancy), and so on. So it isn't that estrogen has a negative effect on the female body; the hormone is simply doing what it was designed to do to preserve the species.

Fortunately, progesterone balances the effects of estrogen for the second half of the cycle. On day fourteen, when ovulation occurs, estrogen wanes and progesterone becomes dominant at about the midpoint of the luteal, or premenstrual, phase. The functions of progesterone include the following:

- Is a precursor of other sex hormones, including estrogen and testosterone

- Maintains the secretory endometrium (uterine lining)

- Is necessary for the survival of the embryo and fetus throughout gestation

- Protects against fibrocystic (lumpy) breasts

- Is a natural diuretic

- Helps use stored body fat for energy

- Functions as a natural antidepressant

- Helps thyroid-hormone action

- Normalizes blood clotting

- Restores sex drive

- Helps normalize blood sugar levels

- Normalizes zinc and copper levels

- Has a thermogenic (temperature-raising) effect

- Protects against endometrial (uterine) cancer

- Helps protect against breast cancer

- Builds bone and is protective against osteoporosis
- Is a precursor of cortisol synthesis in the adrenal glands

Notice how many of these benefits relate to weight management. It is important to maintain optimum levels of progesterone so we do not remain estrogen dominant throughout the entire cycle. Progesterone is a "pro-gestation" hormone: if fertilization of the ovum occurs at ovulation, high levels of progesterone are then needed to carry the pregnancy to term.

As you probably know, one of the typical effects of the menstrual cycle is a change in eating habits during the late luteal phase, or the days just preceding the onset of menses. We tend to crave highly energizing foods like chocolate, other sweets, and other carbohydrates. One possible explanation is that the body is anticipating pregnancy, and an increased appetite would help accumulate the extra calories needed to sustain a pregnancy. Notice that although the metabolic rate increases, this does not offset the additional calories; but that would also be expected, considering that the body would "want" to deposit extra calories in the form of fat tissue as an added energy source for the pregnancy. Most of the time, pregnancy does not occur, and so the extra water weight and fat weight normally disappear, leaving the body to resume its normal twenty-eight-day cycle.

Normal Isn't Normal Nowadays

Over the past few decades, many environmental, dietary, and social changes have thrown the menstrual cycle into chaos, and we seldom experience normal cycles anymore. You just learned in Lesson III-2, for example, how hypothyroidism skews the hormonal system, generally in the direction of estrogen dominance. Later in this curriculum, you will learn about the influence of thousands of environmental toxins that produce estrogenic effects in the body, and about how stress also influences hormone imbalance.

Many women use synthetic estrogens in birth control pills and hormone replacement therapy (HRT). When oral contraceptives or HRT render ovulation impossible, a structure called the corpus luteum cannot produce the progesterone that it should. These and other influences tend to create relative estrogen dominance throughout the cycle, as progesterone is not present to confer a balancing hormonal effect. If you refer to the list of estrogen's effects, it is easy to see why this hormone imbalance produces weight gain, whether through retained water (edema), added fat deposition, or other mechanisms. Excess estrogen (either natural or supplemental) greatly increases production of the adrenal hormone cortisol, which is directly linked to increased weight deposition. (You will learn about cortisol and weight in Lesson III-4.)

The Luteal Phase and Premenstrual Syndrome (PMS)

Many women gain weight during the premenstrual days. The body's metabolic rate actually increases during the luteal phase by up to 9 percent, increasing the amount of energy utilized by the body; most women, however, tend to crave sugar and chocolate around this time of the month, so the increase in metabolic rate is offset by the increased calories consumed.

Women with PMS significantly increase their caloric intake during the late luteal phase, generally with high-carb junk foods. Eating a carbohydrate-rich, protein-poor meal in the late luteal phase decreases premenstrual depression, tension, anger, confusion, sadness, and fatigue, while simultaneously increasing alertness and calmness scores.

The body tends to hang on to water just before menses, partially because the body is preparing for a potential pregnancy, when added water stores are required.

Female hormone elevations pull down the thyroid gland, which can cause symptoms typical of hypothyroidism, particularly for women using oral contraceptives.

Female hormones increase the appetite during the luteal phase (again, perhaps to help prepare the body for potential pregnancy), decreasing it again after the period has subsided (when pregnancy is no longer currently possible and there is no immediate need for added food stores).

According to one small study, the number of calories consumed did not increase in women with PMS, but the types of foods eaten premenstrually changed. The balance of calories among proteins, carbohydrates, and fats remained about the same, but the women with PMS ate more dairy products, more refined sugar, and more refined carbohydrates than women who did not suffer from PMS. The women with PMS also consumed twice as much sodium as the control group did, and their daily intake of B-complex vitamins (such as thiamine, riboflavin, niacin, pantothenic acid, and pyridoxine) was less. The excess sodium would, of course, cause added fluid retention, which is common in women just prior to

Yes, Women Are Very Different from Men

In centuries past, a rounder, fuller woman was a desirable marriage partner because her apparent "health" made her a likelier candidate to carry a man's child to term and give birth to robust offspring. Estrogen tends to shape the softer, curvier figure that we associate with femininity; men tend to be more angular.

Testosterone is highly beneficial in the weight-management process because it causes the body to lay down more muscle tissue, increases metabolism and body heat, and so on. (Men are lucky, aren't they?) Hormones, in fact, are responsible for numerous and often subtle differences between men and women when it comes to physiology and weight management. These differences include:

- Men carry their excess weight in their upper bodies, or all over their bodies, or in the stomach region (potbelly or beer belly).

- Women tend to carry their excess weight between the waist and the knees (primarily in the hips, thighs, and buttocks); they also carry more weight in the breasts. Part of this weight distribution is an effect of estrogen. Weight below the waist is difficult to lose; weight above the waist is easier to lose, probably because hormones do not so easily influence it.

- Women's bodies tend to accumulate less lean muscle mass and more extracellular fluids than men's do.

- Women accumulate more body fat, making it more difficult to burn calories at rest because their bodies contain, pound for pound, more metabolically inert fat tissue.

- If a man and a woman, both with normal hormone levels, engage in an identical exercise program, the man will typically lay down more lean muscle tissue and lose more body fat than the woman because of the influence of testosterone.

- When women exercise, they burn fat less efficiently than men, and they burn less fat around the abdominal region than men do.

- As men lose weight, their metabolic rate increases, making it easier to lose more weight and keep it off.

- Excessive weight loss actually decreases a woman's metabolic rate, possibly the body's way of conserving energy in order to produce children.

Who said that life is fair?

the onset of their periods. Remember that estrogen itself causes the body to sequester sodium, in turn adding water weight.

Chocolate cravings are so common in women that we think of them as part of the normal female psychology, but these cravings are physiological in nature, possibly driven by nutrient deficiencies. Chocolate cravings can fluctuate with hormonal changes just before and after menses. Women with PMS are often deficient in magnesium, a calming mineral, and a magnesium deficiency often drives the need to consume chocolate or other forms of sugar.

One study notes that chocolate cravings might occur due to such dietary deficiencies or to balance low levels of neurotransmitters, such as serotonin or dopamine, which are involved in the regulation of mood, food intake, and compulsive behavior. In other words, eating chocolate and other sweets may be an attempt to self-medicate against depression or other emotional upsets. The researchers point out that chocolate affects physiology as any other addictive substance does.

Women experiencing PMS tend to eat more junk food to compensate for a bad mood. In fact, in one study, the consumption of chocolate, alcoholic beverages, fruit juice, and caffeine-free cola was prevalent among women with the most severe symptoms. The more coffee you drink, the more severe your PMS symptoms tend to be.

It all sounds dauntingly complex, doesn't it? To make it simpler, remember that female hormones cause physiological changes that drive the psychology of the woman—not the other way around. These hormonal stimuli are very real and very powerful.

Symptoms of Menopause, Progesterone Deficiency, and PMS

Symptoms of menopause may begin to show at a very young age in some women (from thirty years old upward), and may include the following:

- Hot flashes
- High cholesterol
- Mood changes
- High blood pressure
- Sleep disturbances
- Coronary heart disease
- Heart palpitations
- Osteoporosis

- Dizziness

- Skin dryness

- Nausea

- Memory loss

- Abnormal hair growth (for example, on the chin and upper lip)

- Vaginal dryness

- Abnormal uterine bleeding

- Urinary tract infections

- Fatigue

- Decreased sex drive

- Stress to the adrenal glands, resulting in a reduced ability to handle stress

- Change in body shape (more weight to the lower body, with thinning in the upper body)

- Migraine headaches

- Weight gain

- Aches and pains

- Abnormal sensations in hands and feet

- Decrease in glucose tolerance or more difficulty balancing blood sugar

Symptoms of progesterone deficiency or PMS include the following:

- Fatigue

- Depression

- Weight gain

- Water retention

- Headaches

- Loss of sex drive

- Mood swings

- Inability to handle stress

- Irritability

- Fibrocystic breasts

- Uterine fibroids

- Endometriosis

- Low metabolism

- Symptoms of hypothyroidism with normal T3 and T4 levels

- Unstable blood sugar level

- Cravings for caffeine, sweets, and carbohydrates

- Morning sluggishness

CARE AND FEEDING OF THE FEMALE HORMONAL SYSTEM

With a greater understanding of some of the problems inherent to female physiology, we are better able to address our particular situations. We may not be able to totally bring the body back into perfect hormonal balance, but there is much we can do to normalize the menstrual cycle and/or help us get through menopause without so many uncomfortable symptoms. We can certainly alter our way of eating.

NORMALIZING YOUR CYCLE

Before we deal with the hormonal food issues, here are some natural ways to help normalize the female cycle:

- Adopt a high-fiber diet, including up to 35 grams or more of fiber per day (Lesson II-8). It is unlikely that this amount of fiber will be provided by the average diet, so you will wish to use a good-quality fiber supplement, available from your Wings nutritionist (at www.flywithwings.com/pnc.html, click on MyProConnect) or at your local health food store.

- Increase your consumption of all types of plant foods except grains, as the Wings Program encourages. Fruits and vegetables are high in fiber and other nutrients that are beneficial to hormone balance, but grains are highly addictive for many women. Bread and pasta, which are common comfort foods (especially during PMS periods), rapidly stack on unwanted weight.

- Keep the consumption of red meat, or other animal proteins that contain synthetic hormones or growth hormones, as low as possible. Always choose organic meat and eggs when available.

- Remember that the Wings Program discourages the consumption of dairy products, which can aggravate hormonal problems.

- Keep the fats natural! Enjoy olive oil, butter, and foods that contain beneficial fats. Eliminate all processed fats; processed fats increase PMS symptoms.

- Avoid caffeine and sugar, which aggravates PMS symptoms.

- Drink plenty of water to help flush used estrogens out of your body.

- Avoid environmental sources of xenoestrogens as much as possible. For example, avoid drinking water from plastic bottles that may have been sitting in hot temperatures for extended periods of time (Lesson III-11).

- Avoid foods high in salt, particularly processed foods. Remember that estrogen dominance causes salt and water retention.

- Do an internal body cleansing at least twice per year to help rid the body of xenoestrogens and other chemicals that can mimic estrogenic action. (I highly recommend the Wings protocols in Lessons II-6 and II-7 for a complete internal cleanse and healing.)

- Make sure your diet is very high in B-complex vitamins, zinc, and magnesium. Remember that oral contraceptives cause deficiencies of these nutrients and that nutrient deficiencies can underlie symptoms of PMS or menopause. Vitamin B_6 is particularly noted for relieving many PMS symptoms, including emotional symptoms and water retention. Vitamin E is also helpful in relieving many hormonal symptoms.

- Herbs like chaste tree are helpful for PMS symptoms. The herb blue cohosh is often used for menopausal symptoms. You may be interested in the VRP HerBalance II product described at www.vrp.com. Please consult a physician who uses herbal and other natural remedies in his/her medical practice; balancing female hormones is not a do-it-yourself project.

- If your physician recommends that you use supplementary hormones, ask him/her to prescribe them through a compounding pharmacist who can custom formulate your hormones from natural forms of estrogen and progesterone. Many physicians use the following method for testing hormone levels: because estrogen is naturally dominant on the seventh day of the cycle and progesterone is naturally dominant on the twenty-first day, blood draws for those hormones are taken on those days for more accurate results. These results can then be compared to normal values, and your prescription formulated accordingly.

Keep in mind that if you are struggling with hypothyroidism, it will be difficult to achieve hormone balance until your thyroid function is optimal. Start by fixing the thyroid (Lesson III-2), and often the female hormones fall right into line. All of the endocrine organs communicate with one another: the adrenal gland influences hormones and thyroid function; the pancreas gets involved as well, as do some of the endocrine organs higher in the system, as you will learn in a subsequent lesson. Lesson III-4 will show how stress influences the endocrine system, and this information may need to be factored into the equation as well. Yes, it is complicated—but you can accomplish a great deal just by feeding the body properly. Then take one step at a time to bring your body back into beautiful balance!

Eating for Your Cycle

Now that you know you tend to eat more calories the week prior to your period, and that the extra calories are likely to be junk-food calories, you can be on the lookout for these types of eating behaviors and "head them off at the pass."

Because your body tends to utilize more magnesium during the week prior to the onset of your period, use supplemental magnesium throughout the month to increase your overall magnesium stores. Magnesium-deficiency symptoms are, ironically, nearly identical to typical PMS or menopause symptoms (compare the lists on pages 20 and 130–131).

Make sure that your blood sugar remains stable throughout the day. Most women find that, if they have a high-carbohydrate meal at some point in the day (particularly for breakfast), they will then snack and graze on processed carbohydrates throughout the day. But if they eat a well-balanced breakfast that contains adequate amounts of protein and no grains, they tend to remain satisfied throughout the day, and grazing on junk foods is greatly diminished. Use the Wings Breakfast Drink for the first meal of the day to stabilize your blood sugar and satisfy your appetite for several hours.

You can't solve the premenstrual eating pattern in just the week prior to your period. You really have to address these issues all month long. Get in the habit of eating well-balanced meals and it will be easier to stick to your program at premenstrual time.

After you have taken all these steps and have followed this program for at least three months, if you find that you are still eating junky calories during "that time of the month," go back and revisit the information in this section. Seek the counsel of a nutritionally trained physician for more help in balancing your hormones. And check your stress levels! You will find that stress plays a key role in female (and male) hormone balance. You may need to deal with this important part of life before you achieve real balance.

While you address these complicated issues, stay confident in your progress. You are taking yet another pivotal step in achieving real hormonal and dietary balance and long-lasting weight management.

And now, go to page 272 for your new recipes!

 ## TODAY'S ASSIGNMENT

LADIES, ADDRESS YOUR HORMONAL ISSUES

If you gained weight after beginning to take oral contraceptives, review your birth-control options. If you choose to continue using oral contraceptives, make sure your diet supplies adequate B-complex vitamins, zinc, and magnesium.

If you are currently using HRT or have used it in the past and your weight gain followed, work with your holistic physician or naturopathic physician to normalize your hormone levels. Consider herbal alternatives, if possible, and also consider using progesterone cream to restore the normal estrogen-to-progesterone ratio. Check the health of your thyroid gland, too, because HRT can contribute to hypothyroidism.

Make sure your diet is adequate in all the nutrients, and at meals, balance your food among protein, carbohydrates, and fats to optimize blood sugar (following the Wings eating plan does this for you). Be aware, in particular, that blood sugar problems can accompany the use of synthetic estrogens. Get plenty of rest, as rest is critically important for the thyroid and the female hormone system.

And finally, give yourself grace this week. This lesson's information may not be a surprise—but it may not be good news either. Perhaps you used synthetic estrogen to improve your health and then gained weight on it, and that is frustrating. Keep in mind, however, that although your weight challenges may be more difficult because of a female hormone issue, they are not impossible to overcome. Work hard to balance your hormones naturally and to enhance your overall health. Engage in moderate, enjoyable forms of exercise to stimulate your metabolism. Keep working at it, girl!

LESSON III-3 STUDY GUIDE

1. Explain the normal menstrual cycle and how it affects short-term weight management.

2. What factors tend to throw off the normal estrogen-progesterone balance?

3. What dietary habits or cravings are influenced by the female cycle?

4. What are some physiological differences between men and women (beyond the obvious)?

5. What are some dietary strategies to help reduce cyclical weight gain and deal with PMS?

HEALTH TIP

NAILS AND HAIR

According to Dr. James Balch and Phyllis Balch, authors of *Prescription for Nutritional Healing* (New York, NY: Avery Publishing Group, 1997), specific nutritional deficiencies can produce changes in the nails as follows:

- Lack of protein, folic acid, and vitamin C can cause hangnails.

- White bands across the nails may indicate protein deficiency.

- Lack of vitamin A and calcium causes dryness and brittleness.

- Deficiency of B-complex vitamins causes fragility, with horizontal and vertical ridges.

- Deficiency of vitamin B_{12} leads to dry, very rounded and curved nail ends, and darkened nails.

- Iron deficiency results in spoon nails (nails with a concave shape) and/or vertical ridges.

- Zinc deficiency may cause white spots on the nails.

- Lack of friendly bacteria in the intestines can result in fungus under and around the nails.

- Lack of HCl contributes to splitting nails.

You want gorgeous, strong fingernails and hair? Start with good nutrition:

- Provide all forty-plus micronutrients and enhance your nutrition by using digestive enzymes.

- If you do not secrete enough hydrochloric acid to assist in protein digestion, use supplemental HCl to improve protein digestion and mineral absorption (see the Health Tip on page 96).

- Supplement the diet with herbs like alfalfa, burdock root, dandelion, and yellow dock to provide minerals and vitamins for the nails.

- Use good oils like olive oil and flaxseed oil to nourish the nails and hair.

- Fresh carrot juice is good for the nails.

- For a nice nail treatment, mix equal parts of honey, avocado oil, and egg yolk, and add a pinch of salt. Rub the mixture into the nails and cuticles; leave on for half an hour, and then rinse off. Repeat this treatment daily. You should see results in about two weeks.

- Soak nails in warm olive oil or cider vinegar for ten to twenty minutes daily.

- Don't use your nails as a tool.

✐ ADDITIONAL NOTES

Lesson III-4. Stress Will Make You Overweight

Today's lesson is for both men and women. We have heard about the negative effects of stress for many years, but it is not commonly known that stress can, indeed, make us fat. Let's look at the physiological effects of stress, and how it contributes to overweight.

? **TODAY'S QUESTION**

How stressed are you?

_____

_____

_____

Put a check beside each stress event that you have experienced over the past year, and then add up the points to determine your score.

❏ Death of spouse	100
❏ Divorce	73
❏ Marital separation	65
❏ Jail term	63
❏ Death of close family member	63
❏ Personal injury or illness	53
❏ Marriage	50

❏ Fired from work	47
❏ Marital reconciliation	45
❏ Retirement	45
❏ Change in health of family member	44
❏ Pregnancy	40
❏ Sex difficulties	39
❏ Gained new family member	39
❏ Business readjustment	39
❏ Change of financial state	39
❏ Death of close friend	37
❏ Change to different line of work	36
❏ Change in number of arguments with spouse	35
❏ Mortgage over $120,000	31
❏ Change in responsibilities at work	29
❏ Son or daughter leaving home	29
❏ Trouble with in-laws	29
❏ Outstanding personal achievement	28
❏ Beginning or ending school	26
❏ Change in living conditions	25
❏ Revision of personal habits	24
❏ Trouble with boss	23
❏ Change in working hours or conditions	20
❏ Change in residence	20
❏ Change in schools	20
❏ Change in recreation	19
❏ Change in church activities	19

✎ **NOTES**

_____

_____

_____

_____

_____

❑ Change in social activities 18

❑ Change in sleeping habits 16

❑ Change in number of family get-togethers 15

❑ Change in eating habits 15

❑ Vacation 13

❑ Christmas 12

❑ Minor violation of the law 11

Total points _____

If you scored over 200, it is likely that stress is negatively impacting your health and your ability to lose weight.

STRESS: FRIEND OR FOE

Stress can be either harmful or beneficial. It can kill us, or it can revitalize us.

Harmful stressors are pressures that we cannot control or resolve: a physically or emotionally toxic work environment, work that we dislike or find meaningless, illness, death and other losses, marital problems, financial difficulties, and so on. Beneficial stressors, by contrast, are issues of life over which we can exercise control or authority. Beneficial stressors may include sixteen-hour workdays in a profession we enjoy, raising our children, engaging in hobbies, travel, social events . . . In other words, we may be stressed by being busy, but if we enjoy the activity, the stress energizes us. It keeps us excited and motivated. It doesn't harm us—and it doesn't stack on unwanted weight.

The Stress Response

The physiological stress response is a life-protective reaction to a threat to personal safety. Our ancestors' lives were threatened by wild animals, food shortages, and sudden illness. Such stress-inducing events, thankfully, did not generally last very long. Stress is meant to be a temporary event.

The body reacts to sudden emergencies by secreting adrenal hormones. When a mother bear chases us up a tree, our adrenal glands secrete hormones like adrenaline and cortisol, causing an elevated heart rate, elevated blood pressure, and other intense reactions. The purpose of the hormone rush is to equip our bodies to run fast or fight to save our lives. Digestive activity is put on hold for the stress response; who needs to digest a meal when we may die at any moment? The work of our immune and reproductive systems is similarly disabled because this work is not a priority during a stressful incident. After the emergency is over, adrenaline levels fall, as do heart rate and blood pressure. The body rapidly returns to homeostasis. No harm has been done. That is a normal stress event—and a normal stress response.

Our modern, twenty-first-century stress is not like that. Rather than being the same type of short-lived, intense stress that our ancestors faced, our stress is typically milder—but chronic. In other words, we may not often feel that our lives are in jeopardy, but we are very often uncomfortable. We seldom face intense, life-threatening emergencies, but we are seldom at peace. Our less-intense stress goes on day after day. It is relentless.

The body reacts to this chronic pressure with a lower, constant stress response. We do not necessarily feel an adrenaline rush (although some people seek out that type of "high"), but our bodies do physiologically react to long-term stress with a less-intense but real adrenaline "push." As adrenaline and cortisol are released daily in small, measured amounts, heart rate increases, blood pressure elevates, and digestive, immune, and reproductive systems are less efficient. Our bodies can actually handle short-term, intense stressors much more efficiently than long-term stres-

---

Stress Is Different from Work

Who doesn't feel that life is just a little (or a lot) out of control? I recently contemplated my overfull life and complained, "Shouldn't life be a little easier? Should I be working this hard?" Then I thought, "My life is full of work—blessed work! My life is full of family—blessed family! A full, busy life is a blessing!" Let's make the most of our time here on Earth, ministering to bless the people around us. Work is good. Enjoy life by working hard!

We can work hard without suffering the consequences of negative stress. Stress can energize us when it is kept within reasonable boundaries, or when the stressors are pleasant. I, for example, enjoy work very much, and even though my life is often overbusy, nothing excites or energizes me more than taking on a big project. I love the challenge of the task. If I do not have meaningful work to do (in other words, if life is too calm), I feel a "negative stress" that causes me severe depression and anxiety.

So hard work, in itself, is not necessarily negative, and may not be stressful. Perhaps we should not dream of retirement in the belief that indolence is good—the thought of retiring to do nothing but relax is terribly stressful to me!

sors. Chronic, lasting stress is deadly in many ways that we have not considered before.

Stages of Stress

Here is a more complete picture of how the stress response affects the body and the psyche over time.

1. The initial, acute reaction to stress is called the stage of alarm. We see imminent danger: Our boss has just yelled at us! Our spouse did it again! Our bank account is overdrawn! Traffic is stalled and we will be late! The body's defense systems go on full alert. We feel intense symptoms including sensations of anxiety and heightened mental awareness. Our hearts pound. We breathe faster. Our minds race to determine the best course of action. We are intensely focused. We perspire heavily. Our stomachs are upset and we feel nauseated.

   Unfortunately, when one stress-generating event clears, another appears, and so the stress does not abate. We know we have to deal with the stress, but our lives are not in danger. Now the body begins to actually adapt to the stress, and resistance sets in.

2. People in the resistance stage often deny that they are even under stress because they are used to living this way. On the surface, they seem to have adjusted to the continued tension; nonetheless, the body responds to the continuing stress, at a deeper level. Stress hormones are still being released in small amounts, depressing the immune system, decreasing bone strength, compromising brain functions such as memory, and decreasing energy. Headaches, insomnia, irritability, and stiff muscles are all signs that the body is responding in this way.

   Several years ago, I was under an enormous amount of emotional stress and physical exhaustion. I was working more than sixteen hours a day, juggling several jobs at once. At first, I felt exhilarated, and thought, "Who says that stress is harmful? This feels energizing! I can handle this!" I actually thought I could go on forever that way. But within a few weeks, exhaustion set in and I began to experience the severely negative effects of relentless, extreme stress. I soon realized that if I didn't make big changes in my lifestyle, I would collapse, because the next stage of the stress response had begun to unfold. When the resistance stage is exhausted, *we* are exhausted.

3. The final stage of the stress response is exhaustion or burnout. The symptoms of exhaustion are similar to those of the alarm stage, but the repercus-

sions are much more severe because the body's strength has been depleted by weeks, months, or perhaps years of excessive wear and tear. Some people, stimulated by the intensity of the stress and dependent on reserves of hereditary strength, can sustain resistance for a very long time. However, most people without relief from stress eventually break down, even to the point of nervous breakdown. Individuals who reach the stage of exhaustion may age prematurely and risk developing life-threatening diseases such as cancer, heart disease, and diabetes. (See *Stress and Natural Healing* by Christopher Hobbs [Loveland, CO: Interweave Press, Inc., 1997].)

How Stress Affects Weight

Stress causes all of the effects discussed above, but it also causes weight gain—and isn't that a stressful piece of news! How does stress affect weight? First, stress can increase body fat by promoting unhealthful eating behaviors (primarily, cravings for carbohydrates, salt, fat, crunchy foods, and caffeine). Second, stress can derail the body's hormonal regulation and metabolism.

Under stressful circumstances, we tend to eat for comfort or to increase energy production. Stress is extremely exhausting, and we find that we are constantly tired (fatigue, by the way, is one of the leading causes of visits to the doctor's office). Because we have a schedule to keep up and cannot indulge our need for rest, we use stimulating foods to regain our energy. We drink coffee, soft drinks, and other caffeinated beverages; we eat pasta and sweets; we self-medicate with sugar. Salt is highly energizing, so we crave salty foods like potato chips or corn chips. Eating crunchy foods can also seem calming at times: might this represent a psychological way of crushing our enemies between our teeth?

Weight gain as a consequence of stress, however, is not just a matter of food choice and consumption. The body itself responds to stress by dysregulating important weight-management systems. When first confronted with an intense stress, we often lose weight: we often feel that we cannot eat (remember how stress hormones affect the digestive system?), so caloric intake is reduced. Research shows, however, that after the initial weight-loss period of several days or even weeks, the body then begins to gain weight rapidly. Once the stage of resistance sets in, eating becomes a way of compensating for lost energy or nutrient stores. Although we couldn't eat when the

What Happens Internally When You Are Under Stress?

Although it may feel more emotional or mental, the body's stress response is a physiological event. The adrenal glands (part of the endocrine system, a messenger system of the body) are our primary stress organs. They release epinephrine and norepinephrine, the hormonal messengers necessary to "ramp up" the body for action. These hormones intensify and prolong the following effects of the sympathetic nervous system on respiration, circulation, metabolism, and other systems:

- Breathing is more rapid and shallow

- Bronchioles dilate for faster air movement in and out of the lungs

- Heart rate, force of cardiac contraction, and blood pressure increase

- Blood vessels of organs involved in fleeing or fighting off danger dilate to allow faster blood flow (in the skeletal muscles, cardiac muscle, liver, and adipose tissue, for example)

- Blood vessels of organs that are nonessential to the fight-or-flight response (such as the skin and certain internal organs) constrict

- The liver converts sugar stored as glycogen into glucose for immediate energy

- Blood sugar levels increase

- Brown adipose tissue splits triglycerides into fatty acids to generate ATP for cellular energy

- "Nonessential" functions (such as digestion and reproduction) are slowed or stopped

stress first hit, now we *must* eat. We are exhausted, so we eat sugary and salty foods. These eating behaviors are all part of the stress response; they are the body's way of trying to adapt to an intense stress, and to increase body energy.

I experienced this phenomenon during a severe family crisis. At first, I found that I could not eat. The thought of food was revolting, my stomach was upset, and I wasn't hungry. But several weeks into the emergency, I was drawn to sugary foods, and I started drinking coffee. The sweets and caffeine were my body's defense against severe fatigue: my body craved sugar (in this case, cherry pie) and coffee because I

had to boost my energy enough to function. Understanding what was happening, I gave myself a little grace to get through the stressful time. I lost weight at the beginning of the crisis, but within two months, I had gained an additional 10 pounds in my waist and abdomen—a common type of weight distribution in stress-related overweight.

Extra eating, or eating sugary foods, may serve as a *temporary* fix to the problem of acute, severe stress, but it should never be used as a long-term solution to chronic stress. Again, however, disordered eating is not the only reason for stress-related weight gain. Stress wields its own fat-depositing effects. Note these functions of stress hormones:

- Dysregulates the thyroid hormones

- Dysregulates the sex hormones

- Increases the deposition of fat in the upper body (face, neck, trunk, and abdomen)

- Increases the breakdown of lean muscle tissue

- Dysregulates blood sugar

Here is an alarming piece of news: your morning cup of coffee may be making you gain weight or making it more difficult for you to lose weight. Coffee is the number-one psychoactive addictive drug in the world. Because we are tired from the stress in our lives, we drink enormous amounts of coffee as a way of increasing physical and mental energy—but long-term coffee consumption has the same effect as stress itself: it increases the production and release of adrenaline. By drinking coffee, we actually increase the physiological stress response.

Remember that the organs of the endocrine system communicate with one another, and that when we struggle through long-term stress, our sex hormones are affected (reproduction is not a priority in the face of life-endangering events). Stress has the ability to dysregulate the female hormonal milieu; you learned in Lesson III-3 how female hormone imbalances affect weight management. It is similarly difficult to control our blood sugar when we are stressed. (You will learn in Lesson III-10 how blood sugar affects weight management.)

Stress has an impact on the thyroid gland; on the other hand, when thyroid function is low, the body can use stress hormones to increase energy, leading to a long-term stress (adrenaline) response.

As already noted, one of the effects of long-term stress is an increased breakdown of lean muscle mass and an increased accumulation of fat tissue, primarily in the waist (the "spare tire") and abdomen. The long-term effect of decreased lean body mass and increased fat mass is lowered metabolism, thereby decreasing the number of calories burned in normal activities. Lowered metabolism means difficulty in losing weight!

It is clear from this information that if we want to lose weight and keep it off, we must learn to manage our lives better to reduce the amount of stress we experience.

PRACTICAL SOLUTIONS FOR YOUR STRESS PROBLEM

Solving the problem of stress is not easy. We all need to take a serious look at our lives. What are our primary sources of stress? Today's assignment will ask you to take a serious inventory of your life, and then write a plan for reducing your negative stress. Some things we cannot change; other things we can. We can learn different strategies for dealing with stress points. We may even need professional help, but remember: We always have choices! We always have options! We are not victims of our lives. We can learn to take charge.

Here are some suggestions for reducing your body's physiological reaction to stress:

- Teach your body to calm down by practicing good stress-reduction techniques. What activities (other than eating) will calm you and give you pleasure? Do you enjoy walking? Biking? Sewing? Reading? Drinking tea? Visiting friends? Massage? Swimming? Bathing? Whatever gives you a calm feeling of pleasure, indulge in it. Indulging such feelings is not self-indulgent or narcissistic: rather, it is an important part of your healthcare program. Give yourself some happiness today!

- Take charge of your life. This is not easily done, but it is so important. Stress is negative when we lose our sense of control. Do you need to make significant life changes? Construct a plan for making necessary changes. If you need help regaining control over your life, consult a pastor, life coach, or counselor.

At the risk of offending my male audience, let me make this generalization: men are more reluctant to seek professional help, especially for emotional or psychological needs. Perhaps they feel they should be able to solve their own problems, or they are too embarrassed to ask for help. Whatever the reason, reluctance to receive counsel may harm your health. Everyone needs help at times; it is not shameful to seek it.

Marital difficulties are extremely stressful. Women often postpone getting help in dealing with a difficult spouse because of embarrassment or, sadly, because they do not feel safe doing so. Both men and women can live in a toxic home environment for so long that they eventually lose sight of what a normal, healthy marriage looks like. If you are in a difficult home situation, do not feel ashamed. Do not feel that you have lost your chance to take control of your life. Do not feel that you have no options, or that there are no solutions to your problem. Seek professional help from someone who will be able to provide you with options and then support you as you make lifestyle changes.

Whatever your difficult life situation is, it is not hopeless. Get help and take charge!

- Perhaps you eat to deal with your stress. What types of foods do you crave during stressful periods? Salty, sweet, fatty, crunchy? Devise a strategy for changing these habits: don't simply grit your teeth and say, "I won't eat it! I won't eat it!" because eventually you will lose the battle and you will eat it. Use other activities or strategies to comfort yourself during stressful times.

The important thing is to make a plan now, while your life is (relatively speaking) under control: don't wait until a stressful period hits. What will give you pleasure (in the place of a chocolate-chip cookie)? Gardening? Painting? Napping? Playing with your children? Remember that doing what you enjoy is an important part of self-care!

- Use herbs to calm the body's stress response. Holy basil (not to be confused with the culinary varieties of basil) actually reduces the production of cortisol, and is soothing and healing to the adrenal gland. The herb rhodiola reduces the physiological stress response and also increases the production of the mood-calming hormone serotonin. Purchase these herbs from your local health food store.

- Nourish your adrenal glands. The following nutrients are helpful in compensating for the extra "nutrient burn" of stress, and will also help relieve stress-related eating patterns:

  • Vitamin C: 5,000+ milligrams (mg) per day

- Pantothenic acid: up to 1,000 mg per day

- Magnesium: 300+ mg per day

- Potassium: 99 mg per day (or more; check with a physician)

- B-complex vitamins: a high-potency supplement that provides 100 mg of each of the main B-complex vitamins

- Zinc: up to 50 mg per day

▪ Eat regular, small, well-balanced meals that keep your blood sugar steady. Remember that cortisol unbalances blood sugar. Stress burns more calories and protein, but hastens the deposition of fat tissue and the breakdown of lean muscle mass. Make sure you eat the right amount of protein for your body and your stress level. Add lots of fresh vegetables and fruits that nourish the body. Do not shortcut nutrition because of time constraints or because you "don't feel like it." Eat slowly and relax. Stop eating just before you feel satisfied, not full. In other words, follow the Wings Program! Now is the time to maximize your nutrition, not compromise because it seems too difficult.

▪ Sip a cup of chamomile or peppermint tea before meals to calm your stomach. Drink a cup of ginger tea before each meal to prepare your body to receive food. Consider using natural digestive aids (Eclectic Institute's Neutralizing Cordial, for example) to correct stress-impaired digestion.

▪ Moderate amounts of exercise are helpful, but make sure that you do not stimulate a cortisol response by plunging into an excessive exercise regimen. Engage in exercise activities that calm the mind and give you pleasure (Lessons II-9 and II-10).

▪ Get plenty of sleep each night! Make rest a real priority. This is important enough to repeat: get plenty of sleep each night. Begin sleeping prior to 10:00 P.M., and make sure the room is dark so you sleep deeply.

The important thing is to take care of yourself. Indulge in a little pampering. Believe it or not, pampering is healthful—do it often.

WILL YOU LOSE YOUR STRESS FAT?

"Stress fat" centers on the waist and abdomen, and is one of the most difficult forms of fat to lose. This type of fat is only indirectly related to dietary intake. It will be shed more slowly, and only as your physiological stress response is reduced. Be patient: it will come off,

and even if you still carry a spare tire around for a time, you are restoring your health and vitality by dealing with the stress in your life.

Measuring Up

It's that time again . . . Weigh yourself, and then take five girth measurements: bust at the largest point, waist at two inches above the navel, hips at the largest point, and right and left thigh circumference at the point where your extended fingertips reach with your arms hanging down at your sides. Record these figures, and your calculated BMI value, on your Progress Chart.

And now, go to page 273 for your new recipes!

 TODAY'S ASSIGNMENT

STRATEGIZE TO REDUCE STRESS

Takde the following six steps to reduce stress in your life:

1. Take a careful inventory of your life. What are your major stressors? What strategies can be used to reduce your stress response? Do you need help? Call a counselor this week and make an appointment. Do not delay! Do it today!

2. Find alternatives for stress eating and make a plan for doing them. What are your favorite comfort foods? What are some good substitutes (think in terms of activities as well as food)? Write out your plan and put it to work immediately.

3. Go to the health food store for holy basil and rhodiola, herbs that will lower your cortisol response.

4. While you are at the health food store, stock up on nutrients that nourish the adrenal glands. Start taking these supplements today!

5. Get plenty of rest this week. Wouldn't you enjoy a warm bath and a cup of hot tea? Indulge!

6. Stop drinking coffee (slowly) and replace it with soothing herbal tea. Replace sugary and salty foods with fresh vegetables and fruits. This may take some time, so give yourself a little grace, but be relentless in your pursuit of health.

If you don't take care of your stress, your stress will "do you in"! If you do take care of your stress and your body, it will respond with delight. You'll feel your natural energy returning and you'll start to feel good again.

And now, go take a nap . . .

LESSON III-4 STUDY GUIDE

1. Review the physiological stress response.

2. How does stress influence weight?

3. What are some possible reasons that people crave sugar, caffeine, and/or salty foods during periods of stress?

4. List the three stages of stress and the physiological consequences/symptoms of each.

5. What are some dietary strategies for dealing with stress?

6. What lifestyle changes may be necessary to lower stress levels?

7. Where does stress-related weight tend to accumulate?

8. What two herbs may be helpful in reducing the release of cortisol?

9. What nutrients may be helpful in nourishing the adrenal gland?

HEALTH TIP

NOSEBLEEDS

Does your nose bleed at the slightest touch? There are a number of reasons for frequent nosebleeds, including warm air that dries the nasal passages, causing the nasal membranes to crack and bleed. Obviously, a blow to the nose can cause bleeding, as can foreign objects (including fingers) in the nose. A change in atmospheric pressure, or even blowing the nose too forcefully, can also cause bleeding.

When a nosebleed starts, blow the clots gently out both nostrils. Lean forward in a chair (do not tilt backward). Pinch the soft parts of the nose together firmly for ten minutes. Apply an ice pack to the nose, neck, and cheeks. Do not blow your nose again for at least twelve hours. Refrain from vigorous activity for at least two days, if possible. (If you suspect a posterior nosebleed, or a nosebleed in the back of the nose, consult your healthcare practitioner.)

Nosebleeds can signal underlying illness such as arteriosclerosis, high blood pressure, malaria, sinusitis, and typhoid fever. Hemophilia, leukemia, thrombocytopenia, aplastic anemia, and liver disease are other conditions associated with nosebleeds. But for average, garden-variety nosebleeds, try the following tips to strengthen the nasal membranes naturally:

- Take a bioflavonoid complex supplement, 2,000 mg or more per day, along with vitamin C to promote healing.

- Take quercetin thirty minutes prior to each meal (it also reduces nasal allergies).

- Use a comfrey ointment or apply vitamin E topically to soothe dried-out nasal passages. Marigold ointment is particularly good for healing the tissue.

- Eat plenty of kale and other sources of vitamin K to assist in blood clotting.

- Avoid aspirin, tea, and coffee.

- Use a cool-mist humidifier, a vaporizer, or a pan of water on a radiator in the winter to humidify the air.

- Use nasal irrigation.

- Your local health food store should carry nasal sprays that strengthen the nasal membranes.

If you continue to have frequent nosebleeds, consult your physician.

ADDITIONAL NOTES

Lesson III-5. WAT, BAT, and Other Fats

We abhor the fat that makes our clothes bulge—we are trying to get rid of it, aren't we? Excess body fat, of course, is harmful to our physical health and also to our mental health. Being overweight mars our self-image: we don't feel that we look good when we are overweight. I've heard people say, "I wish I could take a vacuum and suck all the fat out of my body!" This is spoken in a moment of frustration, certainly, but it shows that we misunderstand something crucial. Fat, in itself, is not bad—not even body fat.

? TODAY'S QUESTION

Can fat make you thin?

Yes, it is a riddle!

When we consume more calories than the body can immediately use (or store in the liver as glycogen), they are stored as fat, in case of a shortage of calories later. Fat is an energetically dense nutrient, providing more than 9 calories of energy per gram; it is a major source of stored energy, and even a buffer for times of famine. A certain amount of body fat is essential and plays important structural and functional roles. For example, fat is deposited in cell membranes and participates in their metabolic activity. Saturated fats make the cell membrane firm so it is not crushed by the pressure of the surrounding cells; unsaturated fats make the membrane permeable so nutrients can pass into the cell and waste materials can be excreted. Fats are also used to synthesize male and female hormones and other hormones—and so on. Fats are very important!

THE WHITE AND THE BROWN

The problem with fat arises when too much fluffy white body fat is encasing the internal organs. Many people have millions of stored calories in "fat-storage depot sites" throughout the body, far more than they could ever use. When they go on a diet to rid themselves of their extra fat, they are trying to lose white adipose tissue (WAT), or white fat, also known as triglycerides.

Subcellular structures called mitochondria are the "furnaces" of cells, and it is the presence and number of mitochondria that determine a cell's metabolic activity. Muscle cells, for example, have many mitochondria; thus, they are metabolically active and burn many calories. White fat, however, is relatively inert, as it has only one or two mitochondria per cell, just enough to keep the cell alive and functional as storage. Because white fat is metabolically inactive, bodies that have more white fat than lean muscle tissue have the disadvantage of a lowered metabolism, which makes them even more likely to store ingested calories as body fat. They lose the ability to burn calories efficiently and become fatter as time goes on—unless they break the cycle by losing the fat.

NOTES

Another type of body fat, however, actually assists in the weight-loss battle: brown adipose tissue (BAT), also called brown fat, which is metabolically active. Whoever would have thought that fat could make you thin?

Brown fat has two primary purposes. Because it contains many mitochondria, it is a heat source for the core of the body. BAT tends to nestle around organs of high metabolic activity such as the adrenal glands, kidneys, and liver, and keeps them at a constant 98.6°F, the temperature at which their enzymes work most efficiently. Under the influence of the thyroid gland and certain hormones released from the adrenal gland, BAT serves as fuel to mitochondria, which "uncouple" BAT and oxidize it to produce body heat. Having sufficient levels of active brown fat is important in maintaining normal body temperature.

The second function of BAT is to waste calories—a very important task! We never know exactly how many calories we'll need for our daily activities. Plus, our caloric requirements change from day to day, depending on many factors, including temperatures in the surrounding environment, immune system activity, illness or fever, levels of physical activity, stress, and so on. If we eat more calories than we need on a given day or at a given meal, our BAT burns off the excess calories as heat. If it did not, we would inexorably gain weight from just a few extra calories per day! But active brown fat generally works efficiently to keep weight stable, so most people do not have to concern themselves with a few extra calories here and there.

BROWN FAT THERMOGENESIS

Did you know that babies do not shiver? Babies have a lot of brown fat nestled up against the back of the neck and clustered around organs of high metabolic activity. When babies are cold, their brown fat keeps their organs warm: this function is called non-shivering thermogenesis. As we age, however, our stores of BAT tend to shrink.

Age isn't the only factor that diminishes BAT activity. When the thyroid gland is active and "burning hot," brown fat burns hot too. When thyroid function is diminished, brown fat activity is reduced proportionately. Hypothyroidism blunts the effect of norepinephrine, an adrenal hormone that stimulates brown fat thermogenesis (heat production). This is one of the main reasons that hypothyroidism results in a colder body temperature, particularly in men; in women, low body temperature is often a consequence of hypothyroidism, but can also be caused by estrogen dominance or low progesterone.

When we gain excess weight, we essentially gather a large "blanket" of white fat around our upper body, which stores heat. The more body fat we have in this insulating blanket, the less we need brown fat, as we simply don't require as much heat generation to keep our internal organs warm. We can lose the function (that is, the benefits) of BAT, which may even change into WAT. This unfortunate loss or change is known to be caused by such things as excessive exercising, fasting, pregnancy, breastfeeding, diabetes, dressing too warmly, fever, and hypothalamic lesions. (Depressing, isn't it?)

Stress inhibits brown fat thermogenesis. Infrequent food consumption (only eating once or twice per day) or eating large meals likewise inhibits brown fat activity. A high-sugar diet down-regulates brown fat thermogenesis, as does a low-fat diet, especially one deficient in the class of fats called the omega-3 fatty acids.

ACTIVE BROWN FAT IS THE DIETER'S FRIEND

How can we encourage the thermogenic activity of our stores of BAT?

- A diet rich in omega-3 fatty acids promotes brown fat activity. Omega-3 fatty acids are found in deep-sea fish and are also provided by flaxseed oil and olive oil. I encourage you to enjoy several servings of ocean-raised fish per week, and use omega-3 fatty acid supplements (I recommend taking at least 5 grams of fish oil per day), to ensure you are getting enough of these valuable oils. Among their many functions, omega-3 fats are protective of the heart, anti-inflammatory, and good for the brain.

- Prolonged exposure to cool temperatures may be helpful, although if the ambient temperature drops low enough or stays low for long periods of time, BAT activity will be "cooled off." Keep the temperature in your home and workplace a little on the cool side; don't bundle up so warmly in the winter. When your body is cool, it is forced to produce heat, thereby burning more calories.

- Certain components in green tea (not the caffeine) stimulate brown fat thermogenesis. Drinking one cup of green tea with breakfast, lunch, and dinner significantly increases twenty-four-hour energy expenditure.

■ The dietary supplement coenzyme Q_{10} (CoQ_{10}) (available in health food stores) may increase the "uncoupling protein" I mentioned earlier, which increases BAT activity. CoQ_{10} is good for the heart and helps increase mental and physical energy. I recommend taking at least 100 milligrams (mg) of this valuable coenzyme per day, or more if you have a family or personal history of heart disease.

■ Moderate amounts of exercise heat up the furnace. Too much exercise, however, can be too stressful on the adrenal glands and can slow down the activity of brown fat. The key word? Moderation.

■ The Wings Program food plan, being a little lower in protein and higher in carbohydrates, also helps stimulate BAT activity.

And now, go to page 274 for your new recipes!

TODAY'S ASSIGNMENT

KEEP YOUR BROWN FAT ACTIVE AND HEALTHY

Take your body temperature several times during a couple days this week, using the basal temperature test procedure on page 124. Does your temperature run normal or low? A low body temperature may be due to low thyroid function, a low progesterone level, or low BAT activity. Try "washcloth therapy" for your thyroid (page 125) several times in a day to kick in some heat production. Review your lifestyle and diet. Are you encouraging your BAT activity, or unwittingly lowering it?

LESSON III-5 STUDY GUIDE

1. What is the function of white adipose tissue (WAT)?

_____

_____

_____

_____

2. What is the function of brown adipose tissue (BAT)?

_____

_____

_____

_____

HEALTH TIP

ORAL HYGIENE

Bleeding gums, periodontal disease, and gingivitis can be serious health problems that should be addressed naturally—and vigorously. Here are some tips for promoting a healthy mouth:

• Use the antioxidant coenzyme Q_{10} (CoQ_{10}) to increase gum health and tissue oxygenation.

• Do an ascorbic acid flush (pages 8–9), and then take vitamin C at a daily dosage of 75 percent of your flushing level, along with 1,000–2,000 milligrams of bioflavonoids daily (in divided doses).

• To increase healing of irritated oral tissue, put a few drops of nonalcohol goldenseal extract (available at health food stores) in a little water, and swish the mixture around in your mouth for a few minutes; do this oral rinse once or twice daily.

• If the gums become inflamed, place a few drops of nonalcohol goldenseal extract on a gauze ball and place it directly on the inflamed area for a few minutes; repeat this several times a day.

• Avoid alcohol, soft drinks, coffee, and other strong beverages. Drink water or herbal teas.

• Toothbrushes accumulate bacteria, so change your toothbrush frequently. Keep your toothbrush clean by soaking it nightly in a mixture of water and a few drops of grapefruit-seed extract.

• Treat your gums gently. Stimulate the gums by lightly brushing them with a soft toothbrush, but do not press too hard or you will injure the delicate tissue.

• Floss daily.

Lesson III-6. Review of the Past Few Lessons

Over the past few weeks, in exploring weight loss from a physiological rather than a dietary perspective, we have gone deeply into some very complex material. Following through on this information requires you to do some medical "homework."

? TODAY'S QUESTION

Have you done your homework?

_____

_____

_____

_____

In this lesson, you will stop and catch your breath. You may not have had an opportunity to pull your personal health information together and get in to see your physician with your findings. Sometimes life can be very intrusive, can't it?

So before we push ahead to other huge issues, we will review those covered in the past five lessons, dig a little deeper, and help you formulate a plan of action. After all, my purpose is not simply to inform: my purpose is to provide you with meaningful information, and then help you put it to practical use. If I succeed in this, you succeed in achieving your health goals!

ENDOCRINE COMMUNICATORS

We have discussed the role and significance of three endocrine organs in health and weight maintenance: the thyroid, the gonads, and the adrenal glands. Each of these organs communicates via hormones, and each influences the maintenance and functionality of brown adipose tissue (BAT).

Other endocrine organs, such as the hypothalamus, help regulate the activities of these organs and keep them in balance. When one organ is out of balance, the balance of all the endocrine organs is upset, much like an entire mobile wobbles when just one piece is knocked by the wind. When female or male hormones are out of balance, the thyroid gland is affected. For example, when estrogen is dominant over progesterone, the activity of the thyroid is diminished, setting the stage for hypothyroidism. When stress is prolonged, the female and male hormones become unbalanced, throwing the thyroid gland off-kilter.

Most people have found themselves, at one time or another, dealing with thyroid or other hormonal problems. For many of us, unrelenting stress has become a major life issue. The reality is this: if you struggle with endocrine imbalance in one area (thyroid, adrenals, or gonads), you will likely struggle with it in at least two others. And we've just learned that hypothyroidism, estrogen-progesterone imbalance, or hypoadrenalism (low adrenal output, possibly due to chronic stress) will down-regulate the activity of brown fat, causing low body temperature—which further reduces the metabolic rate—and turning brown fat into metabolically inert white fat. It almost feels that you can't win this contest, doesn't it?

WHERE TO START

If you have any endocrine system problems, you prob-

✐ NOTES

_____

_____

_____

_____

_____

_____

ably have at least two of them, so let's prioritize them and put a plan together. Which of your endocrine issues seems to be the most pressing: thyroid function, female hormones, or stress? Go over the symptom lists for each to see where you "scored the most points," and start there.

1. If you plan to start with the thyroid gland, assemble the following:

   ▪ A body-temperature chart for at least five days (follow the instructions on page 124).

   ▪ A list of any of the symptoms of hypothyroidism (Lesson III-2) that pertain to you.

   Make an appointment with your physician, take the above information with you, and ask for a blood test for hypothyroidism. Remember that the T3 and T4 tests may not always be diagnostic; if you have all the symptoms of hypothyroidism but those tests come back normal, request additional evaluation such as measurement of TSH (thyroid stimulating hormone) or thyroid antibodies.

2. If you plan to start with female hormones, identify your symptoms as listed on pages 130–131 in Lesson III-3. Make an appointment with your family physician or obstetrician-gynecologist, take this information with you, and ask for a saliva test to check your estrogen-to-progesterone ratio. *Note:* Often, as the thyroid gland is nourished, levels of female hormones normalize.

3. If stress seems to be your overriding health and weight-management issue, review the information in Lesson III-4. Devise your stress-reduction strategies and put them in place. Write a plan for nourishing your adrenal glands, and start today. *Note:* Stress reduction diminishes stress on the thyroid gland as well, making it easier to resolve thyroid and female hormone problems.

4. Have you done tasks 1–3 already and brought your endocrine system into balance, but are still not losing weight? Is your weight stuck? Revisit the allergy/intolerance information in Lesson I-10. Also revisit the BAT issue, as discussed in Lesson III-5:

   ▪ Get moderate amounts of exercise.

   ▪ Readjust your diet to include plenty of natural fats and a balance of protein and carbohydrates.

   ▪ Adjust thermostats to a cooler setting and leave your sweater at home.

   ▪ Drink several cups of green tea per day to stimulate brown fat activity.

Bringing your body back into hormonal balance will not be achieved overnight. Follow your plan for at least three months before reevaluating its effectiveness. As your body begins to respond, revisit your plan periodically. How is it working? What adjustments need to be made?

I strongly encourage you to work closely with a nutritionally trained doctor through this process. If he/she does not understand what you are doing and refuses to work with you, find a new doctor! Remember that your doctor should be part of your team, not your health dictator. Your pursuit of health is an organic, dynamic process that requires active participation by several players: you, your physician or other healthcare practitioner, your nutritionist, and your family.

Keep in mind that health is a journey, not a destination. Layer by layer, you are building good health. As good health develops, the weight will drop. You will achieve your goals.

And now, go to page 275 for your new recipes!

 TODAY'S ASSIGNMENT

REVIEW AND REST

There is no need for an additional assignment: do the work described above. If it turns out that you do not have to pursue any of these issues, take a rest this week. Believe it or not, rest is good for weight loss!

LESSON III-6 STUDY GUIDE

Review the study questions for Lessons III-1 through III-5. If there are sections you don't understand, review the material. Start reading the books recommended in the text and in the Resource Guide. Become fully informed about each of the issues we've discussed!

 HEALTH TIP

ROSACEA

Rosacea is a chronic skin disorder affecting the forehead, nose, cheekbones, and chin. The skin on these parts of the face develops blotchy red areas with small bumps; it can swell and thicken, and it may become tender and sensitive. Factors that can trigger an outbreak of rosacea include certain foods, alcohol, hot liquids, exposure to sunlight, extremes of temperature, irritating skin-care products, stress, and nutrient deficiencies.

Here are several tips for healing your skin from rosacea naturally:

- Do the pulse test (pages 47–48) to determine any food allergies you may have, and remove all allergens from your diet.

- Avoid all the Wings "no-no's": coffee, cheese, chocolate, sugar, spicy foods, and so on.

- Do not drink hot beverages. Avoid saunas, spas, steam baths, and hot tubs.

- Take 25,000 international units (IU) of vitamin A daily for six months, and then reduce the daily dose to 15,000 IU. Take your vitamin A along with 15–30 milligrams (mg) (or more) of zinc. *Caution:* If there is a possibility of pregnancy, do not consume more than 7,500 IU of vitamin A per day.

- Take a double dose of your daily B-complex vitamins.

- Take 75 percent of your "flushing level" (page 9) of vitamin C daily, along with 2,000–3,000 mg daily of a bioflavonoid complex to strengthen the capillaries in the skin.

- Herbs that are healing to the skin when taken internally include burdock root, red clover, ginger, dandelion root, yellow dock, and stinging nettles (don't worry, the nettles are in capsule form!).

- Evening primrose oil is also healing to the skin (take 1,500 mg per day).

- The amino acid L-cysteine contains sulfur, a mineral that is good for the skin and reduces chemical toxicity in the liver.

- Keep your liver clean by following the Wings body-cleansing protocol (Lesson II-6) at least quarterly.

- Alfalfa is a good source of chlorophyll, which helps detoxify the liver, and the herb provides minerals and vitamins as well.

- Consider taking the herbs dandelion or milk thistle daily to help support liver function.

- Apply *Aloe vera* gel or juice directly to irritated skin.

- Use natural makeup that nourishes the skin (I like products by Aubrey, Annemarie Borlind, and Zia, among others). Make sure all cleansing, moisturizing, and makeup products are "clean"—that is, do not contain chemicals of any kind.

- If an infection develops, consult your healthcare practitioner.

ADDITIONAL NOTES

Lesson III-7. How Prescription Medications Make You Overweight

"Here is your prescription, Mrs. Jones." You walk out of the doctor's office with a bottle of pills in your hand: just the thing to "cure" your medical problem. Unfortunately, that little bottle may lead to a significant amount of unwanted weight. Chances are you were never told about the possible weight consequences—and it probably wouldn't have made any difference if you had been told, as your doctor believed the prescribed medications were necessary for your physical condition. But if you had known ahead of time, you could have prepared yourself mentally for the added pounds, and perhaps adjusted your diet or lifestyle to avoid gaining the weight.

Is it possible to lose the weight while continuing to take the drugs? Sometimes yes, sometimes no. This lesson will present information on the medications that commonly cause weight gain; drug-discontinuation strategies to discuss with your physician; and solutions to a medication-induced weight problem. I may be able to point you toward a more natural approach to health care that will help you, for the most part, to reduce or avoid your use of medications. According to United States government calculations, up to 80 percent of all health conditions could be prevented by making simple dietary and/or lifestyle changes—that is very exciting news! Perhaps for the first time, you can truly take charge of your health.

? TODAY'S QUESTION

Are medications making you fat?

_____

_____

_____

_____

List all prescription medications you are using now or have used in the past. Did you begin gaining weight when you began taking them? One Wings student gained more than 25 pounds after starting a popular cholesterol-lowering drug. She is still working to get the weight off, years after discontinuing the medication. (Ironically, her cholesterol levels started to normalize within weeks of beginning the Wings Program!)

Drugs generally cause weight gain by two different mechanisms: water retention and increased fat deposition. The body may use fat tissue to sequester the foreign material (the medication), or the medication may alter metabolism. Altered metabolism may lead to metabolic syndrome, impaired glucose tolerance, or increased carbohydrate sensitivity (explored further in Lesson III-10.)

Put impaired glucose tolerance because of prescription medications together with increased consumption of sugary, fatty foods (so common in our culture, especially in individuals prone to depression, PMS, or other disorders), and you have a formula for disaster in terms of overall health, weight, and vitality. We, as a culture, are rapidly headed downhill toward greater and greater health challenges, which

✒ NOTES

_____

_____

_____

_____

_____

_____

will "require" more and more medications . . . See where this is going? As we take more drugs, we'll need more drugs—and we'll gain weight as a result.

DRUGS THAT CAUSE WEIGHT GAIN— AND WHAT YOU CAN DO ABOUT IT

A research article about obesity relates:

> While usually not the only factor in obese patients, prescription medications, which may increase appetite or body weight, can be important in some individuals. Most reports of medication-induced weight gain are anecdotal or gleaned from clinical trials. Notable offenders include hormones (especially corticosteroids and insulinotropic agents) and psychoactive antipsychotics . . . Medication-related increases in appetite and body weight are under-recognized and cause noncompliance with pharmacotherapy. (L. J. Cheskin, S. J. Barlett, R. Zayas, et al., "Prescription Medications: a Modifiable Contributor to Obesity," *Southern Medical Journal* 1999, Vol. 92:898–904.)

In the Wings Program, it is my passionate desire to spiral my students' health upward. I aim to focus your attention away from the mentality of "a pill for every ill" and entice you to pursue natural approaches to health care instead. In doing so, you will greatly enhance your health *and* lose weight naturally! I will suggest lifestyle and dietary modifications that may reduce your need for the prescription medications described in this section. As noted above, the vast majority of health problems can be prevented if we make simple changes—and that is what Wings is all about.

Caution

Please keep in mind that if your physician has prescribed a medication, you must continue to use the medication until your physician gives you permission to stop taking it. It is dangerous to discontinue the use of a medication without proper supervision.

What types of medication commonly cause weight gain?

- Psychotropic medications (drugs that exert an effect upon the mind or modify mental activity)

- Cardiovascular medications (such as cholesterol-lowering drugs)
- Hormone replacements or regulators
- Anti-inflammatory and steroidal medications

These four categories comprise most of the commonly used prescription medications on the market. This is not, however, a complete list of all medications that cause weight gain.

You may not be able to discontinue the use of your medications, as they may be medically essential, but knowing that weight gain may result may help set your mind at ease. You shouldn't feel guilty about weight gain caused by a medical problem or therapy.

Psychotropic Medications

The use of mind-altering prescription pharmaceuticals is increasing. Psychotropic medications include antidepressants, antianxiety medications, antipsychotics, and others, most of which are expected to cause some amount of weight gain. Some of the more commonly prescribed psychotropics are Depakote, Effexor, Elavil, lithium (can cause significant weight gain), Paxil (can cause either weight loss or weight gain), Prozac (can cause anorexia and weight loss in underweight patients), Sonata, Thorazine, Wellbutrin, and Zoloft.

Women who take antipsychotic drugs display lower serum levels of estrogen and progesterone; they also tend to lose testosterone. The imbalance between the three hormones can actually cause a type of hyperandrogenism, or excess testosterone in relation to the female hormones, but these women nevertheless lose the weight-management advantage normally conferred by testosterone. Men who use antipsychotic drugs also secrete significantly lower levels of testosterone than they normally would. Researchers note, "These endocrine abnormalities may contribute to the excessive weight gain observed after AP (antipsychotic) treatment." (T. Baptista, D. Reyes, and L. Hernanez, "Antipsychotic Drugs and Reproductive Hormones: Relationship to Body Weight Regulation," *Pharmacology, Biochemistry, and Behavior* 1999, Vol. 62:409–417.)

One journal article notes that antipsychotic-treated patients "who tend to take combinations of psychotropic agents that may cause weight gain are at special risk for the problems associated with being overweight or obese." (G. L. Blackburn, "Weight Gain and Antipsychotic Medication," *Journal of Clinical Psychiatry* 2000, Vol. 61, Supp. 8:36–41, discussion 42.)

Practical Tips for People Using Psychotropic Drugs

▨ Blood sugar abnormalities may occur due to the use of psychotropics, so if you are using one of these medications, you will need to be particularly careful to eat frequent, small meals to maintain a level blood sugar. (In other words, follow the Wings Program!)

▨ Supplement your diet with magnesium, zinc, and the B-complex vitamins to help stabilize blood sugar and to resolve eating behaviors that stimulate insulin resistance. As it happens, all three of these nutrients are "antidepressant" as well!

▨ Chromium (the GTF form) is very helpful in balancing blood sugar; use up to 1,000 micrograms per day for added insurance.

▨ If weight gain is unavoidable due to the nature of the prescribed medication, you need to be particularly careful to balance your proteins, carbohydrates, and fats to minimize the risk of developing metabolic syndrome (Syndrome X).

▨ Because anticipated or actual weight gain is a common reason for noncompliance with prescribed antidepressants, you should speak with your doctor about this important issue. (For an in-depth discussion of the nutritional implications of mental and/or emotional illness, read my book *The Crazy Makers: How the Food Industry Is Destroying Our Brains and Harming Our Children* [New York, NY: Jeremy P. Tarcher/Penguin, 2000].)

The subject of mood, weight, and natural therapies as alternatives to antidepressant pharmaceuticals will be presented in Lesson III-8. Several wonderful natural remedies work well to ease most mild-to-moderate depression and other mood disorders. Occasionally, however, these remedies are insufficient; sometimes, particularly in the case of severe depression, medication is necessary.

Cholesterol-Lowering Medications

There is a huge controversy in the medical community about whether or not cholesterol is the major culprit in cardiovascular disease. Many other factors are as important—or more important—than total serum cholesterol. Nevertheless, many physicians still feel that cholesterol-lowering medications are necessary, and they are commonly prescribed for cardiovascular purposes.

The cholesterol-lowering medication that most often causes weight gain is Lipitor. Lipitor affects the liver, which is the organ responsible for detoxifying the body, producing thousands of enzymes, and hundreds of other vital functions. The medical literature does not provide clues to the exact cause of weight gain when taking Lipitor, but we should suspect metabolic causes such as altered blood-sugar regulation or lowered metabolism.

If you begin to gain weight after going on Lipitor, speak with your doctor immediately, and ask whether another medication may work better for you. Make sure your liver enzymes are checked regularly, as Lipitor has been linked with sudden death. And if you experience any side effects from the drug, make sure your doctor is aware of them and is dealing with them appropriately. Do not be afraid to seek a second opinion, if necessary: you are responsible for your own good health!

If you are taking a statin drug, speak with your physician about the tendency of the statin drugs to lower the production of CoQ_{10} (a coenzyme that promotes heart health). Discuss how you can protect your tissues from CoQ_{10} deficiency.

Important Considerations in Heart Health

If you have a personal or family history of heart disease, let me recommend my book *A Woman's Guide to a Healthy Heart* (New York, NY: Contemporary Books, 2004). One chapter is devoted solely to female concerns, but the rest of the book is appropriate for both men and women; it provides valuable information on how to protect and heal the heart, including lowering elevated cholesterol and/or triglyceride levels. Following is a brief outline of information that can help reduce your dependence on cardiovascular medications:

▨ Elevated homocysteine, a protein-like metabolite of the amino acid L-methionine, is an important marker for heart disease. Fortunately, several of the B-complex vitamins can be used to lower elevated homocysteine levels, and a good-quality multivitamin-mineral supplement contains adequate amounts of B-complex vitamins for this purpose; I particularly recommend 400–800 micrograms of folic acid.

▨ C-reactive protein is a marker for inflammation. It is now known that inflammation can be at the root of many forms of cardiovascular disease. A blood test for the level of C-reactive protein provides you and your physician with a good indicator of your risk of developing cardiovascular (and other) diseases. C-reactive protein levels can be lowered by reducing inflammation in the body. Fish oil, for example, is an excellent anti-inflammatory nutrient and also helps thin the blood, reducing the tendency for blood clotting. Turmeric (curcumin), bromelain (a pineapple enzyme), and ginger are beneficial against inflammation as well.

- You may also wish to use a supplement called a lipotropic, available at health food stores. Lipotropics contain a combination of nutrients (including choline, inositol, and methionine) that are very helpful in normalizing fat levels in the bloodstream.

- Consider using dandelion and silymarin, two herbs that are traditionally held in high esteem for their liver-supportive properties.

- Drink plenty of water.

- And, oh yes . . . don't eat sugar! Your body converts sugar into cholesterol and triglycerides!

Follow the Wings Program for a Healthy Heart

With very few exceptions, following the Wings food plan will bring cholesterol down to a healthy level and help balance the ratio of LDL (low-density lipoprotein, or "bad cholesterol") to HDL (high-density lipoprotein, or "good cholesterol"), providing protection to the heart. The Wings food plan will also normalize triglycerides (white fat or WAT, discussed in Lesson III-5).

If your serum cholesterol level remains high after you've been on the Wings Program for three months or more, or your LDL-to-HDL ratio remains high, I highly recommend that you use the Wings cleansing protocol (Lesson II-6) to keep your liver and other organs of detoxification clean.

Do not be tempted to abandon the Wings Program for a low-fat or low-cholesterol diet unless your cholesterol levels are extremely high and have not been reduced by any other means; and in this case, follow the low-fat protocol for a short period only! In the absence of adequate amounts of dietary fat and cholesterol, your liver will produce even more cholesterol itself, which is far more damaging than the intake of dietary cholesterol.

Hormone Replacement Therapies and Contraceptives

Hormone replacement therapy (HRT), estrogen replacement therapy (ERT), and birth-control pills have been aggressively marketed to the female population over the past forty years; more than 20 million American women may be using synthetic hormonal replacement or contraception. A common consequence of any form of synthetic hormone replacement is weight gain. Using ERT or oral contraceptives, for example, can cause an individual to retain 35 or more pounds of excess water!

As discussed in Lesson III-3, hormone replacement alters the natural estrogen-to-progesterone balance. Estrogen dominance, often caused by supplementing with estrogen or synthetic progesterone, also contributes to hypothyroidism. According to Dr. John Lee, "No hormone works in isolation from other hormones; they all function within a complex, subtle web of interconnectedness. If thyroid is low, cortisol and sex hormone production lag. Estrogen inhibits thyroid hormone activity and thus exacerbates thyroid deficiency . . . Persistent estrogen dominance . . . creates a cycle of lowered thyroid function . . . " (John R. Lee, M.D. *What Your Doctor May Not Tell You about Breast Cancer.* New York, NY: Warner Books, 2002, page 68.)

A review of four common menopause therapies (Alora, Climera, Premarin, and Vivelle) shows the same listed side effects: weight gain, impaired glucose tolerance, and fluid retention. Every type of HRT or hormone-based contraceptive, in fact, causes weight gain as well as increased fat deposition. Most of the excess weight gained from these metabolic changes will be extremely difficult to lose once the drug therapy is begun, even after use of the drug has been discontinued. Glucose intolerance keeps circulating insulin at high levels while decreasing the sensitivity of insulin's receptor sites. High levels of insulin in the bloodstream predispose an individual to weight gain, because insulin increases water retention and fat deposition.

Synthetic estrogens and progesterones may also affect weight and health via other mechanisms not covered in the primary medical literature. Dr. Lee writes, "Synthetic progestins such as Provera and those found in some birth control pills have been shown to increase insulin resistance." (Lee, 2002, page 64.) Insulin resistance inevitably leads to weight gain (the roles of insulin and glucagon in weight management are further discussed in Lesson III-10).

You Have Options

Unfortunately, weight gain caused by hormone imbalance, and particularly by hormone therapy or contraception, is difficult (though not impossible) to resolve. Even after the medications are discontinued, their effects don't just vanish when you take the last pill. It isn't that you cannot lose the weight once it appears; it is that you now have to correct the underlying, ongoing metabolic problem created by the synthetic hormones.

This information in this lesson is problematic for women who wish to use hormonal contraceptives. Please consult a naturally oriented physician about alternate (nonhormonal) forms of birth control. A barrier method (such as condoms or a diaphragm) may be appropriate for you, or perhaps your spouse can take care of the contraception issue himself.

Many women use synthetic HRT or ERT therapies, not for any particular health reason, but simply because they are in the menopausal age bracket. I encourage you to discuss this with your physician, who should be able to suggest more natural approaches to managing menopausal symptoms. Remember: menopause is not a disease and should not be medicated as such! Review Lesson III-3 for strategies to normalize your female hormones.

The Skinny on Natural Progesterone

In a personal conversation with Dr. Lee, I asked him what women who have used synthetic hormones can do about their weight struggle. He said that, in his clinical experience, using natural progesterone not only helps restore the natural estrogen-to-progesterone balance but helps normalize weight as well. Compared to synthetic progestin, natural progesterone is more thermogenic (burns calories in the form of heat), increases metabolism, and resolves many hormone-driven eating behaviors. His final word was, "Yes! They can lose their excess weight by using natural progesterone." Dr. Lee has tested scores of natural progesterone creams on the market. His several excellent books and other materials provide a list of creams that contain the best sources and dosage of natural progesterone.

Anti-Inflammatory Medications

Anti-inflammatories are another class of medications that frequently cause weight gain, particularly if they contain cortisone, an adrenal hormone that promotes weight gain through edema (water retention) and increased fat deposition (particularly in the face, upper body, and abdomen). Common anti-inflammatories include Cortone, Hydrocortone, and Pediapred, but there are many others on the market. Other side effects of hydrocortisone (a cortisone compound) may include the following:

- Blood sugar dysregulation
- Loss of muscle protein (loss of lean muscle tissue) and muscle wasting
- Congestive heart failure
- Mild hirsutism (unwanted hair growth) in women
- Adrenal atrophy
- Impaired wound healing
- Muscle weakness
- Osteoporosis
- Emotional disturbances

Fortunately, much of the weight gained through steroid use is water weight, most of which is easily lost when the medication is discontinued. So your problem may be solved—*if* you nourish your adrenal glands on the other side of the steroid treatment. Steroids inevitably cause adrenal dysfunction; it is critically important to restore the health of the adrenal glands (see the following inset, Adrenal Nourishment), or other weight-management issues will soon follow.

Adrenal Nourishment

The adrenal glands are often overworked as a result of our stressed lifestyle. When anti-inflammatories that contain cortisone are used, these important glands are in even greater jeopardy of exhaustion. Symptoms of adrenal exhaustion include depression, fatigue, impaired immune function, and so on.

If you have used prednisone or other steroid hormones, nourish your adrenal glands by supplementing with vitamin C and pantothenic acid. Some natural physicians also recommend using "raw adrenal" products, which are available through health food stores. Unless the strength of the adrenal glands is restored, it will be difficult to resolve the side effects of using steroid medications.

AN IMPORTANT REMINDER

I will not (cannot!) recommend that you discontinue using your prescription medications. As tempting as it may seem to stop taking them immediately, you must consult your physician regarding the important issues raised in this chapter. It is likely that your physician believes the medications are necessary for your well-being, or he/she wouldn't have prescribed them. Seek his/her counsel on the best way to maintain a healthful weight, especially if you simply must use medication. Meanwhile, explore your options for improving your health through lifestyle and dietary changes.

And now, go to page 276 for your new recipes!

 ## TODAY'S ASSIGNMENT

GO THROUGH YOUR MEDICINE CABINET

What drugs do you use? How do they affect weight? Do you have over-the-counter medications that you could get rid of or replace with natural alternatives? Learn more about natural medicine so you can reduce your dependence on drugs (see the Resource Guide for books to assist you in your self-education). The more you know about the workings and magnificence of your body, the more you'll want to take care of it, naturally. The healthier you become, the fewer drugs you require—and that's always a good thing.

LESSON III-7 STUDY GUIDE

1. What four categories of drugs often lead to weight gain?

2. Describe the issues surrounding the use of antidepressants or other psychotropics and weight gain.

3. Discuss the issues surrounding the use of cholesterol-lowering medications and weight gain.

4. Discuss the issues surrounding the use of synthetic hormones and weight gain.

5. Discuss the issues surrounding the use of anti-inflammatories and weight gain.

6. In light of the above issues, discuss natural alternatives for each of these drug categories.

HEALTH TIP

SINUS TROUBLE

Sinusitis can be very painful! Fortunately, much can be done naturally to reduce the frequency of sinus infections or heal them once they start.

- Eliminate all possible allergens, particularly dairy products, and keep the body free of mucus (dairy products form mucus).

- Do an ascorbic acid flush (pages 8–9), and maintain your daily intake of vitamin C at 75 percent of your flushing level.

- Use extra vitamin A—10,000 international units (IU) daily or more (unless pregnancy is possible, in which case you should take no more than 7,500 IU per day)—along with extra zinc (30 milligrams or so).

- Nature's Way Fenu-Thyme and Enzymatic Therapy SinuGuard, among others, are excellent herbal products that support nasal and sinus health.

- Quercetin plus bromelain, taken on an empty stomach several times per day, strengthen and protect the mucous passages.

- Teas of anise, fenugreek, marshmallow, or red clover help loosen phlegm and clear congestion.

- Use a nasal rinse with saltwater, a drop of grapefruit-seed extract, and glycerin several times per day to clear infection. Goldenseal can also be used as a nasal rinse to clear infection.

- Use a nasal spray with grapefruit-seed extract.

- Use a menthol or eucalyptus pack over the sinuses to relieve pressure.

- To relieve congestion in the nose, keep the air moisturized, or sit in a steam bath.

- Do a cayenne pepper treatment several times a day: bring a pot of water to a boil; add a little cayenne pepper to the water; put a towel over your head and breathe the vapor in; and use warm compresses over the sinuses to encourage drainage.

- Avoid smoke!

- If you notice swelling around the eyes, consult your healthcare practitioner immediately.

ADDITIONAL NOTES

Lesson III-8. Mood and Food

We have discussed the marvelous interplay between the systems of the body and how they "talk" to one another through hormones secreted by the organs of the endocrine system. Think of your body as an intricate mobile. Your cells, organs, and systems perform their work elegantly and interdependently, separate from each other and yet intimately connected to every other cell, organ, and system. In a mobile, the separate pieces dangle on different strings, but are connected at the top, so when one piece is moved, the other pieces change positions to compensate. Your "separate pieces" are connected by your brain and central nervous system. The body remains in delicate balance—unless something disturbs that balance.

When something happens in one cell, organ, or system, the rest of your body is affected and must compensate for the weaker member. What happens when you break a fingernail down too close to the quick? Your entire body concentrates on favoring that finger until the nail grows out to protect the sensitive skin in the nail bed. This is true of your mental condition as well. When you do not feel well mentally, various physiological changes take place to compensate. You will learn about some of those compensatory mechanisms in this lesson.

❓ TODAY'S QUESTION

How good—or how bad—is your mood?

_____

_____

_____

_____

Are you depressed? Check out this list of common symptoms of major depression:

- ❏ Feelings of guilt and inadequacy
- ❏ Fearful, overwhelmed feelings
- ❏ Onset of a fear of being alone
- ❏ Diurnal (that is, depending on the time of day) variation in mood
- ❏ Preoccupation with failure, illness, or other unpleasant themes (which may become obsessive thoughts)
- ❏ Nightmares, especially with themes of loss, pain, or death
- ❏ Anhedonia (loss of ability to experience pleasure)
- ❏ Indecision
- ❏ Onset of unexplained anxiety, panic attacks
- ❏ Sleep disturbance (too much or too little, especially with early morning awakening)
- ❏ Appetite disturbance (increased or decreased, usually enough to cause weight change)
- ❏ Fatigue, low energy
- ❏ Vague aches and pains, heaviness in the chest
- ❏ Constipation
- ❏ Loss of interest in sex
- ❏ Poor concentration, slowed thinking

Perhaps you thought you were depressed because you were overweight—actually, the reverse may be true. You may be overweight because you are depressed! Now that is depressing news . . . as is the fact that if you are taking (or have taken) an antidepressant or other psychoactive drug, the drug itself may have caused weight gain. Please review the information on that issue in Lesson III-7.

✒ NOTES

_____

_____

_____

_____

CAUSES OF DEPRESSION

Sometimes life presents challenges that can be too much for our coping mechanisms to handle: unrelenting stress, a problematic marriage, a frustrating work environment, tight finances, disappointments and failures, physical illness or injury (our own, or of someone we love and care for). These situations can overwhelm even the strongest person and can lead to depression. But although difficult circumstances may make life more . . . well, difficult, true depression is a physiological state, not just a life event. Lowered mood is a function of brain biochemistry and should be treated accordingly.

What, then, are the physiological causes of depression? The long and varied list of contributing factors includes deficiencies in critical nutrients (magnesium, B-complex vitamins, iron, zinc, essential fatty acids, protein, and so on), hypoglycemia, hypothyroidism, other biochemical imbalances such as neurotransmitter deficiencies, food or environmental allergies, heavy metal accumulation, candida (yeast) overgrowth, systemic parasites, and more. Adrenal exhaustion, which may be the consequence of long-term, unrelenting stress, is another common cause of depression.

The incidence of mental/emotional disorders is growing, even in our affluent society. Up to one-quarter of all visits to healthcare professionals are for mental illness, and up to one-third of the population has struggled with or will experience depression at some point in life. Depression has been called the "common cold of mental disorders," but it must be taken seriously. It can be life threatening, especially if it strikes a very young or a very old person. Suicide is now the number-two cause of death among teenagers in many states and is also becoming more common in the elderly. Depression is often difficult to diagnose, especially in young children or adolescents who may not appear to have any striking "reason" to be depressed; imbalanced hormones and other physical and emotional stressors, however, can frequently throw a susceptible teenager or child into true clinical depression.

Depression Can Alter Eating Behaviors

People with depression often turn to specific foods for comfort. As adults, we tend to select the foods that comforted us in childhood, when food was often used as a "security blanket." For example, Mom might have made chocolate-chip cookies when we encountered a difficult situation in school. Common comfort foods include macaroni and cheese, tomato or chicken-noodle soup, grilled cheese sandwiches, potato chips, chocolate, fatty foods (like ice cream), hot chocolate, bread, and many others. Unfortunately, comfort foods are seldom good for the waistline! They almost always cause weight gain—which may make you more depressed.

Your eating behaviors are not just a matter of habit or childhood, however. They are often very much under the control of hormones and neurotransmitters in your brain. Neurotransmitters, as you know, are special compounds that serve as messengers to nerve cells. Some neurotransmitters are stimulatory, others are calming or inhibiting. The neurotransmitters most commonly thought to be involved in depression and/or other mood disorders and associated unhealthful eating behaviors include serotonin, dopamine, GABA, acetylcholine, and the adrenal catecholamines epinephrine and norepinephrine.

Research has shown, for example, that when our brains are deficient in the calming neurotransmitter serotonin, we crave sugar, chocolate, and other high-energy, sugary foods because high-carbohydrate meals actually increase serotonin production. In other words, we tend to self-medicate with chocolate when low moods hit—this is particularly true for women who struggle with PMS. Dopamine is the "pleasure neurotransmitter," and dopamine deficiency can trigger depression. That deficiency similarly causes food cravings, possibly in an attempt to elevate mood. People who produce low levels of dopamine often crave foods or take mood-elevating drugs in an attempt to stimulate their dopamine receptor sites. (There may also be a connection between nicotine addiction and dopamine deficiency; smoking may be the body's way to elevate dopamine levels to bring on a feeling of comfort or satisfaction.)

Melatonin is a neurotransmitter released in the evening as the light diminishes and causes the body to slow down and go to sleep. Melatonin then converts to serotonin, a calming neurotransmitter. People who live in darker, northern regions often do not produce as much melatonin as those who live in sunnier climates because we need light to normalize our melatonin levels. Light deprivation tends to increase cravings for carbohydrates, possibly because of the connection between melatonin and serotonin. Seasonal affective disorder, or SAD, is a subtype of depression triggered by low levels of natural light. SAD is very common in areas of the world that have long, dark winters with fewer days of bright sunshine.

You see that your brain chemistry is influenced by the foods you eat and that, by the same logic, your brain chemicals influence the types—and quantities—of foods you typically consume. It is very important to understand the role of brain chemicals in mood and food, because these powerful chemicals affect your eating behaviors at a level deeper than conscious thought. Although you may believe that you can defeat food cravings if you just muster up enough will and grit your teeth ("I will not eat it . . . I will not eat it . . . "), it is virtually impossible to conquer the food cravings caused by disordered brain chemistry for very long. Eventually, the disordered chemicals in your brain win the contest.

Which Comes First: Depression or Excess Weight?

It seems that overweight individuals tend more toward depression, which tends to increase their consumption of carbohydrate-rich foods—leading to more weight gain. As one study suggests, many individuals who fail to maintain a normal weight may be susceptible to daily, monthly, or seasonal disturbances in mood that result in an excessive intake of carbohydrate-rich foods and a resistance to engaging in physical activity. In other words, these individuals tend to eat well *normally*, but frequent or occasional problems with depression or other mood disorders triggers food cravings that cannot be overcome, leading to increased weight. The weight (or the poor control over eating behaviors) then, is not the result of a weak will but stems directly from the mood problem—and with that information, we can stop blaming ourselves for being "out of control."

We often think that we are depressed because we are overweight. We can think of a thousand reasons why our excess weight, and our depression, is our fault: we lack self-control, we are not attractive, our clothes don't look right. We pummel ourselves with negative thoughts constantly. But we now see that our ability to control the types and quantities of food we eat, and our overall mood, is not necessarily under our control. We can stop beating ourselves up!

Is It Low Thyroid Function?

As already mentioned, hypothyroidism is a common cause of depression (thyroid function was discussed in Lesson III-2). Consider this domino effect:

- Hypothyroidism results in low levels of thyroid hormone, causing fatigue, depression, a lowered metabolism, and difficulty in maintaining a healthful weight.

- The depression caused by the hypothyroidism produces cravings for sugary foods in an attempt to (1) increase physical or mental energy, or (2) increase brain serotonin or dopamine levels.

- Consuming sugary foods further contributes to depression because the nutrients needed to maintain a happy mood are also used to metabolize the sugars. Unless the diet is extremely plentiful in these nutrients (magnesium, B-complex vitamins, zinc, and chromium), deficiencies soon result, leading to an even lower mood—and causing a rebound in eating high-sugar foods to elevate mood.

- When you eat sugary comfort foods, you experience a surge in energy that rapidly dissipates, resulting in functional hypoglycemia, another common cause of depression. The individual is again depressed and fatigued—and overweight, a condition that is now difficult to resolve because of the hypothyroidism. This vicious cycle is not easily interrupted.

- The fatigue of hypothyroidism and depression that leads to sugar cravings may also stimulate cravings for coffee or other stimulants as an attempt to boost flagging energy levels.

It is important to remember that if depression seems to be unrelated to life circumstances, thyroid function should be assessed first. Resolving hypothyroidism can quickly and easily elevate one's mood.

Is It Hormonal, Ma'am?

One of the most common symptoms of estrogen dominance is depression. You may have found that resolving your female hormone issue eased your depression; or, you may still be trying to achieve hormonal balance. If you suspect you are estrogen dominant, continue working to correct that, and you'll probably find that it will become easier to deal with your mood. Remember, it takes at least three months to resolve a hormone problem: don't give up! (Review Lesson III-3.)

Is It That Time of Year?

I mentioned earlier that periods of prolonged darkness can affect the brain's neurotransmitters and trigger the seasonal type of depression called SAD. SAD can often be effectively treated with light therapy. You may obtain further information about light therapy from your local public library, your physician, or Internet sources.

Is It an Allergy?

Sensitivity to certain food or environmental triggers can often trigger depression. Unfortunately, few people recognize the power of a cerebral allergy (one that attacks the brain). Some healthcare practitioners believe that food allergies and food intolerances are a much more common cause of depression than we imagine; although this idea still generates some controversy in the medical profession, a number of doctors who incorporate nutritional therapies in their medical practice have written extensively on the subject. The most common allergic triggers for depression and other mental symptoms are grains and dairy, but as we've previously discussed, an allergy or intolerance to any food can trigger any type of symptom, including depression and other mood disorders.

Food and Mood: Client Stories

Several years ago, a client came to me with a complaint of severe depression. She had been using antidepressant medications for many years and was still deeply depressed. After analyzing her weekly Food Diary for commonly consumed foods, I recommended that she eliminate all wheat and other gluten-containing grains from her diet for a period of four weeks to determine whether these foods were triggering her allergies. She was reluctant to eliminate grains; she and her husband had recently purchased a bread-making machine and they enjoyed fresh-baked bread nearly every day. However, she was eager to resolve the depression, and took my counsel. Within just a few days, her depression began to lift and by the end of the month, it had resolved itself to the point that she was able to greatly reduce her antidepressant medications (with her doctor's supervision, of course).

A young child who presented with a great deal of emotional instability was similarly found to be sensitive to grains, especially when they were eaten in combination with dairy (pizza, for example). Once we eliminated the grains for a period of time, her emotions settled down nicely.

How can you tell if an allergy is causing your mood disorder? Food allergies can be dauntingly difficult to discover. Review Lesson I-10. There are several tests that can help determine the presence or influence of allergies. Many doctors recommend an IgG or IgE blood test that measures these specific immune bodies that indicate a problem with either immediate or delayed reactivities to foods. Ask your doctor which test he/she prefers. You may also choose to do the pulse test (see pages 47–48), either with or without the blood work. If your mood disorder is partially caused by allergies or intolerance to food, you'll want to solve that problem.

You are keeping a Food Diary, aren't you? Because any food can be problematic, you need to keep careful records of everything you eat and drink. Note any symptoms, especially mental or emotional symptoms, in your Food Diary, and study it weekly to see whether you can track a trend in a specific food or combination of foods.

If you believe you have discovered a potential link between a food and a mood, eliminate that food for at least seven days and see whether your mood improves. If it does, reintroduce a small amount of the suspected food to see whether it again triggers a mood problem. If it does, you will want to eliminate that food completely for at least six months to clear your system of it totally. Sometimes people are able to then eat small amounts of the food without suffering a relapse in their mood disorder, but this outcome varies from person to person.

If you find that you cannot successfully do this detective work, get a professional to help you. Seek the counsel of a nutritionally trained physician or a nutritionist who has experience working with food allergies and intolerances. And don't be embarrassed if you cannot figure it out yourself. It can be difficult!

NATURAL STRATEGIES FOR IMPROVING MOOD

Whoever declares that a weight challenge is simply a matter of eating too much food, or the wrong kinds of food, has no idea! It really is very complicated. But that does not mean you cannot solve your particular issue(s). If you have been doing your weekly assignments, you have probably already discovered many of your triggers and are well on your way to resolving them. This lesson is simply another step in your journey toward good health. Just learning that depression can lead to becoming overweight is half of the battle—let's finish it.

Earlier, this lesson briefly listed some of the common causes of depression and other mood disorders. Many of those causes are related to nutrition and/or lifestyle. The good news is that you can do a great deal to improve your mood! Take these steps toward improved mental health:

1. Follow the Wings meal plan! In other words, eat

several small, well-balanced meals per day to maintain steady blood sugar. Hypoglycemia is a common cause of depression, and, is easily resolved by good nutritional habits. If necessary, follow the Two-Hour Diet protocol (pages 253–255 in the Menus and Recipes section) for even better blood sugar control.

2. Nutrient deficiencies or imbalances often cause depression. Some of the common culprits are magnesium deficiency, zinc deficiency (or excessive copper in relation to zinc, described in #5 below), B-complex vitamin deficiency, and/or essential fatty acid deficiency. Ask your Wings nutritionist (at www.flywithwings.com/pnc.html, click on MyPro Connect) to recommend a supplement that can help ease mild-to-moderate depression, and include these nutrients in your supplement program:

   ▪ Magnesium citrate or Krebs cycle metabolites (300+ milligrams per day)

   ▪ Zinc citrate (30–50 milligrams per day)

   ▪ B-complex vitamins (a well-rounded supple-

Don't Take Too Much

Check the labels on all your supplements and add up the amount of each nutrient you are taking in order not to exceed the levels given above (unless you are under the care of a nutritionally trained physician or nutritionist).

- If you are taking too much magnesium, you will get diarrhea.

- If you are taking too much zinc, or taking it with too little food, you will feel nauseated.

- Taking B-complex vitamins can often cause a "niacin flush," which makes the skin on your face, neck, arms, and hands tingle and turn red—a harmless but uncomfortable sensation. Always take your B-complex vitamins with food to avoid a niacin flush.

- If you take too much vitamin C at one time, you will feel gassy or get diarrhea. This is harmless and passes quickly.

- If you are taking a blood-thinning medication, be careful not to overuse salmon-body oil, because it is a natural blood thinner.

- If you are scheduled for any type of surgery, please inform your doctor that you are taking these supplements, in order to avoid excessive bleeding or any other complications.

ment with at least 50 milligrams per microgram of each nutrient)

   ▪ Vitamin C (buffered, 2,000–5,000 milligrams, in divided doses)

   ▪ Salmon-body oil and/or flaxseed oil (3–5 grams) in addition to olive oil (2–3 tablespoons), daily

3. I strongly urge you to seek the professional counsel of a nutritionist who can help you determine the presence of food and/or environmental allergies, and/or other nutrient imbalances. If you do not know of a nutritionist in your area, see the Resource Guide to find one.

4. Ask your doctor to test your blood for iron deficiency, a common cause of lowered mood.

5. Accumulated toxic metals can cause mood disorders. Lead, for example, has been causally linked to learning disorders and several mood disorders. Mercury lodges in nerve tissue and has been causally linked to several types of mental and/or emotional disorders. Generally, the best tests to identify the presence of toxic metals and learn your toxic metal load are a hair analysis and a packed-erythrocyte test. See the Resource Guide to find laboratories that can perform these tests or a physician in your area who can treat you. Seek the help of a physician who is board certified in chelation therapy, which removes toxic metals.

   Although copper is an essential nutrient, when copper becomes dominant over zinc (as is typical in estrogen dominance or in severe mental disorders), severe mood disorders can result. Symptoms of copper-to-zinc imbalance include aggression, hostility, extreme depression to the point of suicidal ideation, food and other allergies, white spots on the fingernails, distaste for protein foods (and cravings for bread and pasta), and learning disabilities. If you, or someone you love, display several of these characteristics, get professional help immediately. Correcting a zinc-to-copper imbalance requires the assistance of a competent nutritionist or a nutritionally trained physician (not all physicians recognize the significance of this imbalance).

6. As you learned in Module II, mild-to-moderate aerobic exercise can be as effective in reducing depression as many antidepressant medications. Aerobic exercise also stimulates the production of endorphins, our feel-good hormones. Want to get some endorphins flowing? Exercise! If you don't

A Note of Warning about Depression

If you are truly depressed, you may not have the physical or mental energy to take care of yourself. Depression can manifest itself as an inability to care for oneself. If you feel you cannot take the steps outlined in the following material, give this section to a loved one who can understand it, support you (not criticize you), and help you through it. He/she can help facilitate your journey toward mental health and vitality.

If you have had thoughts of suicide or of otherwise harming yourself, please seek professional help immediately. Don't take chances with your life. You may not feel that life is worth living, but take heart: when your mind is working better, when you are not as depressed, you will find that you can take a great deal of pleasure in life. Seek help today!

enjoy exercise, do it with a friend or spouse who will help you stick to your commitment.

7. If you have not resolved your stress issues, start working on that today. To what activities can you say no? How can you bring your stress—and your life—under control? Unrelenting stress can actually cause a form of depression. Nourish your adrenal glands, as discussed in Lesson III-4; when your adrenals begin to recover their vibrant energy, your mood will lift and life will feel like it is worth living again.

8. Start going to bed each night before 10:00 P.M., sleep in a pitch-dark room, and get at least eight hours of sleep per night. There is nothing to be gained by staying up later than you should. Sleep deprivation is a common cause of depression and a common cause (believe it or not) of weight gain. Take a nap! Insomnia and fatigue are serious problems; if you struggle with a sleep disorder, seek professional help.

9. If you suspect that you may suffer from SAD, check the Internet or the library for information on light therapy. For a very small amount of money, you can greatly improve your mental well-being, simply by spending a few minutes each day in bright light.

10. Depression and other mood disorders can be caused by hypothyroidism or an estrogen-to-progesterone imbalance. Have you resolved these issues yet, or are you at least working on them? Hormonal problems usually won't be solved by psychotherapy. Follow the suggestions given in Lessons III-2 through III-6 for balancing your endocrine organs.

11. Last, but very important, although these suggestions are very powerful and very effective in solving most forms of mood disorder, some people suffer from depression for which the cause is unknown. After working your way through each of the steps above, re-evaluate your mood. If you are still depressed, please seek professional help immediately. If you know someone who suffers from a mood disorder and has been unable to resolve it following these steps, please take him/her for professional help. Depression can be life threatening. Sometimes prescription medications are necessary; sometimes people are better served by counseling. There is no reason to continue to suffer when help is available.

Well, that is about it—but that is a lot, isn't it? Whew!

Measuring Up

It's that time again . . . Weigh yourself, and then take five girth measurements: bust at the largest point, waist at two inches above the navel, hips at the largest point, and right and left thigh circumference at the point where your extended fingertips reach with your arms hanging down at your sides. Record these figures, and your calculated BMI value, on your Progress Chart.

And now, go to page 277 for your new recipes!

 TODAY'S ASSIGNMENT

TAKE CARE OF YOURSELF

Go through the list of depression symptoms at the beginning of this week's lesson. If you feel that you are suffering from depression, follow the natural antidepressant strategies listed above. Start today! After working on each of these strategies (alone or with a helper), you should feel empowered to take control of your mood and your health. I am excited to present this information to you because I know that, as you follow these suggestions, your health will improve. Your mind will clear. You will feel better than you have felt in years—and you'll take another giant step forward in resolving your weight issues. How good is that?!

Depression is exhausting. Depressed individuals often do not have the emotional or mental strength to take the suggestions listed above. If you are depressed but do not feel that you have the ability to "do the work," please show this chapter to your accountability partner, a loved one, or someone else who can help you.

LESSON III-8 STUDY GUIDE

1. List five or more common causes of depression.

2. How does depression affect weight management?

3. Briefly explain the (complex) role of nutrition in depression.

4. List some strategies for resolving the nutritional issues in depression.

5. What is SAD and how does it influence eating behavior?

6. Explain how neurotransmitters influence eating behaviors, and how eating behaviors influence the balance of neurotransmitters.

7. Go back to Lesson III-7 and review how antidepressant medications affect weight management.

8. Explain how food allergies can cause depression, and list the foods most commonly linked to mood disorders.

9. List ten natural strategies for reducing depression.

HEALTH TIP

LET'S CLEAR THE AIR

We all know that we should stop smoking; we all know the dangers. But quitting can be more difficult than "just saying no." Nicotine is very addictive! There is some evidence that nicotine is even more addictive to women than men, and women may find it even more difficult to quit. The good news, however, is that many natural products can help you break the habit.

- Try taking the herb *Avena sativa* to relieve nicotine cravings.

- The amino acid L-glutamine is also good for relieving addiction to nicotine or other substances.

- Increase your intake of vitamin C, vitamin A, and zinc to support the immune system and heal the mucous membranes in the lungs. If you have smoked for a long time, it is particularly important to increase your vitamin C levels, as each cigarette "burns" 120 milligrams of vitamin C.

- Drink lots of water to wash the lungs.

- Use a good antioxidant supplement to help repair damaged lung tissue.

- The herb slippery elm helps relieve congestion in the lungs.

- The herbs dandelion and milk thistle protect and heal the liver and help relieve liver congestion.

- Take daily hot showers or use a sauna to help detoxify the body.

- Use the Wings cleansing protocol (Lesson II-6) to clear toxins out of the body, and take several tablespoons of fiber supplement daily (Nature's Secret Ultimate Fiber is one of my favorites).

- I strongly urge you to try Juice Plus+, a fruit and vegetable supplement that has been clinically shown to make it easier to stop smoking.

ADDITIONAL NOTES

Lesson III-9. Leptin, Human Growth Hormone, and Cortisol

Research results are often published in the mainstream press long before the claims have been thoroughly tested and reviewed by the scientific community. Because being overweight is such a huge problem in our society, the pharmaceutical company that actually concocts a magic pill to reduce weight will make a staggering amount of money. So don't be surprised if you read in your favorite women's magazine that someone finally found it—the pill that will make it all go away without diet or exercise or lifestyle changes. But (more so) don't be surprised when you read a few weeks later that (1) it didn't work, or (2) people were injured or killed by using it. Remember fen-phen?

?   **TODAY'S QUESTION**

How gullible are you?

_____

_____

_____

_____

How desperate are you to lose weight? Enough to buy into the latest "cure" that hits the market? If someone offered you a magic pill or lotion to make your fat melt off your body like butter on a hot sum-mer day, would you buy it? How much would you be willing to spend?

Hardly a week goes by that someone, somewhere, doesn't offer a new lotion or potion to cause weight loss, usually with "no lifestyle changes necessary." How silly is that?! And yet, the American consumer must be gullible enough to purchase these products, because they keep appearing in the marketplace. Equally frustrating is the supermarket's magazine section: virtually every magazine on the shelf offers a new weight-loss theory on the front cover, usually right next to a picture of a new junk food. Dreadful!

When will we learn that weight loss and health management are achieved by making significant lifestyle changes, and that we promote good health by good food and lifestyle choices? There are no short-cuts! Despite the millions of dollars spent in the research laboratory, it really all comes back to the same thing: Satisfy the needs of the body. Heal the body. Restore strength and vitality to the body so it can lose weight naturally. Granted, there isn't a lot of money to be made in selling organic produce and ocean-raised fish! But the health benefits to you are enormous.

One of the goals of the Wings Program is to teach you about your body so you are not vulnerable to the weight-loss sales pitches that flood the market. Today's lesson will explore a couple of weight-loss research projects that, so far, haven't resulted in much success—and one interesting research project that is actually very promising.

LEPTIN

The hormone leptin is synthesized and secreted by fat cells (adipocytes). Leptin is believed to regulate the amount of body fat, as leptin's concentration seems to

✒ NOTES

_____

_____

_____

_____

_____

_____

be in proportion to the level of body fat in humans. This hormone is the communication link between adipose tissue and the central nervous system: it provides information about satiety (telling the body when it has received enough food) and quiets the appetite. The higher one's leptin level, the lower one's appetite and food intake. Perhaps you are thinking, "How helpful!" But because leptin is secreted by fat cells, less and less leptin is released as you lose weight, thereby increasing your appetite and your tendency to regain the weight. That is definitely not helpful!

Given that high levels of leptin are beneficial for reducing appetite, researchers have hoped that they could provide supplemental leptin in pill form, much like supplementary estrogen or thyroid hormone. The supplement was constructed, and experiments with animals proceeded to human studies. Although it worked moderately well in rats, it hasn't worked well in humans; so at this point, it is not possible to take leptin orally to reduce appetite. Increase your leptin levels naturally, then!

What stimulates leptin production?

- Eating several small meals per day, rather than three (or fewer) larger meals

- Healthy brown fat (helps maintain healthful leptin levels)

- A low-sugar diet (keeps insulin levels down; insulin disrupts leptin production)

- Body fat (sadly)

- Adequate sleep

Conversely, what lowers leptin production?

- Eating larger, infrequent meals (as in one or two large meals per day) or skipping meals

- Loss of body fat (unfortunately)

- A high-sugar diet (stimulates an insulin response)

- A high-fat diet (at least in rats)

- Estrogen (leptin is reduced, for example, in overweight menopausal women)

- Excess male hormone

HUMAN GROWTH HORMONE

Human growth hormone (hGH), also known as somatotropin, is secreted by the pituitary gland. Adequate levels of hGH inhibit the breakdown of lean muscle tissue, help maintain bone size, promote tissue repair, and increase the ability of the body to burn fat (instead of carbohydrates and protein) for energy. The many functions of hGH include the following:

- Causes body cell growth

- Stimulates protein synthesis and inhibits protein breakdown

- Encourages anabolism (increases the rate at which amino acids enter cells and are used to synthesize proteins)

- In childhood and adolescence, increases the growth rate of the skeleton and skeletal muscles

- In adulthood, helps maintain muscle and bone size and promotes tissue repair

- Retards the use of blood sugar for ATP production (cellular energy)

- Stimulates fat catabolism (causes cells to switch from burning carbohydrates and proteins to burning fats for cellular energy)

- Stimulates lipolysis (the breakdown of triglycerides into fatty acids and glycerol) in fat tissue, and encourages other cells to use the fatty acids for energy production, especially during periods of starvation (dieting!)

That may sound like a lot of scientific mumbo jumbo, but notice how many of those functions relate to weight management! Adequate levels of hGH are clearly very important to the dieter.

We naturally produce hGH as children, but its production is diminished as we age. Many characteristics associated with aging are directly related to the amount of hGH available to the body, and can be positively affected if the body's hGH level is increased. The activities of hGH and its mediator, insulin-like growth factor-1 (IGF1), may actually help alter the blueprint of aging by keeping the cells in as healthy a state as possible. It is obvious, then, that we want to maximize our hGH.

Factors that increase hGH production are as follows:

- Low blood sugar

- Decreased fatty acids and increased amino acids in the bloodstream

- Deep sleep (non-REM sleep stages 3 and 4)

- Increased activity of the sympathetic division of the autonomic nervous system

- Vigorous physical exercise

- The hormones glucagon, estrogen, cortisol, and insulin

From that list, you can see that we can increase hGH by keeping our blood sugar on the low side but not too low, allowing ourselves to become hungry before we eat, and eating balanced meals (that is, by following the Wings Program); by getting a good night's sleep; and so on. The only one of the above factors over which we exert little control is the activity of the sympathetic nervous system, such as the stress response (Lesson III-4).

Various factors diminish the production and release of hGH—but aside from growing older, we have some level of control over most of them:

- Increased fatty acids and decreased amino acids in the bloodstream (in other words, eating high-fat, low-protein meals)

- Insulin release and sugar intake

- Increasing age

- REM sleep

- Emotional deprivation

- Obesity

- Hypothyroidism

- The hormone itself, through negative feedback (a negative feedback loop is the body's way of controlling each one of its hormones: when hormone production increases to optimum levels, the negative feedback loop shuts down further production until the hormone falls below a certain minimal level, at which point the negative feedback loop again stimulates the hormone's production)

An item on this last list warrants further explanation: emotional deprivation. Scientists studying the impact of emotional deprivation on babies and young children have found that children who are deprived of a nurturing relationship with a loving caregiver do not grow normally; if the deprivation is severe enough, they can actually die. I wonder how many overweight adults go through life without hugs . . . So many people do not enjoy loving support and face life alone. It has been said that we need twenty hugs per day to be truly healthy. That may be true, and the absence or loss of emotional support may be, for some of us, an issue in our being overweight.

It is known that people who are in a loving, supportive marriage live longer and healthier (on the other hand, being in a "toxic" marriage reduces lifespan). It is known that people who actively participate in religious activities or other forms of fellowship enjoy better health, and that even caring for a pet confers a longer and happier life. So there is something important here for all of us: we all need to participate in community. Actively participating in community also increases the production of hGH, which makes it easier to lose and maintain weight. Amazing!

How can you tell if you are deficient in hGH? Symptoms may include:

- Fatigue

- Increased weight and abdominal obesity

- Decreased lean body mass and decreased muscle mass

- Decreased strength

- Poor sleep

- Impaired sense of well-being

- Reduced exercise capacity and physical performance

- Reduced cardiac performance

Researchers are exploring the use of a pill form of hGH to increase body levels of this important hormone, but the side effects make supplementing with hGH both impractical and potentially unsafe. A concern that has been insufficiently addressed in clinical trials is whether supplemental hGH could stimulate the growth of cancer. There is no way to know whether cancer is developing in a patient's body before clinical work reveals its presence, so it is critically important to avoid using a product that could unwittingly promote tumor growth. (No physician would prescribe hGH to a known cancer patient.)

There is, however, some promising news. Some clinicians recommend taking the hGH precursors arginine and orthinine, amino acids they have found to stimulate muscle growth. Biomed Comm, Inc. has been working on a homeopathic form of hGH that is, apparently, a safe way to encourage the body's own production of the hormone. I encourage you to explore the concept of homeopathic medicine in general, and the use of homeopathic hGH in particular. This particular application of homeopathy is fairly unusual, and the body of research is not large. However, the preliminary research conducted by Biomed Comm, Inc. looks good, so I have started to use their homeopathic hGH in my clinical practice. Safe alternatives to increasing hGH may buffer some of the damaging effects listed above that reduce our body's normal hGH production. (For more information, go to the website www.biomedcomm.com.)

CORTISOL

Cortisol is another major hormone that negatively influences weight management: it pulls down leptin and hGH production, hastens the breakdown of lean muscle tissue, increases the deposition of fat, causes water retention, and has many other side effects. Lesson III-4 covered the problems associated with cortisol and stress in some detail, so there is no need to reiterate them here. Just remember how important it is to minimize stress, get plenty of rest, and reduce your cortisol output.

And now, go to page 277 for your new recipes!

 TODAY'S ASSIGNMENT

INCREASE AND DECREASE

Again, it is time to make a plan. What can you do to increase your production of leptin? Review your Food Diary to make sure you are still following the Wings Program faithfully. If you have reached a weight-loss plateau, increase your number of daily meals while simultaneously keeping the calorie count the same or a little lower. Small, frequent meals increase leptin production and often stimulate weight loss when other techniques have failed. Make sure you avoid all processed sugar, and increase (slightly) the amount of healthful fats like olive oil or avocados. Have you removed all potential allergens from your diet?

What can you do to increase your levels of growth hormone? Consider using the amino acid precursors to hGH. Check out the information on homeopathic hGH at www.biomedcomm.com; you can review the scientific literature and download the company's research to take to your physician for input on the product. The benefits can be very gratifying, particularly if you are over the age of fifty.

Meanwhile, review your lifestyle to consider changes that could boost hGH production. For example, get plenty of rest each night. Rest has many benefits, including increased hGH and reduced cortisol production. Do you retire for the evening no later than 10:00 P.M. and sleep in a pitch-dark room? Improve the quality and duration of your sleep and watch your health improve! Get moderate amounts of exercise, particularly exercise designed to increase lean muscle mass in the large muscles of the body.

1. What is leptin and what function does it serve?

2. Have human trials shown that supplementing leptin increases fat loss?

3. What is hGH and what functions does it serve?

4. What lifestyle and dietary factors reduce the production of hGH?

5. What lifestyle and dietary factors increase the production of hGH?

6. What are the weight and health consequences of producing too much cortisol?

HEALTH TIP

SORE THROAT

Did you wake up this morning with a sore throat? Not to worry! Tackle it head-on with remedies from Mother Nature:

- If your sore throat is a sign of an impending bout of influenza, use a homeopathic flu-preventive remedy (such as Oscillococcinum from Boiron or Flu Solution from Dolisos; Boericke and Tafel Cough and Bronchial Syrup is also a helpful product).

- Do an ascorbic acid flush (pages 8–9) and maintain high levels of vitamin C, vitamin A, and zinc for immune system support.

- Bee propolis (available at health food stores) helps protect mucous membranes and supports immune system function.

- Mushrooms like maitake, shiitake, and reishi are also excellent for the immune system.

- Make an onion-and-garlic tea (recipe on page 181) and sip several cups throughout the day.

- Gargle with a tea of fenugreek or goldenseal root, or with some warm water containing three to four drops of grapefruit-seed extract (goldenseal and grapefruit-seed extract are both intensely bitter but excellent for sore throats).

- Use zinc lozenges throughout the day to kill bacteria lining the throat passage.

- If the sore throat persists for more than a few days, consult your healthcare practitioner.

ADDITIONAL NOTES

Lesson III-10. Squabbling Sisters, Insulin Resistance, and Syndrome X

If you grew up in a family with sisters, you know the petty bickering that can result from borrowed clothes, stolen friends, or a serious case of PMS. I have four daughters, all of whom (at one time or another) have seen themselves as the queen; in fact, one wore a sweatshirt that begged, "All I ask is that you treat me no differently than you treat the Queen . . . " It seems that sisters are always fighting for supremacy. Unfortunately (or thankfully!), they can't all be queen at the same time, and have to take turns. And that is why they fight.

Your body may be going through the same struggle. At different times, under different circumstances, your various hormones rise and fall. Today we will discuss two hormonal "sisters" that wield a huge influence over your health and weight: insulin and glucagon. Each gets to be dominant sometimes; at other times, recessive. They are both important—but they can't both be "queen" at the same time.

? TODAY'S QUESTION

What is your family health history?

_____

_____

_____

Look back into your family tree. How many of your ancestors died from diabetes, heart disease, or cancer (the "Big Three")? How many alcoholics are in your family? Is there any family history of hypoglycemia or other blood sugar problems? Have any family illnesses played out in your personal history?

THE COMPETITION BETWEEN INSULIN AND GLUCAGON

Insulin, a powerful hormone secreted by the beta cells of the pancreas, signals the body's cells to receive blood sugar. Insulin promotes the storage of nutrients as body fat. Insulin causes nutrients to be stored in the liver, muscles, and adipose tissue. The liver is the main site for sugars to be stored as glycogen; when the liver's capacity is reached, the remaining excess sugars are pulled into fat cells and converted into triglycerides for storage. By promoting anabolism, or the synthesis of proteins and triglycerides, insulin increases the deposition of muscle tissue and builds adipose tissue. Insulin also pulls blood sugar into muscle cells for energy production.

Glucagon, secreted by the alpha cells of the pancreas, is insulin's sister hormone and has opposing effects. Glucagon stimulates the breakdown of stored sugars to raise the blood sugar level when it falls below the desired point. By locking onto receptor sites on the liver, glucagon stimulates liver cells to release their glycogen for conversion into glucose, or blood sugar; once the liver's supply of glycogen is exhausted, glucagon stimulates fat cells to release triglycerides for conversion into blood sugar. In this way, glucagon makes stored energy (sugar and fat) available to body tissues at times (such as between meals) when food is not immediately available for absorption.

Insulin and glucagon, working in the proper bal-

🖊 NOTES

_____

_____

_____

_____

_____

_____

The Mother of All Blood Sugar Disorders: Diabetes

Diabetes is the third leading cause of death in the United States, and there are strong indications that the problem is getting worse. We are in the middle of a rising epidemic of type II "adult-onset" diabetes in children—a frightening look at the future.

Signs and symptoms of diabetes are:

- Frequent urination

- Thirst that does not go away

- Frequent eating

- Rapid weight loss

- High blood sugar levels

- Increased susceptibility to infection

- Fatigue or weakness

- Blurred vision

- Itching, numbness, and tingling in the hands and feet

- Leg cramps

Factors that increase your risk of type II diabetes are:

- Overweight

- A sedentary lifestyle

- A diet that is high in fat and calories

- Aging (over the age of forty)

- A family history of diabetes or endocrine diseases

ance with each other, respond to fluctuations in blood sugar between and during meals to help maintain a steady blood sugar level throughout the day. Let's do a quick review: When blood sugar is suddenly high (such as after a high-sugar/high-carbohydrate meal or snack), the pancreas secretes large amounts of insulin to pull excess sugar out of circulation and signal its uptake into the liver and fat cells for storage, and glucagon release is suppressed. When blood sugar falls too low, the pancreas secretes glucagon to pull glycogen out of the liver (and later, triglycerides out of fat cells) to raise bloodstream glucose to an appropriate level, and insulin release is suppressed.

Why is this balancing act so critical? For one thing, maintaining a fairly constant blood sugar level is extremely important to brain function. The brain uses about 20 percent of the available sugar in the bloodstream as its primary fuel; if circulating glucose is too high, the excess can damage the delicate brain tissue. Conversely, low blood sugar, or hypoglycemia, often results when sugars are pulled rapidly from the bloodstream by insulin, which deprives both the brain and the body of fuel. The body can only do two things with excess blood sugar: either burn it immediately for energy or store it as glycogen and body fat.

Stimulation and Suppression Summary

- The major stimulus of insulin release is high blood sugar, although just eating a large meal will also stimulate insulin release.

- Exercise and fasting help suppress insulin release.

- The major stimulus of glucagon release is low blood sugar, although other stimuli include ingestion of the amino acid alanine and release of some of the catecholamines (certain adrenal hormones).

- Eating a high-fat meal suppresses glucagon secretion.

It Really Is Simple . . .

Think back on the information in Module I about how to eat. These principles are so straightforward that we are tempted to doubt their simplicity and to pursue something much harder! Or, to people who don't want to eat real food and have always relied on "meals in a box" or other processed foods, the principles seem complicated simply because they require putting more effort and thought into meal choices. Some "experts" go so far as to say that we must avoid fat—or calories, or protein, or carbohydrates, or whatever—in our attempt to lose weight, but you can see from our discussion of insulin and glucagon that none of these approaches will work.

We've also been told that it doesn't matter what kind of carbohydrates you eat, which is, of course, ridiculous. They will all ultimately affect blood sugar, so whether you choose to eat broccoli or Snicker's bars, as long as you eat the right amount of calories, doesn't really matter—or so they say. Well, that "logic" flies in the face of biochemistry, and of *good* logic, because it actually does make a great deal of difference!

What types of carbohydrates are particularly noted for dysregulating blood sugar levels? Typically, the types discouraged in the Wings Program are sugar, soft drinks, grains, white potatoes, and other proc-

AN ABBREVIATED GLYCEMIC INDEX (GI)

This chart, adapted from a textbook called *Food, Nutrition and Diet Therapy* by Kathleen Mahan and Marian Arlin (Philadelphia, PA: W.B. Saunders Company, 1992), is based on the GI standard of white bread, which is 100. The higher the number is, the faster the blood sugar response is—and the worse the food is for blood sugar stability. (There are probably some surprises in this list!)

Food	Mean GI
White bread	100
Whole-grain bread	100
White spaghetti	45
Whole-grain spaghetti	61
Brown rice	81
White rice	79–84
Sweet corn	80–84
All-Bran cereal	74
Cornflakes	115
Muesli	96
Shredded Wheat	97
Oatmeal cookies	78
Mashed potato	100
Baked russet potato	128
Sweet potato	70
Baked beans, canned	60
Kidney beans	45–56
Peanuts	15
Green peas, frozen	65
Apple	53
Banana	84–91
Orange juice	67
Fructose	31–33
Honey	126
Sucrose	89–91
Potato chips	77
Corn chips	99
Ice cream	52
Skim milk	46

essed starchy foods. The chart on the left shows the relative positions of various foods on the glycemic index (GI), a numerical system measuring how rapidly a carbohydrate food triggers an elevation in circulating blood sugar.

Keep in mind that a food allergy can cause an insulin surge that is unrelated to that food's position on the glycemic index. Cow's milk, though low on the index, is high on the list of common allergenic foods, and consumption of cow's milk has been linked to the development of Syndrome X. There is similar bad news about wheat: some clinicians believe that grains, by causing inflammation of the pancreas, lead directly to an insulin response.

Balancing Your Insulin and Glucagon Responses

Let's look at some basic nutrition principles in light of what we've learned about insulin and glucagon:

1. Natural carbohydrate foods like fresh fruits and vegetables (and to a lesser extent, grains) contain fibers that slow digestion. Because these foods are digested slowly, they are not rapidly converted into sugars, and so these sugars are released slowly into the bloodstream. Therefore, blood sugar does not rise to the point where an insulin response is stimulated.

2. Natural carbohydrate foods contain nutrients like magnesium, chromium, and the B-complex vitamins that help metabolize sugars. Because eating these foods brings those helpful nutrients along with them, the body does not have to "rob" them from other tissues to handle the sudden glut of sugars entering the body.

3. High-fat meals (as in a high-protein or meat diet, for example) slow the release of glucagon.

4. Most refined carbohydrates, including whole-grain and juiced products, stimulate a rapid insulin response; therefore, consuming whole-grain breads and pastas, as well as fruit juices, causes weight gain. *Note:* Read that a few times and let it sink in.

Now let's look at insulin and glucagon in the context of the American diet:

1. We are carbohydrate addicts! If you are a "health nut," your carbohydrates of choice are whole-grain products like bread and pasta; if you aren't, you probably "junk out" on soft drinks, desserts, breakfast cereals, and so on.

2. The typical American breakfast (cereal, toast, and juice) is a high-carbohydrate meal that is sure to stimulate an insulin response.

3. If you are a devotee of the high-protein breakfast (steak, eggs, bacon, and the like), you'll be sure to stimulate a fat-building response, because the release of glucagon is suppressed by a high-fat meal—and when glucagon is low, insulin is high.

4. Coffee, another big part of the American breakfast, has been shown to stimulate an insulin response as well.

Finally, let's look at dieting models: low-fat, high-carbohydrate, or high-protein/high-fat diets all contribute to problems with the "squabbling sisters," insulin and glucagon. From what you now know of these two competing hormones, it should be apparent that you want to encourage the release of glucagon and suppress the release of insulin for healthful weight loss and management. Fortunately, the Wings food plan is designed to do that!

SYNDROME X

Our culture is experiencing an epidemic of insulin-based health challenges. This epidemic leads to a cluster of diseases like heart disease, diabetes, arthritis, and cancer—and at the base of the cluster is our hunger for foods that contain large amounts of sugars, artificial fats, and processed carbohydrates.

One of the first researchers to look at the condition now called Syndrome X was Dr. Gerald Reaven, who noticed in 1988 that many of his patients had a common group of symptoms, including excess weight in the abdomen and upper body, high serum cholesterol, and high serum triglycerides. He called this group of symptoms metabolic syndrome, or Syndrome X, for the unknown factor in the blood sugar dysregulation that he and other doctors were seeing in their patients.

CAUSES AND CONSEQUENCES

Dr. Reaven discovered that in individuals with Syndrome X, the insulin receptor sites on the cell membranes cannot receive the signal from insulin to pull sugar into the cells, so the cells don't pull sugar in, and therefore the blood sugar level spirals upward. The pancreas secretes enough insulin to overcome the resistance, and then high levels of insulin are left to circulate in the bloodstream.

Syndrome X Risk Factors

- Impaired glucose tolerance
- High insulin level (hyperinsulinemia)
- Elevated triglyceride level
- Low level of HDL (the "good" cholesterol)
- Exaggerated postprandial lipemia (slow clearance of fat from the bloodstream after eating)
- Smaller, denser particles of LDL (the "bad" cholesterol)
- Increased propensity of the blood to form clots
- Decreased ability to dissolve blood clots
- Elevated blood pressure

Lifestyle factors that worsen Syndrome X:

- Obesity
- Lack of physical activity
- The wrong diet
- Cigarette smoking

(Adapted from Gerald Reaven, M.D., *Syndrome X* [New York, NY: Simon & Schuster, 2000], 22)

In addition to the Syndrome X risk factors listed in the inset above are eating foods that are high on the glycemic index; lack of exercise; smoking; family history of heart disease, hypertension, or diabetes; and (not stated in Dr. Reaven's literature) deficiencies in the nutrients that are key for balancing blood sugar (B-complex vitamins, magnesium, zinc, chromium, and vanadium). The chronic high levels of insulin produce the cluster of Syndrome X symptoms and lead directly to heart disease.

Understand that insulin is merely trying to do its job: to normalize blood sugar. The real problem is that, because the receptor sites on the cell walls develop insulin resistance and refuse to accept the hormonal message, more and more insulin is produced by the pancreas in a desperate attempt to lower the level of glucose in the bloodstream. Excess insulin, unfortunately, is one in a series of events that triggers the damage to arteries that leads to a heart attack.

In his book *Syndrome X*, Dr. Reaven describes the disease process:

This deadly heart ailment begins in the bloodstream, shortly after we eat. That's not a startling idea, for we know that eating fatty or cholesterol-laden foods can be bad for our hearts. However, the Syndrome X culprit isn't red meat or butter, it's carbohydrates . . . Insulin acts like a shepherd, herding its precious flock into the cellular corrals. Unfortunately, in many of us, glucose behaves like a group of errant sheep, stubbornly refusing to go where the shepherd directs. When that happens, the pancreas pumps out more and more insulin. That's the biochemical equivalent of sending out more and more shepherds to get the sheep into the corrals. Imagine hundreds of shepherds chasing thousands of sheep across a pristine field covered with thick, beautiful green grass. Those hundreds of feet and thousands of hoofs will quickly tear up the field, ripping out or flattening down clumps of grass. Soon, the field that once looked so green and lush will be trampled and scarred, brown and dirty.

Something similar happens inside your body when glucose refuses to move into the storage cells at insulin's command. The interior linings of your arteries, like the grassy field, are ripped and trampled as the body attempts to overcome this problem . . . The damage sets the stage for heart disease. (Gerald Reaven, M.D., *Syndrome X* [New York, NY: Simon & Schuster, 2000], 18–19)

One study notes that the low-fat, high-carbohydrate diet currently recommended by many nutritionists in the United States may not help prevent coronary disease, as it has been purported to do. In fact, eating low-fat, high-carbohydrate foods increases the potential for developing insulin resistance or Syndrome X, thereby increasing the risk of developing heart disease—shocking news for many people! The consumption of carbohydrate foods that are high on the glycemic index (such as highly processed sugars, potatoes, and rice) is actually a better indicator than serum cholesterol of the risk of heart disease. The more highly refined carbohydrates you eat, the greater your risk. This risk factor is even more pronounced in overweight women.

Some researchers believe that Syndrome X causes overweight and obesity, but Dr. Reaven believes the opposite: overweight and obesity are one of the causes of Syndrome X. He writes:

When it comes to insulin resistance/sensitivity . . . obesity is not an either-or situation of being either obese and insulin resistant, or slim and insulin sensitive. Not every obese person is insulin resistant, and not all slender people are insulin sensitive. Obesity is but one of the factors interacting with your genes to determine the ability of your tissues to react to insulin. If you are genetically more insulin sensitive to begin with, weight gain will have a less pronounced effect on your risk of developing Syndrome X. Unfortunately, the opposite is equally true. If you are genetically more insulin resistant, becoming obese can create far more damaging effects. (Reaven, 2000, 59)

We do not yet know if Syndrome X is the cause of being overweight or the result, but at this point, does it really matter? We do know from the research that overweight and Syndrome X are causally linked in one direction or the other. We do know that reducing weight reduces insulin resistance and Syndrome X. So we have nothing to lose (but our excess weight!) by following a heart-protective, weight-protective, anti-Syndrome X program like Wings.

BLOOD SUGAR CONTROL FOR PREVENTING AND TREATING DISEASE

The first step in reducing your risk of developing Syndrome X (or its progression) is to eliminate all processed carbohydrates and processed fats and follow the Wings Program. Within days of beginning the Wings meal plan, blood sugar, cholesterol, and triglyceride levels tend to normalize; in virtually every case, sticking to the meal plan results in diminishing each of the risk factors for Syndrome X. Exercise further reduces the risk of Syndrome X and of consequent cardiovascular disease. How powerful this program is!

According to a monograph from Integrative Medicine Access on diabetes mellitus, the following nutritional therapy (along with eating natural foods and maintaining dietary balance among protein, carbohydrates, and fats) can be used to reduce your risk of developing diabetes, and I believe it can also reduce your risk of developing Syndrome X. I encourage you to follow their recommendations for maximizing blood sugar control by taking:

- Fish oil and evening primrose oil (essential fats), to help the body use insulin and help prevent the cardiovascular and neurological complications of diabetes

- Pycnogenol or grapeseed extract, to help support vascular health

- B-complex vitamins, to help control blood sugar levels: biotin (300 micrograms, or mcg), B_1 (50–100 mg), B_2 (50 mg), B_3 (100 mg), B_6 (50–100 mg), B_{12} (100–1,000 mcg), and folate (400 mcg)

- Vitamin C (2–3 grams), to reduce oxidative damage

- Vitamin E (400 IU), possibly to reduce insulin requirements

- Magnesium (400 mg), to help arteries and help maintain blood sugar control

- Manganese (500–1,000 mcg), to help stabilize blood sugar

- Zinc (30 mg), to decrease glucose levels

- Coenzyme Q_{10} (50–100 mg taken twice per day, or up to 200 mg daily)

- Vanadium (5–10 mg), to normalize cholesterol

Coffee (Sorry, folks!)

Coffee is the number-one psychoactive drug used in the world today, and its use is growing (high schools are even starting to install coffee bars—a truly horrific idea). Because I take a strong "water only" position on beverages, I am constantly asked about coffee.

We know that caffeine increases release of the "stress hormone" cortisol (as well as epinephrine and norepinephrine), increased cortisol release leads to increased fat deposition (especially in the face, waist, trunk, and abdomen), and cortisol elevations are also responsible for elevations in blood pressure and stress reactivity. Here is a brief review of some pertinent literature on caffeine and coffee as related to weight, insulin resistance, and heart disease.

- Caffeine ingestion may lead to insulin resistance. In one study, ingestion of fairly small amounts of caffeine by young, fit males resulted in a prolonged insulin elevation that did not result in a lower blood glucose level, as blood glucose levels were 24 percent greater in the caffeine-treated group. (T. E. Graham, P. Sathasivam, M. Rowland, et al., "Caffeine Ingestion Elevates Plasma Insulin Response in Humans during an Oral Glucose Tolerance Test," *Canadian Journal of Physiology and Pharmacology* 2001, Vol. 79: 559–565.)

- Caffeine ingestion may induce an insulin-dependent rise in blood glucose levels. Investigating the effects of 200 milligrams (mg) of caffeine on glucose tolerance, researchers found the glycemic curve (blood sugar elevation) was normal in all participants and similar between the test and control groups until the second hour, when blood sugar continued to rise for four hours in the caffeine-treated group, although blood insulin levels were comparable in both groups. (A. Pizziol, V. Tikhonoff, C. D. Paleari, et al., "Effects of Caffeine on Glucose Tolerance: A Placebo-

Controlled Study." *European Journal of Clinical Nutrition* 1998, Vol. 52:846–849)

- Coffee "has been shown to acutely reduce sensitivity to insulin." (R. M. van Dam, E. J. Reskens, "Coffee Consumption and Risk of Type II Diabetes Mellitus," *Lancet* 2002, Vol. 360:1477–1478) Reduced insulin sensitivity is, of course, a symptom of Syndrome X.

- Researchers found coffee stimulated metabolic rate in both obese and normal-weight individuals, but the normal-weight individuals had greater fat oxidation, which is a causative factor in atherogenesis (buildup of fatty material in the arteries). (K. J. Acheson, B. Zahorska-Markiewicz, P. Pittet, et al., "Caffeine and Coffee: Their Influence on Metabolic Rate and Substrate Utilization in Normal Weight and Obese Individuals" *American Journal of Clinical Nutrition* 1980, Vol. 33:989–997)

- A study found ingesting 500 mg of caffeine (for reference, there is 58–259 mg of caffeine in an average cup of coffee) significantly raised blood pressure, reduced average heart rate by two beats per minute, increased epinephrine levels by 32 percent throughout the day and evening, and amplified increases in blood pressure and heart rate associated with high levels of self-reported stress during the activities of the day. The researchers noted that "effects were undiminished through the evening until bedtime." (J. D. Lane, C. F. Pieper, and B. G. Phillips-Bute, "Caffeine Affects Cardiovascular and Neuroendocrine Activation at Work and Home," *Psychosomatic Medicine* 2002, Vol. 64: 595–603)

These are only a few reasons of the reasons that I discourage drinking coffee if you want to lose weight, avoid cardiovascular disease, and otherwise be healthy!

■ Chromium picolinate (200 mcg), to help normalize sugar metabolism

Note: Don't *add* all of these nutrients to your current supplement program; just make sure that all of your supplement sources *add up* to the listed levels.

The following herbs are helpful as well: garlic, onion, bilberry, and fenugreek. Drink two to four cups of tea from these herbs per day. (For more detail, see the "Diabetes Mellitus Monograph" [Newton, MA: Integrative Medicine Communications, 2000], 979C.) You'll find my recipe for onion-and-garlic tea on page 181; you may also use garlic and onions generously in your general cooking for the same benefits.

And now, go to page 278 for your new recipes!

 ## TODAY'S ASSIGNMENT

REDUCE YOUR RISK

Review your lifestyle, your family health history, and the following Health Tip. Are there indications that you may be at risk for developing Syndrome X, heart disease, or stroke? If you have several of the risk factors for the development of Syndrome X, speak with a nutritionally trained physician so he/she can assist you in lowering your risk.

Cravings for sugar or other processed carbohydrates should diminish greatly or disappear altogether on the supplement program described in this lesson; if they do not, please seek the counsel of your nutritionist to help get those cravings under control. (Contact your Wings nutritionist at www.flywith wings.com/pnc.html by clicking on MyProConnect.)

Review the list on pages 173–174 of the nutrients that help reduce the likelihood of developing Syndrome X. Are you getting enough of them? Be particularly careful about your intake (and dosage) of magnesium, zinc, chromium, and B-complex vitamins, as each of these nutrients is critically important in maintaining stable blood sugar. Remember also that you need about 35 grams of fiber daily.

LESSON III-10 STUDY GUIDE

1. What are the two "squabbling sisters"?

2. Define and describe the symptom profile of Syndrome X.

3. What is the glycemic index? What foods are highest on the index?

4. Describe the roles of insulin and glucagon.

5. How does low blood sugar affect the brain? What about high blood sugar?

6. What is insulin resistance?

7. List some of the effects of caffeine on insulin.

8. Outline the supplement protocol for treating Syndrome X, as taken from the Integrative Medicine Access monograph.

HEALTH TIP

SELF-ASSESSMENT FOR RISK OF SYNDROME X AND HEART ATTACK

Read the following list of risk factors, total your points, and refer to the risk chart to assess your risk of heart attack.

- Fasting glucose level is greater than 100, or your glucose level at two hours into the glucose tolerance test is greater than 140   (3 points) _____

- Fasting triglyceride level is greater than 200   (3 points) _____

- Fasting HDL-cholesterol level is lower than 35   (3 points) _____

- Blood pressure is greater than 145/90 (3 points) _____

- Weight check reveals you are more than 15 pounds overweight   (1 point) _____

- Family has a history of heart disease, high blood pressure (hypertension), or diabetes   (1 point) _____

- Lifestyle is characterized by physical inactivity during both work and leisure time   ($1/2$ point) _____

TOTAL POINTS _____

RISK CHART

If you scored:	Your risk of heart attack triggered by Syndrome X is:
0–4 points	Low
5–8 points	Moderate
9–12 points	High
13 points or more	Very high

Adapted from Gerald Reaven, M.D., *Syndrome X* (New York, NY: Simon & Schuster, 2000, 68).

ADDITIONAL NOTES

Lesson III-11. Environmental Fat Producers

Whether you live in a pristine, pastoral meadow or in the middle of a bustling city, you cannot escape pollution. Pollution is literally everywhere on the planet. Unfortunately, pollutants not only endanger our health by causing birth defects, cancer, mental and emotional disturbances, and more, but they may also increase our risk of gaining weight, and may make it harder to lose unwanted weight. The home is said to be the most polluted place of all. Scary, isn't it? And yet, we are so accustomed to chemicals that we don't realize how intrusive they have become. We cannot even imagine a life without chemicals! But that is not the way we were designed to live: we were designed to live in a beautiful, clean, healthy environment. We've messed it up. This week, we look at the world around us.

? TODAY'S QUESTION

What is the extent of your chemical exposure?

_____

_____

_____

Answer the following questions to get an idea of how many toxic chemicals you are exposed to on a daily basis (it may shock you):

- What kind of toothpaste do you use?
- What kinds of soaps do you use for bathing or face and hand washing?
- What kind of shampoo do you use?
- Do you use bubble-bath products?
- Do you ever use an antidandruff shampoo?
- Is your water fluoridated or chlorinated?
- What kind of dish-washing detergent is used in your home?
- What kind of laundry detergent is used in your home?
- Do you use bleach and/or fabric softeners in your laundry?
- Do you use spray starch on your clothing?
- Do you use chemical pesticides in your home?
- Is your home carpeted?
- What products are used to clean the carpet?
- Is your home damp?
- Is any mold growing in air-conditioning units or air shafts?
- Are your lawn and property chemically treated?
- Do you walk or play on a chemically treated lawn?
- What cleaning products are used in your work or school environment?

✐ NOTES

_____

_____

_____

_____

_____

_____

_____

- What other chemical products are used in your work or school environment?

- Is your work or school facility free from molds and fungus?

- Are pesticides used on the premises of your work or school facility?

- Do any family members wear perfume?

- Do any family members use perfumed skin-care products?

- Do you use perfumed skin-care products?

- Are your clothes professionally dry-cleaned?

- Do you use air fresheners in your home or car?

- Do you use gas heat or a gas kitchen range?

- Do you use a gas fireplace?

- Do you have numerous houseplants? Is mold growing around the plants?

- Do you use art materials?

- Do you use spot-removal products on your carpets or furniture?

- Do you regularly shampoo your furniture?

- Do any of your family members smoke?

- Do you use a woodstove?

- Do you use aluminum or nonstick cookware?

- What types of cleaning products do you use in your home?

- Do you use a chemical oven cleaner?

- Are your cabinets or other furniture made from particleboard?

- Do you use plastic eating utensils?

- Do you use plastic food wraps and/or storage containers?

- Do you use plastics in a microwave oven?

- Do you use rat and mouse killers in the kitchen?

- Do you use silver polish or other metal cleaners?

- Do you eat canned or otherwise packaged foods?

- Do you drink water from plastic containers?

- Does anyone in your home use aerosol hairspray?

- Are any other aerosol products used in the home?

- Is scented toilet paper or facial tissue used in the house?

- Is a vinyl shower curtain used in the bathrooms in your home?

- Is your mattress fireproofed?

- Do you use mothballs in your home?

- Do you use no-iron bedsheets?

- Do you wear permanent-press clothing?

Perhaps a simpler question, to make the same point, might be: Do you live in this world? We cannot avoid these exposures to chemicals unless we leave the world entirely.

Lessons II-6 and II-7 discussed cleaning up our internal environment through body cleansing; today you will discover why internal cleansing is becoming more important. This lesson provides a brief overview of how commonly used synthetic materials affect our health—and our weight. You will also learn about how to eliminate as many chemical exposures as possible in an effort to clean up your personal world for better health.

YOU ARE BEING EXPOSED

Every item on the questionnaire above points to another chemical exposure. We do not even think about most of these items; the chemicals are very familiar parts of our lives. We may not even realize that the products we use are not natural.

It would be helpful to have more specific information about how environmental pollutants cause weight gain. Unfortunately, science is not exploring the health consequences of constant exposure to the vast world of synthetic chemicals. In particular, there is a lack of research on the cumulative effects of these chemicals, that is, the effects of being exposed to thousands of different chemicals at a time.

A growing body of information, however, is pointing an accusing finger at many of the chemicals on which we are so dependent. We may not know *exactly* how they affect us, but we know that they do. From the perspectives of biology and biochemistry, we are beginning to catch a glimpse of an enormous and growing problem. No one really knows how many synthetic chemicals we are exposed to, but it is estimated that tens of thousands are on the market for use in the environment and in food, and that 5,000 new chemicals are designed each year. These chemicals have a variety of effects on living organisms, including us humans.

Synthetic chemicals differ from naturally occurring chemicals in their physiological effects. The body produces enzymes that break down and eliminate endogenous chemicals (that is, those made by the body), and it produces detoxifying proteins that escort toxins out of the tissues and out of the body. The body does not, however, produce enzymes that break down synthetic chemicals, which resist normal breakdown pathways and accumulate in various body tissues. Fat tissue, for example, often serves as a type of "toxic-waste storage-depot site" for chemicals that the body cannot excrete or break down in the liver.

The Damage Done

We are now seeing evidence of damage all over the world, in the animal kingdom and in humans, directly related to chemical exposure. Sometimes the damage shows up in anatomical abnormalities, at other times in behavioral changes, fertility, sexual orientation, or mothering or fathering instincts. Being exposed to these chemicals is like having static on the telephone line, and this static frequently messes up the messages being sent by the endocrine system. Here are some frightening examples:

- Of the 209 compounds classified as PCBs (polychlorinated biphenyls), the 75 dioxins and the 135 furans exert a myriad of endocrine-disrupting effects.

- One researcher noted that dioxin may affect the sexual behavior of male pups exposed early in life, suggesting that it had interfered with the sexual differentiation of the brain. At maturity, these males showed diminished male sexual behavior and increased propensity to exhibit feminized sexual behavior.

- You may be aware that pesticides like DDT have an estrogenic effect; studies have shown that chemicals with estrogenic effects feminize roosters. What do such chemicals do to human males and females?

- Certain types of plastics emit a chemical that gives rise to a compound called nonylphenol that acts like an estrogen, causing rampant growth of breast cancer or causing the lining of the uterus to proliferate. These plastics are used in industrial detergents, pesticides, and personal-care products.

- Other types of plastics (like those found in plastic storage jugs for water) emit an estrogenlike substance called bisphenol A.

- Other chemicals disrupt the enzymes in the brain, particularly affecting acetylcholine, one of the most important transmitters for cognition.

- One class of fungicides inhibits the body's ability to produce the steroid hormones from which estrogen, progesterone, and testosterone are synthesized.

- Another group of compounds depletes steroid hormones by accelerating their breakdown and elimination, leaving the body short of these needed compounds.

- Other chemicals deactivate the enzymes that break down used hormones for excretion.

All in all, such synthetic chemicals wield powerful influences over the human body, especially for infants and children, who are more vulnerable than adults to infinitesimally small amounts. Often, the greatest damage occurs when low doses are used, rather than high doses. The damage may not show up for years or decades, making it virtually impossible to correlate it to chemical exposure. (For more information about the effects of chemicals on weight and weight loss, read Dr. Paula Baillie-Hamilton's book *The Body Restoration Plan: Eliminate Chemical Calories and Repair Your Body's Natural Slimming System* [New York, NY: Avery Publishing Group, 2003]).

WHAT CAN WE DO ABOUT IT?

Because we cannot change the larger world, we'll have to settle for changing our personal worlds. There are many practical steps you can take to reduce your exposure to chemicals in your home, your workplace, and the environments immediately surrounding them.

- Wherever possible, avoid the use of pesticides, herbicides, and fungicides. Seek natural ways of discouraging pests, especially by keeping your home clean and dry.

- Avoid the use of plastics whenever possible.

- Never microwave in plastic containers (you should not use a microwave oven anyway!).

- Cool foods before storing them in plastic containers.

- Do not wrap food in plastics unless it is unavoidable.

- Never chew on plastic material.

- Switch from chemical cleaning materials to natural cleaning products (carried in health food stores) that clean just as effectively as their chemical counterparts. Plain white vinegar is one of the best cleaning agents on the market.

- Never use perfumed or scented products; if you can smell it, molecules of the substance are entering your body.

- Begin converting your personal-care products to more natural alternatives; avoid hairspray, spray deodorants, perfumes, shampoos, and other chemical-laden hygiene and cosmetic products. Shop at health food stores that provide natural substitutes for these items.

- Does your toothpaste contain chemicals? Switch to a natural toothpaste.

- Don't use mouthwash, or switch to a chemical-free product.

- Never use bubble-bath products.

- Use natural soaps without chemicals and artificial scenting agents.

- What is your source of drinking water? Avoid chlorinated and fluoridated water.

- Install a water-purification system in your home that purifies all incoming water, not just your drinking water. A hot shower releases numerous toxic chemicals through the water and into the air, and many are easily absorbed by the body.

- Whenever possible, remove the carpets from your home and replace them with tile or wood floors; carpets can never be truly cleaned, and carpet-cleaning agents contain very dangerous chemicals.

- When installing new furniture, pressboard, flooring, and the like in a home or work environment, leave the windows open and use fans to outgas the fumes. Purchase plants that absorb these gases (spider plants, for example).

- Don't occupy a newly refurbished home until it has outgassed to the point that it no longer carries a smell. Even still, leave the windows open in your sleeping area for several weeks, and blow the air outside the home.

- Keep your home free from mold by keeping it dry. Except for your spider plants, use as few potted plants as possible, because potted plants are a common source of mold. (Although mold is natural, it can cause significant health problems.)

- If you send clothes to the dry-cleaners, let them outgas by removing the plastic wrap before you bring them into your home.

- Don't use chemical air fresheners or scented candles.

- Don't use gas appliances; they leak dangerous fumes.

- Don't use synthetic wood products in an indoor fireplace.

- Don't use aluminum cookware.

Kind of a scary list, isn't it?

Obviously, we cannot "de-chemicalize" our personal worlds overnight. This will be a lifelong process. The benefit, however, will also be lifelong: greatly reduced exposure to chemicals that cause ill health and impede weight loss. Lessening exposure to estrogenic chemicals brings our own hormones into better balance, which helps us with weight management. We will also not have to create so many internal toxic-waste storage-depot sites (fat cells) to deal with the onslaught of materials for which our bodies have no use.

And now, go to page 279 for your new recipes!

 ## TODAY'S ASSIGNMENT

GET RID OF AS MANY CHEMICALS AS POSSIBLE

It was hard enough to break some of your eating habits; now you have to change some lifestyle habits. Keeping in mind your results from this lesson's environmental toxin questionnaire, put a plan together for reducing your chemical exposure. You'll need to attack the list of changes one step at a time, because this is a difficult project. Look at this as a chance to really "clean your house."

LESSON III-11 STUDY GUIDE

1. List five or more of the most common sources of chemical exposure.

   _____

   _____

   _____

   _____

2. What are two significant ways that chemicals "mess up" the endocrine system?

   _____

   _____

   _____

3. List some common problems (in animals and humans) that may be caused by chemical exposure.

_____

_____

_____

4. What effects may PCBs have on the human body?

_____

_____

_____

5. What effects may dioxin have on the human body?

_____

_____

_____

6. List seven or more ways to detoxify your home and work environments.

_____

_____

_____

HEALTH TIP

ONION-AND-GARLIC TEA

This brew is wonderful for supporting your immune system and helping you get over a cold or flu. Place 1 tablespoon of minced onion and 1–2 cloves of minced garlic in a mug, add boiling water, and let the vegetables steep. Drink the "tea" when it is cool enough. Your breath may smell bad, but natural compounds in these vegetables inhibit inflammation, and garlic is also a mild antibiotic.

ADDITIONAL NOTES

_____

_____

_____

_____

_____

_____

_____

_____

_____

_____

_____

_____

_____

Lesson III-12. Don't Forget Your Numbers

Certain lessons are simply too important to learn just once. With all the information covered in Module III, some important health tools from Modules I and II may have gotten lost, so let's refresh your memory by revisiting the issues of pH balance and body temperature.

? **TODAY'S QUESTION**

Does your body need a tune-up?

_____

_____

_____

_____

Your body is a finely tuned machine that works best at very specific settings. Different organs, for example, have precise pH requirements. Saliva should be slightly alkaline, but this varies considerably depending on food consumption and the body's alkaline reserves. Some nutritionists believe that the pH of the first morning saliva is a more reliable test of overall health than the pH of the first morning urine. An ideal salivary pH progression in the morning is 6.8 upon awakening, 7.0 before eating, and 8.5 after breakfast.

Stomach juices, on the other hand, should be highly acidic (around 1.5 pH). Upon exiting a suffi-ciently acidic stomach, chyme (the mass of partially digested food) is then alkalinized by bicarbonate from the pancreas, because during final digestion in the small intestine, proper absorption of the nutrients in the chyme is highly dependent upon alkaline pH.

Urine should be slightly alkaline, and even more importantly, blood needs to be slightly alkaline, with a pH of 7.35–7.45. The pH of the first morning urine, which is indicative of the blood's acidity or alkalinity, should be within a range of about 6.5 to about 7.5, bridging the neutrality point of 7.0—ideally, 7.35–7.45. If the first morning urine is acidic (as is common for people eating a typical American diet), the body's pH is almost certainly out of balance, which can lead to serious health challenges if not corrected. (For a complete picture, you should test your first morning saliva along with your first morning urine, and compare your results to the numbers above.)

MINERALIZE! ALKALINIZE! RESTORE YOUR PH!

Many factors, including diet—and dieting—can keep urine and blood in an undesirably acidic state. All proteins, grains, refined sugars, soft drinks, and so on are foods that leave an acidic residue. Although the Atkins Diet can be a highly effective weight-loss program for many people, it is based almost entirely on acid-producing foods, that is, meat, with minimal amounts of alkalinizing vegetables and fruits. Ironically, vegetarian diets can also be acid-forming if they are based on grains and legumes instead of other vegetables. (It may be hard to believe, but many vegetarians actually eat very few vegetables!)

Stress can quickly acidify the urine, as can fatigue or illness. Perhaps most commonly, however, acidification occurs when buffering minerals like calcium,

✎ **NOTES**

_____

_____

_____

_____

_____

_____

magnesium, and potassium are low. If we live in a perpetual state of subclinical mineral deficiency, our bodies are not able to buffer acidic foods or an acidic internal environment. Some of the consequences of low internal pH are an increased risk of osteoporosis, food allergies, fatigue, damage to the delicate digestive tract, and compromised immune function.

I hope you have been monitoring the pH of your first morning's urine on a regular basis since Lesson I-1, but in case you haven't, it is time to refocus your attention on this important homeostatic function. Refer back to the procedure on page 8, obtain pH tape strips, and test tomorrow morning's urine by comparing the color of the urine-soaked strip to the color chart. If your urinary pH falls below 6.5 (yellow, orange, or red on the strip), focus your energies on restoring an alkaline pH this week and maintaining it through the rest of the program, by taking the following steps:

- Refer to the first week's set of menus in the Menus and Recipes section and follow them carefully until your urine is within the 6.5–7.5 pH range on a regular basis.

- Make sure you get enough sleep.

- Resolve your stress issues as discussed previously in this module (Lesson III-4).

- Take a fully buffered vitamin C (ascorbate) supplement along with a combination of calcium, magnesium, potassium, and zinc to alkalinize and energize your body and rid it of stored toxins.

- If you need more help restoring proper pH, try doing an ascorbic acid flush and following the alkalinizing tips in Lesson I-1.

Be patient and persistent. Your urinary and salivary pH values are indicators of your reserves of alkaline minerals. You didn't become deficient in these minerals overnight, and you won't resolve your overly acidic state overnight. I suggest you continue retesting your pH levels on a regular basis, just to make sure you are staying in the "alkaline zone."

CRANK UP THE HEAT!

For your endogenous enzymes to work efficiently, your core body temperature needs to remain at 98.6°F, and you require a specific number of calories to provide fuel for the energy to maintain this temperature. Why else is 98.6°F important? Your body temperature is a key indicator of your metabolic rate. When your temperature is normal, your metabolism is burning hot,

as it should be, even at rest. But for many reasons including hypothyroidism (Lesson III-2), female hormone imbalance (Lesson III-3), loss of brown fat thermogenesis (Lesson III-5), low muscle mass, and other factors not well understood (like food allergies), your body temperature may not reach the optimal 98.6°F, even in the middle of the day when you are most active.

My temperature has always run on the low side and occasionally hovers around 96.0°F, even in the hot Florida sun. No wonder I struggle with fatigue at times, and sometimes carry an extra 10 pounds that can be difficult to lose. While I'm writing this at 3:47 P.M., my oral temperature is 97.8°F, almost 1 degree colder than it should be! I'm working on raising my body temperature, as you should too if you want to more easily maintain your weight and feel better.

Start by taking your oral temperature several times over the course of the day. Your temperature should naturally be on the low side when you awaken in the morning; it should rise as the morning goes on, peak in the mid-afternoon, and begin to wane again in the evening as you prepare for bed. If your temperature remains on the low side throughout the day, however, here are some tips for elevating it:

- Make sure your diet includes adequate amounts of fat (an important element of the Wings food plan). Use flaxseed oil, olive oil, and fish oil throughout the day. Supplemental conjugated linolenic acid (CLA) has been shown in preliminary research studies to help reduce body fat and increase muscle mass; human trials are ongoing and look promising.

- Make sure you're eating enough calories, and the right kinds of calories. If you have reached a plateau in your weight loss, don't make your body think that famine has struck by cutting calories; instead, increase your metabolism by keeping your caloric intake at optimum levels. Eat only real food (Lesson I-5), and balance your nutrition among proteins, carbohydrates, and fats (the goal of the Wings menus). For optimum health and vitality, you need all three to provide your body with building materials and the fuel for heat and energy.

- Get moderate amounts of exercise (Lessons II-9 and II-10) to increase your metabolic rate and body temperature. Don't overdo it, though, because excessive exercise (beyond your ability to recover quickly) will drain the body and make you tired.

- Turn down the thermostat in your home to keep the ambient temperature a little cooler than you prefer, forcing your body to produce heat to stay warm. Another technique is to soak a washcloth in ice-cold water, wring it out, place it around your neck, and leave it there until it warms up; better yet, soak a bath towel in cold water, wring it out, and wrap it around your entire unclothed body (this isn't as horrible as it sounds). This technique is like putting an ice pack on your thermostat to make the furnace kick in, and it really works.

■ You may need to use a thermogenic product, although I will again express my concerns about using stimulating herbs to boost metabolism. If you intend to use a natural product to raise body temperature and metabolism, do not use anything containing ephedra (ephedra has now been banned by the U.S. Food and Drug Administration), and stay away from guarana and other highly stimulating herbs. Some gentler herbs such as ginger and cayenne are thought to "produce heat" and are safe and beneficial to the body. Make sure you do not use a product that will over-stimulate your central nervous system and jeopardize the health of your heart or adrenal glands. Check with your doctor or with the staff at your local health food store, and please feel free to contact your Wings nutritionist for recommendations or if you have any questions (at www.flywithwings.com/pnc.html, click on My ProConnect).

Measuring Up

It's that time again . . . Weigh yourself, and then take five girth measurements: bust at the largest point, waist at two inches above the navel, hips at the largest point, and right and left thigh circumference at the point where your extended fingertips reach with your arms hanging down at your sides. Record these figures, and your calculated BMI value, on your Progress Chart.

And now, go to page 280 for your new recipes!

 TODAY'S ASSIGNMENT

MIND YOUR NUMBERS

Reassess your pH and your body temperature, and start working on correcting them if necessary. Make your body into a finely tuned machine, functioning at peak levels of efficiency! Taking charge of your own health is a great responsibility, but it is also a great privilege. Go for it! And enjoy the opportunity.

LESSON III-12 STUDY GUIDE

1. What are the ideal salivary pH levels upon awakening, before eating, and after breakfast?

2. What is the ideal pH of the stomach?

3. What is the ideal pH of the blood?

4. What is the desired pH range of the first morning urine?

5. List several foods that leave an acidic residue.

6. List several other factors that can acidify the urine.

7. At what body temperature do enzymes work most efficiently?

8. List three strategies for elevating body temperature.

_____

_____

_____

_____

HEALTH TIP

LET YOUR NOSE
BE YOUR HEALER

Aromatherapy is an ancient healing art that has been revived in a modern form to help promote physical, emotional, and mental well-being. Our sense of smell is a tool that can be used to impart healing and balance to our bodies. Through the simple act of inhaling, numerous scent molecules are transported to the olfactory nerve, which stimulates the brain's limbic system. It is here that many researchers believe emotions, memories, and learned information are stored or processed—and where the right aroma can trigger a desired response (for example, relaxation).

Many high-quality aromatherapy products are available at health food stores. Enjoy experimenting with different companies and varieties to find those that produce the best effects in your body. One of my personal favorites, Nature's Apothecary, offers room sprays that promote calmness (Calm Child), sexual energy (Aphrodisia), and so on. Another line of products, called Bach Flower Remedies, has been used for a couple centuries to help restore emotional balance.

ADDITIONAL NOTES

_____

_____

_____

_____

_____

_____

_____

_____

_____

_____

_____

_____

_____

_____

Lesson III-13. It's a Problem in Your Gut

A couple decades ago, candida overgrowth was the "disease of the year." William Crook, M.D., was one of the first medical doctors to call attention to the problem of chronic yeast overgrowth. Several now well-known books hit the market with a flourish; *The Yeast Connection* by Dr. Orian Truss (New York, NY: Random House, 1983) even preceded Dr. Crook's book and is still one of the top sellers in this category. Candidiasis became a hot topic in medical circles. Some doctors declared that as a natural resident of the human body, candida could pose no problem, so people claiming to be suffering from candida overgrowth were hypochondriacs who needed antidepressants rather than antifungals. Other doctors believed that virtually any unexplained health problems were candida-related and advocated treating patients with aggressive anti-candida protocols.

? TODAY'S QUESTION

Could your weight issues be related to candida?

_____

_____

_____

_____

Read this list of symptoms to see how many of them "sound like you":

- Fatigue
- Frequent headaches
- Depression
- Feeling of "spaciness"
- Muscle aches
- Digestive problems including frequent gas and bloating
- Sugar cravings
- Unusual sensitivity to perfumes or other synthetic fragrances
- Food sensitivities
- Recurrent vaginal or urinary tract yeast infections
- Sexual dysfunction

Do you experience many of the above symptoms? Have you at any time in your life used recurrent prescriptions for antibiotics? Have you indulged in a high-sugar diet, alcoholic beverages, and/or soft drinks? Do you drink chlorinated water? Do you have any health conditions such as hypoglycemia or hypothyroidism that you have been unable to resolve?

If you answered yes to several of those questions, you may have a candida problem. Ask your physician or healthcare practitioner to recommend an appropriate diagnostic test and, if necessary, a treatment protocol (see the Resource Guide to find holistic physicians in your area).

WHAT IS CANDIDA?

You already know that yeasts serve valuable purposes in our lives, especially in our cuisine. To leaven

✒ NOTES

_____

_____

_____

_____

_____

_____

bread, yeast is dispersed throughout dough as it is pounded and kneaded. As the dough warms, the yeast proliferates in the damp environment and produces carbon dioxide that makes the bread rise, giving it a light, airy texture. The organisms also impart the familiar yeasty flavor that we enjoy. Beer and wine are fermented with yeasts that produce alcohol.

In addition to these tiny, single-celled organisms, yeasts also include the entire family of mushrooms and other fungi. Neither animal nor vegetable, yeasts are ubiquitous in the environment, living in the air and on the surfaces of all living things such as fruits, vegetables, grains, and our bodies. *Candida* (from the Latin word meaning "glowing white") is a category of fungi that is part of the normal flora of the skin, mouth, intestinal tract, and vagina. The several species of candida include *albicans* (the usual pathogen) and *tropicalis*, among others.

When our naturally occurring candida population multiplies beyond control, it can cause a variety of infections, including candidiasis, vaginitis, and thrush (yeast in the oral cavity). These are usually superficial infections in the moist areas of the body, particularly in the mouth, esophagus, respiratory tract, and vagina. In individuals with weak or compromised immune systems, however, candida can become systemic; in other words, the yeasts can travel throughout the body, inflicting a great deal of discomfort and even serious illness.

A Modern-Day Plague?

It is easy to understand how candida overgrowth could become epidemic in our culture, given that many of our dietary and lifestyle habits favor the destruction of friendly intestinal bacteria and the overgrowth of pathogenic bacteria and fungi.

For example, the average American consumes over 200 pounds of sugar and artificial sweeteners annually. Sugar feeds yeast and bacteria, and artificial sweeteners may have the same effect. (I am convinced that Splenda feeds yeast, but this has yet to be elucidated in the scientific literature.) In addition, we have overused antibiotics for the past thirty or more years. Antibiotics kill both friendly and unfriendly bacteria and leave the entire gastrointestinal system in disarray, especially from frequent antibiotic use. Children are routinely prescribed antibiotics for minor infections, and by the time they reach adulthood, their digestive systems are very damaged. (A yeast problem often stems from childhood, when we ate "tons" of sugar and went through repeated bouts of infections and antibiotics.)

We also drink chlorinated water from municipal water supplies. Chlorine is not selective in the type of bacteria it kills or where it kills them, and it does not cease its antibiotic activity when it crosses our lips, so it destroys friendly bacteria in the intestinal tract, setting up conditions favorable to yeast overgrowth. The idea that we might have a problem with candida is therefore not that surprising.

In *Modern Day Plagues* (Provo, UT: Woodland Books, 1986), author Louise Tenney writes that candida produces an "intoxifying" alcohol called ethanol, which increases when the yeast has a food source such as white sugar or white flour products. Candida also produces acetaldehyde (a chemical related to formaldehyde) that disrupts collagen production and fatty acid oxidation and blocks normal nerve functions. In fact, Tenney writes, "it interferes with the normal function of the whole body." (Tenney, 1986, page 66.)

Symptoms and Conditions Associated with Candida Overgrowth

According to Drs. Pizzorno and Murray in the *Textbook of Natural Medicine* (London, UK: Churchill Livingston, 1999), the typical candida patient is female, aged fifteen to fifty years, with a history of chronic vaginal yeast infections, chronic antibiotic use for infections or acne, oral birth control usage, and/or oral steroid hormone usage. The list of symptoms is extensive:

- Chronic fatigue
- Loss of energy
- General malaise
- Decreased libido
- Thrush
- Bloating, gas
- Intestinal cramps
- Rectal itching
- Altered bowel function
- Vaginal yeast infection
- Frequent bladder infections
- Depression
- Irritability
- Inability to concentrate
- Allergies
- Chemical sensitivities
- Low immune function
- Premenstrual syndrome
- Sensitivity to foods and chemicals
- Endocrine disturbances
- Eczema
- Psoriasis
- Irritable bowel syndrome
- Craving for foods rich in carbohydrates or yeast

Candida overgrowth can make us very, very ill. References to bloating, intestinal gas, and other digestive problems are sprinkled throughout the medical and popular literature on candida. Individuals with candidiasis often struggle with unrelenting gas that distends the abdomen, and have been unsuccessful in addressing their bloat through increased use of digestive aids; or, they may have been suffering for a long time from a long, often obtuse list of unexplained symptoms that can make diagnosis difficult.

Candida Affects Weight Management

Candida can also cause weight problems, even obesity. Although this issue is not well articulated in the scientific literature, Dr. William Crook believes that the yeast may create problems with metabolism. In *The Yeast Connection Handbook* (Jackson, TN: Professional Books, Inc., 1996, page 207), he writes, "As pointed out by Dr. Orian Truss, individuals with candidiasis develop significant metabolic and biochemical abnormalities. Moreover, Truss and many other observers have noted that sugar craving, fatigue, and other manifestations of hormone dysfunction occur almost uniformly in individuals with yeast-related problems."

According to Dr. Jacqueline Krohn, author of *Natural Detoxification* (Vancouver, BC: Hartley & Marks, 1996), candida produces over eighty known toxins, the most potent of which are the acetaldehyde and ethanol mentioned previously. Acetaldehyde alters the terribly important function of protein synthesis. Remember that hormones, enzymes, neurotransmitters, and all tissues are proteins. Candida, then, could affect virtually any system of the body: disrupting hormone balance (including thyroid hormone), altering the structure and density of muscle tissue, or interfering with any other body process that is critical to weight management.

According to Dr. Nancy Appleton, author of *Lick the Sugar Habit* (New York, NY: Avery Publishing Group, 1996), candida secretes an estrogenlike hormone; although candida's secretion has only a fraction of the potency of real estrogen, it blocks your cells' estrogen receptor sites, preventing your own estrogen from locking onto those sites and preventing your body from receiving the benefits of its own hormone. An article published on the Vitamin Research Products website (www.vrp.com) cites numerous other yeast-associated endocrine problems, including hypoglycemia, hypothyroidism, and adrenal maladaptation, as well as Crohn's disease.

You can easily see from the literature and the clinical evidence that candida overgrowth is something many of us may need to address in order to be successful on our weight-loss path. A number of endocrine issues were covered in Lessons III-2 through III-4; if you are still unable to resolve those problems, you may need to dig deeper and consider the possible involvement of candida.

THE WINGS ANTI-CANDIDA PROTOCOL

If your doctor has determined that you have candidiasis, it is important for you to follow this "candida diet" on top of the "normal" Wings food plan:

1. Eliminate all processed foods, especially sugar or sugar substitutes and soft drinks.

2. Eliminate most starches, including rice, potatoes, and pasta.

3. Eliminate all fermented foods, including alcoholic beverages, tofu, vinegar, malted beverages or sweeteners, pickles, raw mushrooms, soy sauce, cheeses, and yogurt.

4. Eliminate all raw nuts and peanut butter.

5. Eliminate any food with yeast.

6. Severely restrict starches like potatoes, rice, and carrots.

7. Severely restrict fruit intake to no more than one small fruit per day.

8. Do not eat leftovers (they rapidly grow mold).

The goal of this diet is to keep yourself from eating any products that feed yeast (sugars and other high-glycemic carbohydrates) and any products containing yeasts or molds that would further increase the body's yeast burden. Follow this diet protocol until your doctor tells you to resume a "normal" diet; it may take weeks or months, depending on the severity of the problem and how easily your body overcomes it.

Yeast Die-Off

When people who have a yeast problem embark on a diet such as the Wings candida diet, they frequently experience symptoms associated with the death of large numbers of yeasts: headaches, fatigue, gastrointestinal symptoms, intense cravings for sugars and other carbohydrates, and many others that can be extremely unpleasant. Many symptoms of yeast die-off overlap with some symptoms of yeast over-

Candida, Leaky Gut Syndrome, and Food Allergy

One of the most serious problems caused by yeast over-growth (as well as by pathogenic bacteria) is leaky gut syndrome, previously described in Lesson I-8. When candida, which is normally supposed to reside in the bowel, migrates "north" into the intestinal tract, it damages the delicate tissue and creates holes through which partially digested proteins slip into the bloodstream. The body's immune system does not recognize these proteins and stimulates an immune system response to the "invaders," which is one of the prime causes of food allergies. If candidiasis and/or other conditions that wreak havoc with the integrity of the intestinal tract are not addressed, food allergies proceed unabated. No matter how carefully we restrict our intake of offending foods, we keep re-offending, unaware, with the passage of partially digested proteins into the bloodstream. And food allergies, as you know, set the stage for over-weight and obesity.

growth. It's as if the yeasts are "crying out" to be fed! If possible, push through this initial symptomatic period and continue on the candida diet regimen until your physician clears you to relax the restrictions.

Supplements for Yeast Eradication and Bacterial Replenishment

Carefully chosen supplements can be very helpful in eradicating yeast. Some of the most popular herbs used for this purpose are Oregon grape, grapefruit-seed extract, and goldenseal. One of my favorite herbal anti-candida formulas is Renew Life Candi-GONE, a broad-spectrum antifungal and antimicrobial product specifically formulated for individuals experiencing persistent gas, bloating, constipation, joint and muscle pain, chronic fatigue, recurring vaginal yeast infections, sugar cravings, and fingernail and toenail fungus. The formula consists of capsules containing uva ursi, garlic, caprylic acid, grapefruit-seed extract, and other herbs, and a liquid for a topical application containing oregano leaf, orange peel, Oregon grape root, pau d'arco, and others.

Take CandiGONE or another anti-candida product along with 30–40 grams of fiber to absorb toxins and yeast and escort them through the colon for elimination. Good fiber supplements on the market include FibreSMART and Nature's Secret Ultimate

Fiber. Make sure you drink plenty of water with the added fiber so the stool remains soft and is easily passed.

Other supplements are useful for replenishing the intestinal bacteria that normally help reduce the candida population. Take a full-spectrum acidophilus product on an empty stomach each day for several months to make sure these friendly bacteria implant firmly in the gut. Many of my clients have achieved excellent results with Nutrition Now PB8. I also highly recommend DDS acidophilus, which is sold under several brand names in health food stores.

Detoxification and Digestive Recovery

Detoxifying the liver during this die-off time is an excellent idea, as your body is being flooded with the products of yeast decomposition, and the liver is required to handle all such toxins. If your natural detoxification system is a little sluggish, your body may not be able to efficiently get rid of the material, possibly creating more symptoms. Consider redoing the Wings internal cleanse from Lesson II-6 to help you detoxify. Drink plenty of water throughout the day and stay on your program. You'll get through it! The coffee enema (page 83) will help reduce many of the symptoms.

After you get through the initial discomfort of the yeast die-off symptoms, you will notice less bloating around the abdomen. Digestion should improve dramatically, especially as the lining of the intestinal tract begins to heal. Although you have already worked on digestion (in Lesson II-5), now is the time to attend to it again:

- Use the amino acid L-glutamine to help heal the intestinal lining: 2–3 grams per day on an empty stomach is effective for that purpose.

- Use 1–2 teaspoons of *Aloe vera* juice daily to help the intestinal healing process.

- Use digestive enzymes with each meal to aid in the digestion of proteins and carbohydrates.

- If you suspect you do not secrete adequate amounts of hydrochloric acid, consider supplementing with HCl for a few weeks.

If you have any questions about the anti-candida and candida-recovery protocols, please consult a holistic physician who will be able to walk you through this process.

And now, go to page 280 for your new recipes!

TODAY'S ASSIGNMENT

GO WITH YOUR GUT

Go over the list of candida overgrowth symptoms to see how many pertain to you. If you believe you may have a yeast problem, seek the counsel of a nutritionist or a nutritionally trained physician who can help you work out your anti-candida diet and healing protocol, and then set your course. Following the anti-candida diet is not easy, but remember: improved weight and health lie on the other side of the process, and that's worth it!

LESSON III-13 STUDY GUIDE

1. What is candida?

2. What dietary and lifestyle choices increase the risk of candida overgrowth?

3. What are some typical symptoms of candida overgrowth?

4. What are the "do's and don'ts" of the anti-candida diet?

5. Why take fiber during the anti-candida diet?

6. What herbs are helpful in killing yeast?

HEALTH TIP

HEARTBURN

Is it a heart attack, or heartburn? Please make sure! The symptoms of a heart attack can resemble the burning of indigestion. You need to rule out a possible heart attack if you suddenly experience heartburn or other symptoms that could actually indicate a cardiovascular problem.

If it truly is heartburn, there is much you can do to ease the pain naturally:

- Drink 1–2 tablespoons of *Aloe vera* juice several times per day on an empty stomach—very healing for the entire gastrointestinal tract.

- Drink the juice of an unpeeled raw potato, blended with an equal amount of water, immediately after preparation, three times per day.

- Prepare your body for meals by drinking a cup of ginger tea thirty minutes prior to each meal.

- Use a digestive enzyme such as pancreatin, bromelain, or plant-based enzymes. The Prevail products are excellent for additional digestive support. Try Acid-East.

- Do not lie down immediately after eating. Keep your body upright for one or two hours after eating to allow the food to digest and pass through the intestinal tract.

Lesson III-14. Body on Fire

It is a glorious night under the stars. You are camping out in the forest, darkness is descending, and you need to build a fire. You don't want a large fire, just enough to light the immediate area and provide a little warmth against the chilly night air. You assemble a pile of dry leaves, small sticks, and a few larger branches. You strike a match, and instantly the pile blazes into life. "Aaah," you think. "This is beautiful." You walk toward your tent, thinking about heating a pot of soup for supper. But when you turn around, the fire has gone wild! Sparks have burst into the surrounding grass and are burning furiously. You rush over to stamp them out, but your stamping only spreads the fire further. The fire is soon out of control . . .

?   TODAY'S QUESTION

Does your body hurt for "no reason"?

_____

_____

_____

Do you suffer from arthritis-like pains in your joints? Does your back frequently hurt for no apparent reason? Do you notice other aches and pains in other parts of the body? If so, the "fires of inflammation" may be spreading . . . You need a natural fire extinguisher.

I periodically suffer from an inflamed back, and when that inflammation flares, I can gain 5 or 10 pounds overnight, simply from bloating. Apparently, one of the ways the body chooses to deal with inflammation is by flooding the inflamed tissue—an attempt to put out the fire, perhaps?

INFLAMMATION IS BOTH NATURAL AND UNNATURAL

No question about it, inflammation is big news. A recent Internet search turned up over 44,000 articles and books on the topic. Either we are experiencing more inflammation, or the word is just now getting out.

Inflammation *per se* is not unhealthy. It is a normal physiological response to injury and to any pathogen (bacteria, virus, parasite, allergen, and such) that the body perceives as a threat. For example, when you cut yourself, your immune system rushes to the scene, equipped with proteins that seal off the injured area, macrophages (immune system cells) that devour the invading pathogens, and other compounds that carry the "war debris" off the battlefield. The area gets hot and red, and the inflammation event is often accompanied by pain. Then, when the immune system prevails, the swelling subsides, the pain fades as the pressure against nerve tissue is relieved, and everything calms down.

Chronic or long-term inflammation, however, is different; it can become embedded in joints, muscles, or other tissues, creating many symptoms. Pain nearly always accompanies chronic inflammation, but other symptoms can be just as common—and destructive.

Chronic Inflammation and Disease

A list of conditions to which inflammation has been associated illustrates the creative ways that it can present itself in human tissue. Consider the following:

- Chronic inflammation is a causative agent of several diseases of the lungs, among them bronchitis,

✒ NOTES

_____

_____

_____

_____

_____

asthma, and chronic obstructive pulmonary disease (COPD).

■ Chronic inflammation is a causative factor in many neurological disorders, including Alzheimer's disease, multiple sclerosis, certain forms of dementia, depression, schizophrenia, and stroke.

■ Chronic inflammation is associated with rheumatoid arthritis, osteoporosis, and inflammatory bowel disease.

■ It has been known for two decades that metabolic syndrome or Syndrome X, with its cluster of symptoms—including increased blood fats, increased insulin, reduced insulin sensitivity, increased upper body fat, lowered HDL cholesterol (the good kind), and increased blood pressure—is associated with heart and artery disease. Research now indicates that inflammation may accompany the symptoms of this syndrome.

■ Inflammation may link reduced thyroid function to heart disease: preliminary studies show a connection between hypothyroidism and C-reactive protein (a marker for chronic inflammation).

■ Recent research appears to implicate high levels of homocysteine (a byproduct of incomplete metabolization of the amino acid methionine) in the inflammatory process. Homocysteine is also directly linked to increased risk of cardiovascular disease, and scientists are now discovering that homocysteine can be a causative agent in many chronic illnesses such as osteoporosis and depression.

Even obesity is now being linked with chronic inflammation. In fact, it is difficult to discuss any disease process without factoring in chronic or acute inflammation. It would seem that, indeed, our bodies are on fire.

Are We Stoking the Fires?

What has brought us to this place? Any number of dietary, lifestyle, or emotional factors light the fires of inflammation. Food, for instance, can be either pro-inflammatory or anti-inflammatory, and the standard American diet is definitely tilted toward inflammatory foods.

Three types of foods comprise 25 percent of the calories that adults in the United States consume daily: sweets and desserts, soft drinks, and alcoholic beverages. Salty snacks and fruit-flavored drinks make up an additional 5 percent, bringing the caloric energy contributed by nutritionally dead foods to about 30 percent. Each of these categories is pro-inflamma-

tory. Red meats, high in arachidonic acid and low in omega-3 fatty acids, are also pro-inflammatory. By contrast, fruits and vegetables, which are anti-inflammatory, make up a mere 10 percent of caloric intake.

Numerous lifestyle factors can play a major role in inflammation. Mild sleep deprivation, shame, guilt, fear, burn-out, and loneliness are associated with increased inflammation—and, of course, so is stress. Chronic stress tends to "alter the course of inflammatory disease" by "[impairing] the immune system's capacity to respond to hormonal signals that terminate inflammation," according to one study. (G.D. Marshall and S.K. Agarwal, "Stress, immune regulation, and immunity," *Allergy and Asthma Proceedings,* 2000. Jul–Aug, 21[4]:241–246.)

Inflammation and pain can be triggered by structural abnormalities such as tissue, bone, or muscle injury after trauma. Much of the pain of arthritis is caused by bone rubbing against bone when the synovial tissue thins (synovial tissue is the watery cushion between the bones in a joint). If the body cannot fix a structural defect or injury, it may use inflammation as a means of dealing with the misalignment. Sometimes medical treatment is required to put the parts back in place so this sort of immune response is no longer required.

TAKE A HOLISTIC APPROACH TO INFLAMMATION

Chronic inflammation must be addressed with a holistic model. It is tempting to reach for an over-the-counter medication when the pain gets too great, but analgesics cannot solve the problems of inflammation-induced heart disease, osteoporosis, obesity, Crohn's disease, COPD, and other conditions listed above. In fact, analgesics are known to cause liver damage, bleeding in the stomach and intestinal tract, and increasing breakdown of synovial tissue. We might temporarily feel better when we take an analgesic, but the fires rage on, causing tissue destruction and illness. A holistic healing model, however, eliminates the problem by discovering and dealing with the cause.

See Your Doctor

Remember that holistic medicine utilizes standard medical treatment when it is indicated. Do not be afraid to seek the counsel of your personal physician to discover the cause of your inflammation, particularly if you suspect a structural or anatomical problem or a disease process. You may require medical treatment, particularly at the very onset of the problem, to prevent further damage. Because many inflammation-associated conditions (for example, cardiovascular disease) can have life-threatening consequences, it is important to obtain an accurate diagnosis and to follow the treatment protocol from your physician.

As mentioned, hypothyroidism can trigger inflammation, and inflammation can be a causative factor in depression, which is a frequent symptom of a low-functioning thyroid and another trigger of inflammation . . . Yes, it is a downward spiral. See a holistic physician who can accurately assess your thyroid function and treat you for possible hypothyroidism; seek holistic methods of relieving mental and emotional disorders.

Are You Trigger Happy? Remove the Triggers!

If you are following the Wings Program, you have already eliminated most common dietary triggers of inflammation, like grains and dairy. You are also enjoying more fruits and vegetables, which are anti-inflammatory and help restore a normal pH balance. But just in case you still indulge in inflammatory foods like sugar, large amounts of red meats, carbonated beverages, processed foods, or foods to which you are allergic or sensitive, make a plan to completely clean up your diet. Yes, you will have to be strict with yourself, but once you are, you will notice a drastic reduction in your pain, and possibly an increase in your weight loss.

- Don't skimp on vegetables. Remember that fresh vegetables are anti-inflammatory. Plan to include six to seven servings of fresh fruits and vegetables in your daily diet. Strategize ways to do this, as this is not always part of our routine, even on the Wings Program.

- Eating red meat, pork, and shellfish can increase inflammation. Do you feel achy the morning after a steak dinner? Reduce your consumption of red meat, pork, and shellfish, or eliminate them altogether. Replace them with poultry and seafood other than shellfish.

- Keep track of how much water you drink daily; try to drink 1 ounce of water for every 2 pounds of your body weight (for example, if you weigh 150 pounds, you will want to drink 75 ounces of water each day).

- Have several servings of fresh oils each day. Sprinkle 1–2 tablespoons of olive oil on your salad or soup. Supplement your diet with a daily dose of 2–4 grams of fish oil (a wonderful anti-inflammatory agent).

Follow these steps to remove (or at least reduce) common lifestyle triggers of inflammation:

- Get plenty of sleep each night. Remember that even mild sleep deprivation sets you up for inflammation. Go to bed by 10:00 P.M. and sleep soundly for at least seven or eight hours.

- If you feel that you are headed toward burn-out, get some relief. You may need to change jobs or reduce your workload.

- Reduce stress, including emotional stress such as anger, loneliness, shame, guilt, and hostility. Write out your personal program for reducing stress. Seek professional help if you need it.

Supplements Are Important

As you know by now, supplementation helps compensate (not substitute!) for not-so-perfect nutrition. Several supplements reduce inflammation: some of the best known are fish oil, bromelain (an enzyme from the green stem of pineapple), protease (a protein-digesting, plant-based enzyme) ginger, curcumin (turmeric), and the herb cat's claw. Cat's claw, traditionally used by the indigenous people of South America, promotes joint health, mobility, and pain relief, and is a clinically validated natural immunomodulator (substance that adjusts the immune response to an appropriate level) shown to enhance joint flexibility. One milligram daily of folic acid is important in lowering homocysteine levels. Most nat-

A Natural Anti-inflammatory Formula

I highly recommend the SierraSil product Joint Plus, which combines Vincaria (an extract of the cat's claw herb) with a blend of naturally occurring trace minerals.

According to information provided by SierraSil, human clinical trials have shown that Vincaria is an effective treatment for patients diagnosed with osteoarthritis. The results of a multi-center, randomized, double-blind, placebo-controlled study show reduction in both inflammation and pain through the use of this herbal extract. Vincaria appears to regulate the expression of inflammatory genes and provide antioxidant benefits, particularly when combined with minerals. Minerals are very important to the anti-inflammatory process, as they actively participate in every enzymatic function in the body. Many trace minerals increase cellular energy, enhance immune function, and reduce inflammation.

ural anti-inflammatory products should be taken on an empty stomach for best results.

And now, go to page 281 for your new recipes!

TODAY'S ASSIGNMENT

MAKE AN APPOINTMENT

Because inflammation is such a common and serious problem, you may need to make sure you are not suffering from undiagnosed chronic inflammation. If you experience chronic stiffness and pain in any part of your body, make an appointment with your physician and ask for the C-reactive protein test. Then, if an inflammation problem is indicated, make a plan to reduce it naturally, based on the information provided above.

LESSON III-14 STUDY GUIDE

1. Name some common health conditions that have been linked to inflammation.

2. List some possible ways that inflammation can increase weight problems.

3. What common dietary habits increase inflammation?

4. What are some common lifestyle triggers for inflammation?

5. List some supplements that can be helpful in "quenching the fires" of inflammation.

6. List some dietary changes that help reduce inflammation.

HEALTH TIP

HEART HEALTH

If you have a family or personal history of heart disease, there are many natural approaches you can take to reducing your risk of a cardiovascular event:

- Follow the Wings food plan, of course! It is perfect for normalizing blood fats and decreasing inflammation and other markers for heart disease.

- Many cardiologists recommend taking coenzyme Q_{10}, a compound that is used in the production of cellular energy. Depending on your health needs, use 30–240 milligrams or more per day (I prefer the Q-Gel product).

- The amino acid L-carnitine shuttles fatty acids into the mitochondria where they are burned for energy, thereby increasing the energy production of the cell. L-carnitine is particularly good for the heart, as the heart is constantly hungry for energy.

- Magnesium helps to reduce blood pressure and to normalize the heart rhythm. For maximum benefit, take magnesium along with potassium.

- Fish oil lowers the level of C-reactive protein (a risk factor for heart disease) and also helps thin the blood, lower blood pressure, and establish heart rhythm.

- There is not enough space here to list all the dietary and lifestyle factors involved in protecting your heart. I encourage you to obtain a copy of my book *A Woman's Guide to a Healthy Heart* (New York, NY: Contemporary Books, 2004) for a more complete look at cardiovascular health.

MODULE IV
Healing the Heart and the Mind

The past three modules have been exciting and informative, presenting a great deal of valuable information that you have put to use in your life and (hopefully) in the lives of your family members. But we haven't finished! Module IV is another wonderful series of lessons on the emotional and spiritual issues involved in weight management and vibrant health. Again, we'll be covering new territory, and I know that this module will be another exciting segment of your health journey. Don't close the book. Get ready to go . . .

Lesson IV-1. Review of the Food Issues

By this time, you know that weight-management and health are so much bigger than just food and exercise. We have discussed diet issues, lifestyle issues, and medical issues. It is time to explore new territory: how do our minds and emotions affect our ability to manage our weight and health? Before getting into that material, however, I will review the food issues as they relate to your mind and emotions. Never forget that food is a primary healing tool; good health starts at the table.

? TODAY'S QUESTION

What foods do you eat for emotional reasons?

_____

_____

_____

_____

Today's question is intended to direct your thoughts to the larger issue of why you eat what you eat. You know that factors other than hunger are involved. The mind indeed drives the rest of the body, including what, when, and why you choose to eat. "Emotional eating" stacks on weight quicker than nearly anything else. If you are to move forward in health and vitality, you must explore the issue of emotional eating, as you likely are to encounter it repeatedly.

I imagine nearly everyone has, to some extent, eaten because of anger, sadness, frustration, boredom, or whatever else. We needn't beat ourselves up because we do this. We must, however, examine it. Once we understand why we are gobbling a plate of cold spaghetti in front of the open refrigerator door, or hiding a stash of chocolate under the chicken in the freezer, we can begin to solve the problem.

As you proceed through the material in this module, remember that the goal is not to add guilt; rather, the goal is to construct a strategy to deal with your emotional life. So if you eat for reasons that have nothing to do with hunger, thirst, or other physical needs, I understand! We will work together to achieve a more balanced, healthful way of eating.

THE PURPOSE OF FOOD

To kick off today's lesson, I'll summarize the real purpose of food, which was discussed back in the beginning of the Wings curriculum.

The specific and fundamental purpose of food (and eating) is to nourish and strengthen our bodies. Food was designed to satisfy our biochemical needs. Food contains the elements that build the body's structures and perform its functions: proteins that are converted into amino acids, carbohydrates that are converted into blood sugar, fats that perform hundreds of functions, vitamins and minerals that drive thousands of enzymatic and hormonal reactions, and so on. Food is not meant to be a comfort blanket or a tranquilizer—but that is often how it is used.

Common reasons for emotional eating include:

- Sorrow (loss, grief)
- Anger (frustration)
- Fear

✒ NOTES

_____

_____

_____

_____

_____

- Joy (celebration)

- Anxiety (stress)

- Boredom

- Friendship (camaraderie)

- Guilt (or to relieve guilt)

- Pressure from others ("loving saboteurs" are discussed in Lesson IV-9)

- Habit

You can, however, learn how to comfort yourself without grabbing a chocolate-chip cookie or a plate of macaroni and cheese. You can enjoy the company of your friends without expanding your waistline, as long as you understand why you are eating—and have made a plan that accommodates your health needs. You can learn stress-reducing techniques that do not involve potato chips. Hopefully, you began dealing with your stress in Module III and have already abandoned your unhealthful stress relievers; other emotional triggers are explored in Lessons IV-3 and IV-7.

A REVIEW OF THE WINGS FOOD PLAN

Let's incorporate the Wings principles for healthful eating into facing emotional situations, as follows:

1. Eliminate processed foods as much as possible. Enjoy foods that are natural and nutritious. Your body is satisfied on fewer calories of optimum nutrition. This is particularly important for stressful times.

2. When you are tempted to graze on junk food, drink a large glass of water, and while you are sipping it, ask yourself, "What am I hungry for?" Translate your emotional hunger into hunger for nutritious foods instead. (A personal tip: Sometimes when I am tempted to eat sugary or salty foods to deal with my emotions, I opt for a Wings Breakfast Drink; once I finish preparing and drinking it, I am so physically satisfied that I am not as likely to eat something I shouldn't. The nutrient-dense Breakfast Drink is quick and very balancing.)

3. Drink water and non-caffeinated herbal tea. Eliminate all fruit juices, coffee, tea, soft drinks, and other beverages. Water hydrates the body—nothing else does it as well as water!

4. Eliminate grains, with the possible exceptions of millet, rice, spelt, Kamut, or other ancient grains.

These grains can still cause allergy or intolerance problems, however, so please be aware that eating even small amounts of them can lead to weight gain.

5. Eat protein, carbohydrates, fats, water, and fiber at every meal. Get your body accustomed to balance. Eat just until you are satisfied (not full) and then stop eating. Some days you need a little more food, other days you need a little less. Listen to your body!

6. How much protein do you require? Some people need more, others need less. Again, listen to your body. If you are going through a particularly emotional time, increase your protein intake slightly. You will find that additional protein helps the body deal with stress.

7. Eliminate *all* processed sugars and processed wheat products! Once you start nibbling on sugary treats, it is difficult to stop; be firm with yourself and do not start. On the other hand, sweet foods were designed for our enjoyment, so enjoy the dessert recipes in this book to satisfy your sweet tooth without stacking on unwanted pounds.

YOUR EMOTIONAL SIDE

You are embarking on another "chapter" in the Wings curriculum: spiritual and emotional issues. This is an exciting piece in the Wings puzzle. It (again!) presents information seldom covered in other weight-management material.

It is likely that going through these highly personal topics in the next few weeks will stir up unpleasant memories. You may not even be aware that your memories hold such powerful emotional triggers; you have buried them deeply in your psyche, trying to cover the pain. You will find that buried emotions have a great deal to do with eating behaviors and your general health.

Please do not avoid this section out of concern that it may bring unwanted pain to the surface. The purpose of the Wings Program is to bring you to total and complete healing—emotionally and physically. This part of the health journey will not be pleasant for many people, but it is important nonetheless.

If any of these issues "belong" to you, please seek the counsel of a professional who will walk through them with you. Just as dealing with many physical and medical issues is not a do-it-yourself project, healing emotional pain often requires assistance. Do not be afraid to ask for help.

And now, go to page 281 for your new recipes!

TODAY'S ASSIGNMENT

TAKE YOUR EMOTIONAL TEMPERATURE

Have you kept a faithful Food Diary? Review its last two weeks carefully. Put an asterisk beside every "emotional eating" occasion, circle the times that you ate when you were really not hungry, and make a list of any social occasions that called for sugary, processed foods that are not part of your Wings Program.

Do you keep a personal journal? If so, it can help you do some emotional exploration.

- Ponder each emotional eating occasion that you identified in the last two weeks of your Food Diary, and write your thoughts about them in your journal. What released those emotions? Can you write a plan for dealing more appropriately with them?

- Write a paragraph or more in your journal for each of the occasions when you ate when you were not hungry; consider why you ate, and make an alternate plan for the future.

- Consider the social occasions when you indulged in sugary, processed foods. How did you feel when you ate them? Is this a frequent occurrence for you? If so, make a plan: you may need to eat before you go to such events, or bring your own food. What works for you?

- If you feel that professional help would be constructive, make an appointment.

You have done some work on these issues before, but we all slip back easily into old patterns. Break those patterns this week, and take charge of your eating behaviors!

LESSON IV-1 STUDY GUIDE

1. List some nonfood reasons that people eat.

2. What is the purpose of food?

3. List some of your personal strategies to avoid emotional eating.

4. List your comfort foods and then make a list of substitute foods that simultaneously improve health and provide comfort.

5. Write out the concepts of the Wings eating plan.

6. List three new foods that you will try this week. Incorporate these into your shopping list and write a weekly menu that includes these new foods.

HEALTH TIP

WHEN YOU CAN'T BREATHE

If you or someone you love suffers from asthma, you know how terrifying an asthma attack can be. Asthma is potentially life threatening and should never be taken lightly; anyone with asthma must be under a doctor's care.

Certain nutritional factors play a role in asthma. One of the most common causes is allergy. Deficiency in hydrochloric acid production has been linked to juvenile asthma and possibly to adult-onset asthma. Magnesium deficiency has also been linked to asthma. Good nutrition and natural anti-inflammatory agents can be used to reduce the frequency and intensity of asthma attacks.

- Perform the pulse test on all of your commonly consumed foods, and eliminate all of your known or suspected allergens (review the allergy material and test instructions in Lesson I-10).

- Reduce environmental allergens as much as possible. For example, do not allow pets to live in the house, minimize the number of potted plants, and keep the home free from dust. Reduce your chemical exposure as much as possible. (See the list of ways to "de-chemicalize" on pages 179–180.)

- Low stomach acid has been linked to asthma, particularly in childhood. Ask your doctor for a Heidelberg test, which measures the HCl secretion and pH of the stomach; if your stomach acid production is low, consider supplementing with HCl.

- Supplement the diet with 300+ milligrams (mg) of magnesium glycinate daily, to be taken with meals and apart from calcium for better absorption and utilization of both minerals.

- Take 1,000–2,000 mg of a quercetin-bromelain combination daily on an empty stomach. Both quercetin and bromelain are anti-inflammatory and, over time, can reduce the severity of asthma attacks.

- Include many anti-inflammatory foods in your diet and reduce your intake of foods that promote inflammation. In addition to fruits and vegetables, anti-inflammatory foods include seafood that contains omega-3 fatty acids. Pro-inflammatory foods include red meat, sugar, and dairy products (Lesson III-14).

- Supplement the diet with up to 5 grams per day of fish oil. *Caution:* If you are taking anticoagulant drugs, consult your doctor before using fish oil.

- Do the ascorbic acid flush (pages 8–9) on a regular basis, and keep your daily intake of vitamin C at 75 percent of your flushing level.

- Increase your intake of vitamin A and zinc to support the health of the mucous membranes.

- Supplemental N-acetylcysteine helps in thinning mucus and keeping the liver clear.

- Herbs that support lung health include licorice root, wild cherry bark, elecampane, and plantain. Thyme and ginkgo are also excellent for the lungs.

ADDITIONAL NOTES

Lesson IV-2. Review of the Exercise Issues

If you were born several decades or centuries ago, you would not need to exercise. You would get your exercise hoeing the garden, slopping the hogs, and scrubbing clothes on a washboard down at the creek. Our forebears were physically strong because they spent their days on the back end of a shovel. Plowing the field built strong backs and legs. They ate large quantities of food because they needed the calories, and they were not overweight because their daily work burned the calories off. Believe it or not, that was good!

?   **TODAY'S QUESTION**

What keeps you from getting exercise?

_____

_____

_____

_____

Have you written an exercise program for yourself and are you working it? If not, why not? If you are following an exercise program, what is the biggest pleasure you have received from exercising regularly?

Exercise was covered in Module II. If you are like most people, however, you started getting into your program but then got sidetracked by life, and by now you've started slipping back into "couch-potato mode." Welcome to the club! We've all been there—and we may be there still.

Exercise seems to be the hardest part of any good health program, especially for women. Women tend to be more sedentary than men; or perhaps more accurately in some cases, women tend to be involved in so many family activities and spend so much time taking care of the household *and* working a full-time job, they simply don't have time to add another thing to an already hectic schedule. Exercise is usually the last thing on a lengthy to-do list, and it's particularly hard for people who are living on the thin edge of exhaustion.

Lesson III-4 discussed how stress causes physical and emotional exhaustion. Most of us live lives of "controlled stress"; in other words, we know things are a little out of control, but we feel that we're managing them. Sometimes, however, stress boils over in emergencies, family or personal crises, and illness. It is then that we simply must exercise to help relieve the inner tension—but we often find that our internal reserves are gone and we don't have the strength. Personally, I find that a little exercise is good during these times, but I do not try to push myself too hard. A little walking helps clear the mind; swimming is relaxing; dancing is therapeutic. Find a physical activity that you like, and you'll enjoy a brief endorphin release.

You simply must exercise. It is not optional, even—or especially—in our high-tech society. Nowadays we exercise our fingertips on the computer keyboard and our legs by walking to the car to drive our kids to soccer practice. If we belong to a gym, we drive to the gym to work out; if the gym is on the second floor, we take the elevator! Too bad we don't grow our own

✐   **NOTES**

_____

_____

_____

_____

_____

_____

My Personal Exercise Story

I don't like to exercise. I never have. I remember being sedentary even as a little girl; given the choice of riding a bike or reading a book, I chose a book nearly every time. But when the perimenopausal period of life approached and I began to lose muscle tissue rapidly, I had a choice to make: use it or lose it. So I embarked on a ten-year journey toward physical fitness.

I started an exercise program, got interrupted by travel or work or kids, and stopped exercising. A year or so passed. Then, after observing my sagging self in the mirror, I joined a gym and started over, only to be interrupted again. This pattern repeated itself, and each time, my program would come to a halt. When I moved to Florida, a friend asked me to join an early morning aerobics class, which was terrific, because my accountability to her got me out of bed in the morning and kept me going . . . until a major trauma abruptly turned my life upside down, and my exercise program was again on sabbatical, this time for nearly three years.

Age and gravity are not kind to the body. Now that I was fully menopausal, the rapidity at which I lost muscle was frightening. "Old age" began to show in my shape and posture, and I did not look or feel good. I was "losing it"! Interestingly, I was still roughly the same weight, but my clothes no longer fit, and I could tell that fat had replaced muscle.

Once I was on the other side of the trauma, I realized that I would have to commit to a life-long fitness program: I simply had no choice if I wanted to remain healthy throughout my senior years. So even though life still felt out of control most of the time, work was piled high at the end of the day, and I didn't feel like exercising, I made a commitment to exercise for the rest of my life. I started going to bed a little earlier so I could get up earlier and go to the fitness center. I started walking . . . and walking . . . increasing the incline on the treadmill . . . increasing the speed . . . adding weight training . . . and more time . . . Day by day, my fitness returned. I could see it—and I could feel it.

My reward greets me each day. I am rebuilding lost muscle tissue throughout my body. My stamina is increased, my posture is better, my energy is higher, and I am dropping a few pounds of excess weight. Do I enjoy the exercise? Not really. But I *do* enjoy how I feel as a result, and that keeps me going. My fitness program is still interrupted frequently: I sometimes feel so emotionally drained that I spend an extra half hour resting in bed; and because I travel a great deal, I have to be creative to work exercise in. But the commitment is there. If I miss a day or two of my program, I pick it up again the next day. I'm committed for life. If I can do it . . . so can you!

---

food. Not only would we eat more healthfully, but the physical work would do our sedentary bodies a lot of good.

Remind yourself of some of the benefits you will enjoy from regular exercise:

- Regular exercise builds muscles, which helps boost metabolic rate. When you have dense muscle tissue, you burn more calories even when you aren't exercising, for example, while sleeping and doing your daily work. Exercise gets your body working for you instead of against you. (Older women tend to lose muscle as estrogen levels drop, so exercise is especially important for post-menopausal women.)

- Regular exercise significantly relieves depression. Depressed people often eat inappropriately or binge on high-carbohydrate junk foods.

- Exercise cuts the appetite and encourages healthful eating habits. You just don't feel as hungry after a workout as you might think you would.

- Exercise is a great stress releaser, especially when you do something you really enjoy. Choose fun exercise activities like swing dancing, swimming, walking, hiking, bicycling, tennis, or yard work. Anything that turns you on—do it!

Exercise is often best enjoyed in partnership. Find a friend who enjoys the same activity and can play with you. If you laugh while you're doing it, so much the better. Laughter is a good cardiovascular workout! In addition, recent studies show that friendships and physical contact reduce the release of stress hormones; as you may recall, excessive stress hormone release leads to loss of muscle mass and increased fat deposition in the waist and upper body, so combining friends and exercise is a good antidote.

Exercise all the large muscles of the body. If you enjoy aerobics, go for it, but do not forget anaerobic exercise too, to build muscles in the upper and lower body (this helps hold your body upright so you do not develop a "dowager's hump" with age). Remember that you need to burn a significant amount of calories during the week to lose weight: work off up to 2,500 calories per week in your exercise routine (Lessons II-9 and II-10), not counting your daily activities. That is a lot of exercise, but that is when you begin to see huge weight-loss benefits. If you have been under considerable stress, however, and your energy reserves are low, you may not be able to sustain that exercise level without suffering in other ways. Listen to your body and do not overexercise.

If exercise is a struggle because you simply do not have enough energy, then improve your energy production first. Build deep, natural energy by improving your health:

- Remember to take your vitamins and minerals, as these activate enzymes that increase cellular (and whole-body) energy.

- Improve your digestion.

- Get plenty of rest.

- Steer clear of artificial energizers like coffee, soft drinks, herbal uppers (especially ephedra, recently banned by the U.S. Food and Drug Administration), and the like, because although these seem to solve your energy crisis, the fix is temporary and they actually rob the body of long-term energy.

Measuring Up

It's that time again . . . Weigh yourself, and then take five girth measurements: bust at the largest point, waist at two inches above the navel, hips at the largest point, and right and left thigh circumference at the point where your extended fingertips reach with your arms hanging down at your sides. Record these figures, and your calculated BMI value, on your Progress Chart.

And now, go to page 282 for your new recipes!

 ## TODAY'S ASSIGNMENT

DO IT WITH A SMILE!

Have you written your exercise plan yet? I hope you did not skip over that section in Module II, thinking that you would do it later. Well, if you did, it's later—time to get started! Enlist the aid of a personal trainer or another knowledgeable person and put together an exercise plan that works for you. You may start with a

simple program at the beginning to get things going. Then, as habits develop and your strength and endurance improves, increase your physical activities until you burn 2,500 calories per week. Make sure you include exercises that you truly enjoy. Then, after the exercise plan is written, work it! Get started!

LESSON IV-2 STUDY GUIDE

1. Review this lesson's material as well as Lessons II-9 and II-10.

2. List the benefits of exercise (apart from weight management).

3. List some reasons that you are not exercising, and write a strategy for overcoming these obstacles.

4. How much exercise is needed to achieve a fat-burning benefit? How many calories is that per week?

HEALTH TIP

MORE ON CANDIDA

As you know, candida (yeast) inhabits the colon as part of the natural flora and fauna of the digestive system. When you consume sugar on a regular basis, along with using antibiotics frequently, yeast proliferates in your gut, causing damage to the intestinal lining and possibly creating systemic health problems (Lesson III-13).

The Wings dietary protocol is excellent for controlling the overgrowth of internal candida, along with the following natural tips:

- Avoid all fermented products like vinegar, wine, soy sauce, tofu, pickles, and the like. (This obviously entails making some adjustments to the Wings food plan.)

- Avoid dried fruits and fruits that are shipped from overseas, because these often gather mold.

- Keep your vitamin C and vitamin A levels high.

- Increase your intake of the vitamin biotin, which inhibits a specific form of candida that is most irritating to membranes.

- Increase your B-complex vitamin supplementation (make sure to use a yeast-free product).

- Increase your intake of essential fatty acids such as the natural antifungal caprylic acid, available at health food stores.

- Take a probiotic product daily on an empty stomach. If necessary, do a douche or enema using acidophilus.

- The herb pau d'arco bark is an antifungal agent and can be used in a douche.

- Goldenseal, Oregon grape root, and barberry are antifungal herbs and can be used in a sitz bath.

- Use diluted tea tree oil as a topical application.

- Marigold salve is also soothing to the skin and mucous membranes.

✒ ADDITIONAL NOTES

Lesson IV-3. The Most Painful Topic of All

Today's lesson introduces the most difficult topic in the entire Wings curriculum: past sexual, physical, or emotional abuse, and how such events in your life have made it difficult for you to lose or maintain your weight. Because this is a very painful topic for people who have experienced these events, I want to be as gentle as possible in the presentation of this material. I do not want to hurt you again. However, because this issue is so vitally important, I feel that unless it is dealt with here in this safe environment, you may not be as successful in the pursuit of your health goals as you would like to be.

Some of the material provided in this section comes from my personal spiritual perspective. You may have a different spiritual/emotional perspective and should feel free to address the issues contained here in a manner that honors your beliefs.

? TODAY'S QUESTION

Were you abused?

_____

_____

_____

_____

Close your eyes and review the events in your life.

Did you experience any type of physical, sexual, or emotional abuse? Do you feel safe talking about it? Is it safe to remember? Write down what you remember. Did your weight problem begin after the abuse?

You may never have associated these ugly events with your current weight and health struggle. Most people feel that childhood events are in the past; they are trying to forget them and do not wish to revisit them.

YOU ARE NOT ALONE . . .

How common is sexual, emotional, and physical abuse? Frighteningly common. In many studies, more than half of respondents report at least one exposure to childhood abuse, and nearly 25 percent report more than two incidents of childhood abuse. At least 15 to 38 percent of adults have been sexually abused as children; however, only 25 to 50 percent of sexual abuse incidents may come to the attention of authorities, which may make these statistics artificially low. In fact, some experts believe that 50 to 75 percent of adults have been sexually abused as children.

Abuse occurs throughout every stratum of society, from upper to lower class, from highly educated families to families where no one went to college. Several forms of abuse often occur within families or to certain individuals in a family. Emotional abuse stands alone or occurs as a consequence of physical abuse. If sexual abuse is occurring in a home, physical and emotional abuse is likely to occur as well. Most sexual abuse is leveled at females; however, males are also victimized.

Researchers do not all use a common definition of abuse, which leads to some uncertainty in the statistics, but much of the variation in statistics is a result of non-reporting. Most people simply do not report abuse to

✏ NOTES

_____

_____

_____

_____

_____

_____

_____

the authorities or to physicians, for deep personal reasons. Children obviously do not typically report abuse in the home. We really have no way of knowing the magnitude of the problem for certain. But what is known is terribly frightening—and it makes the victims of abuse physically and emotionally sick.

It Doesn't End with Childhood

What are the consequences of past abuse? The following outline of abuse-related physical and emotional problems comes directly out of the primary research. Abused children tend to have higher levels of weight dissatisfaction, purging, and dieting behavior. Abused women experience depression, anxiety, and low self-esteem. Chronic pelvic pain is common in women with histories of severe childhood sexual abuse. A history of abuse also carries an increased risk of lifelong diagnoses of major depression, panic disorder, phobia, and drug abuse.

People who have experienced four or more categories of childhood abuse have a four- to thirteen-fold increase in their risk of alcoholism, drug abuse, depression, and suicide attempt. They have a two- to four-fold increase in tendency for smoking, poor self-rated health, history of more than fifty sexual intercourse partners, and sexually transmitted disease. And there is a 1.4-fold to 1.6-fold increase in severe obesity.

Past abuse often leads to anger problems, and there is a strong connection between anger and weight, especially weight carried around the stomach (the spare tire). Hostile attitudes lead to weight gain in midlife. Chronic stress is associated with excessive production of stress hormone, and this type of stress response leads to development of abdominal body fat (Lesson III-4).

Past sexual abuse leads to later binge-eating disorders. This is because when trauma of this sort occurs in early childhood, an important hindrance to personal growth develops: a disturbance in the beliefs (1) that the world is a reasonably safe place in which to live, and (2) that the individual controls his/her life and body. These disturbances can affect later eating and/or health behaviors. If the world is not a safe place and personal safety (one's health) cannot be reasonably certain, why bother to care for the body or the mental self? The abused individual lost control over his/her body a long time ago, and continues to relinquish control over eating and health behaviors because giving up control becomes a "normal" way of life. Abuse victims were not more powerful than their abusers . . . they are not more

powerful than the chocolate-chip cookie or the bowl of ice cream.

Abused women use food to comfort themselves when stress hits, even later in life. It is possible that eating for comfort is a habit they established long ago, when the abuse occurred, and they are simply carrying on a stress-release tradition. They may also feel that they must control their food as a way of exerting control over their bodies. They eat to gain and maintain this control. They refuse to allow others to dictate how their bodies look or feel.

Sexual and/or emotional survivors show many of the same physiological profiles as male combat veterans diagnosed with post-traumatic stress disorder (PTSD). In one study, members of a PTSD group had significantly elevated daily levels of stress hormones as well as a greater tendency toward obesity, even long after the stress was over. Although these people were no longer experiencing continued trauma, their bodies had developed an ongoing internal coping mechanism for stress. In earlier lessons, you learned that stress hormones increase the rate at which muscle tissue is broken down, decrease the body's ability to build new muscle tissue, dysregulate blood sugar, and pull down the strength of other hormones. Ongoing stress is very difficult for the body to manage in a healthful way.

Being Overweight Can Feel Very Protective

Some overweight abuse survivors use excess body fat as protection against further assault. Have you been successful in losing weight, only to find that as your body became more attractive to the opposite sex, you became afraid? Are you uncomfortable with your new body shape? Now that the weight is coming off, do you again feel vulnerable and uncomfortable around certain people or around members of the opposite sex? It may be difficult for you to pursue weight and health goals if you do not feel safe doing so.

People with a history of sexual abuse typically lose less weight and are more noncompliant than other people in the same weight-loss programs. Dropouts of a weight-loss program are more likely to have reported a history of sexual abuse. Maybe these abuse survivors simply do not feel safe being more sexually attractive. They feel that losing weight will make them more attractive—and, therefore, put them in jeopardy.

AS PAINFUL AS IT MIGHT BE . . .

If sexual, physical, or emotional abuse is part of your history, I encourage you to explore the association(s) between your weight and the abuse. It is possible that unless this issue (however painful) is addressed, it will be difficult to achieve your weight-loss goals. Past studies indicate that until this work is done, weight loss is usually not successful. In a safe environment, however, healing can take place. You can resolve these issues, once and for all, and go on to enjoy life to a depth you never dreamed possible. I encourage you to seek healing by working with a trained counselor.

Spiritual Healing

When you seek help, be sure to work with a spiritual counselor who can guide you toward forgiveness of your abuser. Abuse does not just create a physical or mental problem; it creates a spiritual problem. If you have not forgiven your abuser, the anger and grief you experienced during that time will gnaw away at your soul and spirit, depriving you of the joy of releasing it to God. It is impossible, however, for human beings alone to truly forgive so grievous an injury. We simply cannot let it go because it is so much bigger than us; yet, we cannot heal if we cannot forgive.

Do not think that your forgiveness denies the power of the offense. It does not absolve a victimizer of guilt or responsibility. Forgiveness does not mean that you must reestablish contact or friendship with the abuser. You do not forgive to help abusers, to make them feel better about themselves or what they did: you forgive to release yourself from their power. Forgiveness is the only way to set yourself free. Forgiveness is for you.

A spiritual counselor can help you release your grief and anger to God. God alone is able to remove it from you and bring complete healing. You cannot rush this process. You may have to go through a season of grieving, because you lost something very precious in the abuse. You may need to revisit the damage and acknowledge just how deeply you were hurt. That process is similar to opening up an infected wound so that the infected material can be removed. It is painful, but necessary for healing. In the counsel and care of someone who helps you release your pain to God, you can find safety—and find healing.

And now, go to page 283 for your new recipes.

  TODAY'S ASSIGNMENT

LET YOUR MEMORY BEGIN TO HEAL

Close your eyes and go back over events in your life. Did you experience any type of sexual, emotional, or physical abuse? Have you done the healing work? If not, please seek the counsel of a professional who is trained specifically in this area. Preferably this will be a counselor who can work with you spiritually, but if not, please contact a spiritual advisor who will work with you toward spiritual healing.

This has been a difficult topic, hasn't it? I pray that if you have experienced this type of abuse, over the next few weeks and months, God will restore all those lost years. He will recreate new memories for you—memories of how deeply you are loved by God. He will bring inner healing to you. He will give you rest.

If this topic has spoken to your heart, please look for counselors in your area and make an appointment. There are also many excellent books on this topic; you may wish to do your own private research, or if you do not know where to begin, you may wish to speak with a trusted friend or family member or a spiritual counselor. Whatever you do, do not continue to suffer in silence, hoping that the problem (and the memories) will vanish. There is help for you, and there is hope!

Because childhood or adult abuse may be a continuing stressor, review Lessons III-4 and III-8 for techniques and information on nourishing your body against stress. Consider using holy basil and rhodiola (page 139) to lower your stress response.

How can you make yourself feel loved and honored? Make a plan to care for yourself, and then do it! Remember that you are more than the sum total of the abuse event(s). You are truly stronger than your abuse—and your abuser.

LESSON IV-3 STUDY GUIDE

1. Approximately how many adults may have been abused at some point in their lives?

_____

_____

2. What are some of the physical health consequences of past abuse? What are some emotional or spiritual consequences?

_____

_____

_____

_____

3. How can past abuse affect weight and weight management?

_____

_____

_____

4. Discuss how being overweight feels safe to a victim of abuse.

_____

_____

_____

5. How does forgiveness work to resolve past injuries?

_____

_____

_____

_____

HEALTH TIP

BRAIN FOOD

We would like to approach our senior years with all our "marbles" in place, wouldn't we? We fear dementia even more than being overweight! Symptoms of dementia include memory impairment, language deterioration, motor activity impairment and disturbances, impaired ability to recognize objects, inability to think abstractly, spatial disorientation, suicidal behavior, uninhibited behavior, anxiety, mood and sleep disturbances, hallucinations, incontinence, tremor, seizures, and increased susceptibility to physical stressors such as illness or emotional stressors such as bereavement. Scary list, isn't it?

Fortunately, there are steps you can take to reduce the risk of dementia and support healthy mental functioning into your senior years:

- Make sure that your nutrition is superior and that digestion is enhanced through the use of digestive aids such as digestive enzymes or hydrochloric acid (HCl).

- Drink a cup of ginger tea prior to each meal to enhance the flow of digestive juices.

- Have several sources of antioxidant nutrients in your diet, including several daily servings of brightly colored fruits and vegetables, and supplements. Biotin, the entire B-complex, and vitamin C are often deficient in the senior population.

- Add calcium, magnesium, and zinc to your supplement program.

- Avoid extra manganese and copper.

- Essential fatty acids (omega-3 fatty acids) are anti-inflammatory and good for the brain.

- *Ginkgo biloba* increases circulation to the peripheral tissues, including the brain. Use up to 200 milligrams per day. *Caution:* If you are taking anticoagulants, however, check with your physician before using ginkgo.

- Hawthorn is a circulatory stimulant, as is rosemary, Siberian ginseng, and ginger.

- Drink several glasses of pure water per day.

- Use Juice Plus+ (see the Resource Guide).

- Avoid stress! Stress damages the memory center of the brain.

ADDITIONAL NOTES

_____

_____

_____

_____

Lesson IV-4. How Do I Look?

Get out your paper and pencil. Draw yourself, in your current shape, on the paper. Next to it, draw your "ideal figure." What do you want to look like someday? Next to that picture, draw the body you think your spouse sees in you, and the body your spouse would like to see. Compare the pictures! If you are married, ask your spouse to draw a picture that represents how he/she sees you. Compare the pictures. You may be surprised!

? TODAY'S QUESTION

Do you love your body?

_____

_____

_____

_____

Do you have a picture of the "ideal you" on your refrigerator door? What does that figure look like? How close are you to your ideal weight?

If you are unhappy with the shape or size of your body, you are not alone! Consider these interesting facts:

- Up to 56 percent of surveyed women are dissatisfied with their bodies.

- Some 63 percent of women said that weight often affects how they feel about themselves.

- In women over the age of sixty-two, the fear of weight gain is their second greatest concern, second only to memory loss.

- Men and women are dissatisfied with different parts of their bodies.

- Thirty-two percent of men and 45 percent of women are discontent with their muscle tone.

- Fifty percent of men and 57 percent of women are unhappy with the size of their abdomen.

- When people are unhappy with their body shape and size, they are more likely to develop eating disorders.

- Men think that women like a larger male figure than they actually do.

- Men like a larger female figure than women think they do.

- Women (not men) tend to feel larger than they think they look (that sounds a little confusing, doesn't it?). In other words, women experience a "body feel" that "feels" larger than it looks. Women often express the thought that they take up "more room" than they should, although their mirror image belies that feeling.

- Body-image disturbance is associated with depression, low self-esteem, and history of being teased.

- When overweight individuals lose weight, their perception of body size doesn't decrease proportionately; they still consider themselves fat.

What is your ideal weight? You and your body may disagree. As you know, the body mass index (BMI) is a *rough* estimate of percentage of body fat. The ideal BMI range for women is 22–25. If women are in the perimenopausal period of life, they may be

🖋 NOTES

_____

_____

_____

_____

_____

_____

healthier at the upper end of that range, given the protective nature of body fat during and after menopause (Lesson III-3). The ideal BMI range for men is 18–22. Men who are very muscular will feel better and be healthier at the upper end of that range.

I mentioned earlier in this curriculum that as men and women age, their bodies naturally change shape. I call it the furniture problem: the chest sinks into the drawers! Seriously, though, even if we do not gain weight with age, our body shapes do change. Women tend to get heavier on the bottom; men tend to get a little heavier all over, especially in the upper body. After childbirth, women often gain a few pounds that the body can use for energy during the breastfeeding period. Over time, particularly while passing through menopause, women tend to gain a few extra pounds, especially in the hips, abdomen, and buttocks.

As we get older and our growth hormone (hGH) and leptin levels drop (Lesson III-9), it becomes a little more difficult to maintain lean muscle tissue. It does not mean that we cannot gain new muscle tissue or hold onto our existing musculature; it does mean that we have to work a little harder to maintain muscle tone as our bodies age. Women, in particular, need to work harder to maintain hormone levels that optimize body shape and health.

We can learn to be content with our own body shape even if we are not the "perfect" 36-24-36. Remember Barbie? Barbie was a fictional woman, created in the mind of someone who thought those measurements represented the perfect size. We have been trying to live up to that ideal ever since, to our great detriment.

If I asked, "What shape is a woman?" how would you respond? Most people would draw an hourglass figure, but does that shape really represent the majority of women? Some women are athletic, others rounder. Some are heavier in the chest, others in the hips. Some are tall, some short. We can generalize about what shape women are, but that is all it is: generalization! Which, then, is the "right"—and beautiful—shape for you? It probably is not 36-24-36!

We need to stop idealizing fictitious shapes and affirm the beauty of the female body, in all its various real shapes. We also need to stop idealizing the Arnold Schwarzenegger image for men. How many men can live up to that? Men also come in many shapes and sizes. Some men are tall and lanky, others short and stocky; some are muscular, others naturally slim.

If we exercise regularly to build strong muscles, we will be muscular rather than "fluffy." But genetics play a huge role in body size and shape, as do the male and female hormones. We also know that stress

Your Weight Is Not Your Worth

Weight and health have nothing to do with worth. Why are you valuable?

- You are valuable because you contribute something of value to this Earth.

- Your life is meaningful to your spouse, your children, your coworkers, your neighbors, and others your life touches.

- You are valuable because your life brings beauty, joy, security, and many other gifts to people.

- You are valuable because someone (a spouse, a child, a friend, a neighbor, a mother or father) loves you.

- You are valuable just because you are a person—no other reason is needed!

influences fat deposition and adds weight; even if we want to, we cannot always diminish our stressors to the point that the weight disappears. In short, many factors enter into why we acquire the shape we do.

Why am I saying all of this? Because, frankly, we need to give ourselves grace if we do not reach our target weight goal. Factors beyond our control may keep a few extra pounds hanging on our hips or other places. Remember that a "magic number" on the scale is not very important: your health is the most important thing, and you can be gloriously healthy even if you are 10 or 15 pounds over your goal weight.

Do you need to re-evaluate your perception of what your body shape should be? Can you accept yourself if you are not "perfect"? Can you be happy in a body that doesn't quite match your fondest expectations? What can you do to shift your expectations into the realm of reality—and be happy there?

Weight and health are goals; health is a journey that you will travel the rest of your life. Each decade of life brings with it new health—and weight—challenges. You have learned so much about caring for your body. Learn now to appreciate it. Feed it! Give it rest! And love it!

And now, go to page 284 for your new recipes!

  TODAY'S ASSIGNMENT

REVIEW YOUR WEIGHT AND HEALTH GOALS

How many of your health goals have you achieved? Have you achieved your weight goal? If not, how close are you? Are you satisfied with your body? If not, how can you build satisfaction? Do you need to improve your level of fitness? Join a club? Do you need to revisit your weight goals to make them more realistic?

Let this be a week of introspection. Decide that you will learn to love your body and that you will accept your body for what it is, and be pleased about it. Make a list of everything you love about your body.

LESSON IV-4 STUDY GUIDE

1. What is the target BMI range for women? For men?

2. Write down some interesting facts about weight and body perception. How many of these "belong" to you?

3. What factors influence our personal body shape and size?

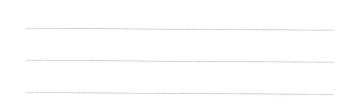

HEALTH TIP

A HOMEOPATHIC MEDICINE CHEST

A well-stocked medicine chest is one of the secrets to natural health. Don't wait for an emergency before racing off to the health food store for herbs and other natural products to ward off illness. As a mother of four, I keep my cabinets well supplied with homeopathic remedies. You will develop your own favorites, but these, for starters, are mine:

- Arnica cream, for muscle strain and sore muscles

- Belladonna, for impending illness and fever

- Bryonia, for dry cough

- *Nux vomica*, for upset stomach and vomiting

- *Apis mellifuca*, for bee stings or the pain of shingles

The "art" of homeopathy is complex; one reference that is a must for your health library is Stephen Cummings and Dana Ullman's book *Everybody's Guide to Homeopathic Medicines* (New York, NY: Jeremy P. Tarcher/Penguin, 1997).

ADDITIONAL NOTES

Lesson IV-5. Does This Make Me Look Fat?

Note to male readers: This lesson is *not* for women only, so don't skip ahead just yet . . .

Even the most "perfectly shaped" person will not look good if he/she dresses funny! Most of us agree that we just look better in clothes—and the more we learn about how to dress, the better we look. No one will even notice that you have a few lumps and bumps here and there if you dress to disguise them. No one will care that your hips are a little wide or that your waistline isn't svelte if you dress to take the focus off your least attractive parts and draw attention to your more gorgeous parts.

? TODAY'S QUESTION

What makes you beautiful?

_____

_____

_____

What is your best feature? What is your worst feature? Look at your spouse. What is his/her best feature?

In the last lesson, you learned to love your body. In this lesson you'll learn more about presenting and dressing your body. Some people may be tempted to postpone focusing on these details if they have not achieved all of their weight and health goals; but if you are still working on some of these goals, now is actually the perfect time to build your self-esteem and make yourself absolutely gorgeous.

BEAUTY STARTS INSIDE

Do you believe the saying, "Beauty is only skin deep"? I don't. True beauty starts on the inside and works its way out to the surface. If we feel beautiful, we look beautiful. Some of the most beautiful people on earth cannot boast of perfect features; they simply know how to present themselves. They glow with an inner beauty that comes from loveliness of the spirit and from self-confidence.

The first step toward building beauty is to allow joy and peace to bubble out, from the inside to the outside. If you feel contented or happy within, let your face know! Practice smiling throughout the day. Some time ago, one of my children commented, "Mom, one thing I've always loved about you is your smile. Whenever one of us talks to you, you automatically smile." What beautiful affirmation—thanks, daughter!

Practice letting your inner beauty shine on your face. We often think that the expression on our faces mirrors our inner emotions, but scientists tell us that the opposite is true: if we smile, even when we don't feel like it, we soon feel happier on the inside. What a wonderful way to relieve stress! Practice smiling today, and let your inner beauty shine.

The second step toward real beauty is walking with confidence. Many overweight people feel embarrassed by their weight, even if they are only carrying an extra 10 pounds. They allow shame to filter through their minds and souls, and they try to hide their overweight by slouching. Stand tall! Practice walking confidently! Do not let a few extra pounds rob you of these abilities. If you are accustomed to walking slumped down, work with a personal trainer to build strong muscles in your back; maintaining them will hold your posture straight and tall.

The third step toward being beautiful is dressing to fit your personal shape and style. Even if you have dressed for beauty in the past, you need to look at

✎ NOTES

_____

_____

_____

_____

_____

your personal style again and bring it up to date. According to Valerie Foley, creator and designer of VenusDivas.com, we tend to find our style and perfect our "look" in our twenties. But then, as we age, even as our body shape and skin coloring change, we retain the same style. It often doesn't work anymore. In our minds we want to look like we did when we were twenty. Some of us never graduated from the 1960s. Or the 1970s. Or the 1980s . . .

As you know, women are especially susceptible to body changes. Many women give birth to their children in their twenties, and body shape almost always changes after childbirth! Women tend to experience another shift in body shape as they approach perimenopause. Why, then, do women continue dressing as we did when we were in our twenties? It is time to update our thinking—and our wardrobe!

DRESS FOR YOUR BODY SHAPE

Are you an apple-shaped person? Follow these tips to flatter your figure:

- Avoid accentuating the upper part of the body with large patterns, large accessories (scarves and jewelry, for example) around the neck and upper chest.

- Wear clothing that flows with the body and doesn't cling tightly to it.

- Choose tops that extend down below the waistline.

- Pants and slacks should be narrow through the sides; skirts should be straight.

- Adopt a linear look; a monochromatic (one-color) scheme makes you look taller and leaner.

- Select tones that are darker on top and lighter on the bottom. White makes you look a little bigger, so whatever part of your body is dressed in white will look larger.

- Avoid large, bulky fabrics and styles! Stay away from heavy sweaters, for example, especially ones that end at the waistline or shortly below it.

- Men should avoid the temptation to wear belts below their protruding stomachs, a practice that only accentuates the abdomen.

Are you a pear-shaped person? (Men usually aren't.) Here are some tips for you:

- Draw attention away from the hips by focusing on the upper body.

- Bring the whole body into visual balance by drawing a vertical line from the shoulders to the hips;

use shoulder pads or accessories to bring the shoulders out in line with the hips.

- If you are wearing clothing with darted seams, make sure the darts lay flat against the fabric so they don't bulge. The clothes should not cup under the buttocks area or blouse out at the abdomen.

- Color should emphasize the waist and upper body. Use a darker color on the bottom of the ensemble; a monochromatic outfit is also good.

- Do not use big, bold prints but select smaller ones with lots of space between the print. The print should be scaled to your body size.

- Scarves are good for bringing emphasis to the neck and upper body. Accessorize!

- Clothing that drapes softly over the shoulder pads and down vertically over the hips is very flattering to the pear-shaped woman, especially when it extends down to the buttocks or lower. It draws attention away from the hips and abdomen, and creates a linear effect.

- Avoid clothing that stops at the waist.

Are you shaped like a banana? Banana-shaped men and women want to look fuller. Wear clothing that adds size to the upper body, and enjoy belts that define the waistline.

If your excess weight is centered in the abdomen, use a longer jacket or sweater and pull the emphasis up to your face so that others will look at the whole you. Disguise your middle by wearing longer clothing over it.

Whatever your body shape is, pick your best feature and focus on that area. Everyone has something wonderful about his/her body—emphasize it!

You may want to browse through magazines to see how the people in the photos are dressed, and get some ideas for yourself. Remember your assignment last week to make a list of your best features? Emphasize them through your clothing or makeup (makeup and skin-care are discussed in next week's lesson). You are beautiful. Let it show!

And now, go to page 285 for your new recipes!

 TODAY'S ASSIGNMENTS

CLEAN OUT YOUR CLOSETS, AND SMILE

This is a big assignment. Remove the following from your closets:

▓ Outdated clothing

▓ Every piece of clothing that doesn't fit anymore (by the time it fits again, it will be outdated)

▓ Every item of clothing that doesn't look good on you

▓ Every item of clothing that reminds you of an unpleasant time in your life

▓ Every item of clothing that is the wrong color

We tend to hang on to clothes of different sizes for fear we'll need them again, that we'll get big again. But keep in mind: If it is too large for you, it will make you look bigger. If it is too small for you, it will make you look bigger (think of sausage in a casing). Hanging on to old things is a way of hanging on to the past, or living in the past. Clean it all out!

I hope you are not left with a bare closet. If so, go shopping! Find a store that offers the services of a personal shopper to help you create a style that accentuates your positive features.

Your second assignment is to practice smiling every day this week. Put a written reminder on your refrigerator, bathroom mirror, computer screen, and car mirror: "Smile!" Let your face take charge of your feelings and see how it lifts your spirits.

LESSON IV-5 STUDY GUIDE

1. What is the first step toward beauty?

2. What is the second step toward beauty?

3. List some tips for dressing an apple-shaped figure (men and women).

4. List some tips for dressing a pear-shaped figure (primarily women).

5. List some tips for dressing a banana-shaped figure (men and women).

HEALTH TIP

AN HERBAL MEDICINE CHEST

Continuing with the theme of the medicine chest, stock up on well-chosen herbs, nature's healers:

• *Aloe vera*, for burns, abrasions, or other skin irritations

• Dandelion, for all sorts of liver ailments and digestion

• St. John's wort, for mild-to-moderate depression

• Echinacea, for immune system support (take "one week on and one week off" during cold and flu season)

• Kava kava and passionflower, for tension and anxiety

• *Panax ginseng*, for an energy boost

• Siberian ginseng, for stress reduction (take along with vitamin C and pantothenic acid)

• Peppermint tea, for calming the stomach or nerves

• Neutralizing cordial, for any type of upset stomach, gassiness, and nervous stomach

To be prepared when my family needs preventive care, I also keep these other natural remedies on hand:

• Zinc lozenges

• Buffered vitamin C crystals

• Melatonin (for sleeping)

• Holy basil and rhodiola (for reducing the stress response)

• Lipotropics and L-cysteine (for liver detoxification)

• Olive leaf (for immune system support, especially against viruses)

Lesson IV-6. Make My Face Beautiful!

Note to male readers: This lesson (except for the section "Nutrition and Skin Care") is mostly relevant to women, so feel free to go to the next lesson if you wish, *but* do see the inset on page 215 ("Measuring Up") and then check out the Health Tip before you skip ahead.

Last week you cleaned out your closets. Was it painful? Do you now know how to dress to accentuate your body's best features? Today we're going to discuss how to make your face look great with attitude, diet, skin care, and a little cosmetic assistance.

? TODAY'S QUESTION

Do you feel beautiful today?

_____

_____

_____

_____

Do you have any great stories to share about a time you embarrassed yourself with your makeup or fashion? Or, a time in your life when you felt really, really gorgeous? What did it? Was it your hair, your makeup, your clothing? Or was it your own self-confidence? Write these stories down and share them with your daughters or a close friend.

As mentioned in Lesson IV-5, we tend to hang on to the look we developed in our twenties, even though our shape, skin color, and other features change as the decades pass. Our skin tends to lighten as we age, making it more essential to add a touch of makeup to make us look healthy. Gently applied makeup enhances our natural beauty by putting color back onto the skin. The goal of wearing makeup is not to make us look like we're wearing makeup but, ironically, to make us look natural.

BEAUTY FROM THE INSIDE OUT

Before starting on skin-care tips, I want to revisit beauty step number one from the last lesson: your smile. Remember that your inner self shines out on your face for the world to see. Facial features are an expression of personality, character, and emotional tone.

A lifetime of frowning physically distorts the muscles in the face, pulling its expression into a permanent frown. By the same token, a lifetime of smiling reshapes the muscles into a permanent smile. When you see laugh lines around the eyes of a friend, you know he/she has been laughing for years, don't you? But when you see brows permanently knitted together in a frown, you know those brows have been frowning for years. It is hard to disguise a disposition when it is etched right on the face.

Change your face today! Do you have a habit of frowning? Change the frown into a smile! Do you have a habit of being sad? Turn your sadness into joy! Remember that your emotions can follow your facial expression, not just the other way around. Put the smile on your face and, before long, you will feel happiness in your heart. Really!

 NOTES

_____

_____

_____

_____

_____

NUTRITION AND SKIN CARE

It is likely that you had to overcome a certain amount of chronic malnutrition by the time you entered the Wings Program. Most dieters have not eaten healthfully for some years, and as a result, malnutrition has taken its toll on their faces, causing the skin and various other facial tissues to lose elasticity. Some loss of muscle tone is a natural part of aging, but poor-quality diets accelerate the process: cheek muscles sag and droop, and muscle tone from forehead to chin can be lost where we didn't even know we had muscles in the first place. Adding to the wrinkle problem, low-fat diets dry out the skin.

Use these tips to bring some beauty back into your skin:

- Never use soap on your facial skin. Use good-quality cleansers that moisturize as they clean.

- Avoid any cleansing or moisturizing products that contain mineral oil or artificial ingredients; these are absorbed into the skin and are damaging to the body.

- Moisturize! Sun and wind dry out the skin on the face, neck, and hands. Rain or shine, your face is exposed to the weather. Use a daily moisturizer that is specifically designed for facial skin. Day creams should be thick enough to protect against damage from weather exposure and environmental toxins. Night creams should add nutrients back into the skin, as tissue repair takes place during sleep.

- Exfoliation creams can be used to dissolve the top layer of dead skin and rejuvenate the underlying tissue. One of my favorite facial products is Zia's Papaya Enzyme Peel, which I encourage you to use at least twice per week; if used frequently, it can help erase acne or other scars, or remove discolored skin.

- To moisturize your skin from within, drink at least eight to ten glasses of fresh water per day and include several tablespoons of fresh oils in your daily diet. One of the benefits of the Wings Program is that it makes the skin look so good—and whatever is good for the skin is good for the rest of the body.

- Get your beauty rest! Remember to get a full eight hours of sleep each night. A tired face is a droopy face. Cleanse your skin thoroughly before retiring for the night (never wear makeup to bed), make your room totally dark to stimulate the production of melatonin (a sleep-promoting hormone), and then sleep soundly. Consider taking a daytime nap for even more beauty rest (napping is not usually advisable, however, for people who struggle with insomnia).

WHAT ABOUT MAKEUP?

If you haven't changed your makeup program or products for several years, ask a professional to design a program for your skin-care needs. When selecting a foundation makeup, choose one with an SPF (sun protection factor) of 30 or higher so the face is not as likely to incur sun damage. Avoid baking in the sun; oxidation and sun hasten the aging of the skin.

What makeup do you enjoy wearing? Some women like eye makeup or lipstick, for example. Experiment to find colors and applications that make you look good. I often enjoy letting a professional makeup artist do my face and learning techniques as I watch; for example, light blush on the cheekbones helps accentuate the cheek line and adds color to the face, making it look younger and healthier. Again, the goal is not to look "made up" but to look natural.

As much as possible, stick to all-natural skin-care and cosmetic products (I love the Annemarie Borlind, Zia, and Aubrey lines). You do not want to absorb chemicals into your skin.

Measuring Up

It's that time again . . . Weigh yourself, and then take five girth measurements: bust at the largest point, waist at two inches above the navel, hips at the largest point, and right and left thigh circumference at the point where your extended fingertips reach with your arms hanging down at your sides. Record these figures, and your calculated BMI value, on your Progress Chart.

And now, go to page 285 for your new recipes!

  TODAY'S ASSIGNMENT

DESIGN THE NEW YOU

Go to a department store that provides an aesthetician and ask her to give you some makeup tips. Don't save your new look for special occasions; if makeup helps you feel good and look good, why not wear it every day?

LESSON IV-6 STUDY GUIDE

1. List some beauty tips.

2. How does dieting affect skin tone and facial musculature?

3. How do attitudes and emotions affect facial appearance?

4. What does "beauty sleep" mean?

5. List some skin-care tips.

HEALTH TIP

BURNS AND OTHER SKIN INJURIES

When a burn or injury occurs, prevent further skin damage by minimizing further trauma. Cool a first-degree or second-degree burn at once to reduce pain and swelling; use cool running water or cool compresses—not ice water or ice, however, as these will further damage the affected area. Remove any clothing or jewelry that is near the area so that blood flow won't be constricted if the tissue swells. Keep the burned area out of the sun and out of hot water when showering or bathing. If there is any sign of infection (odor, pus, or redness), see your physician immediately.

Caution: In a case of a possible third-degree burn, go immediately to the emergency room of the nearest hospital, as serious burns require prompt professional help. Do not attempt to treat it yourself, do not remove clothing that is touching it, and do not put ice or water on it.

Not only are burns and other skin injuries painful, they are potentially dangerous. To prevent them from developing into something more serious, take care of them—naturally. These topical applications are helpful:

- Cooling *Aloe vera* gel can be applied to a burn to ease the pain and promote healing.

- For other skin injuries, bathe the area in a tea of goldenseal root several times per day to prevent infection.

- Vitamin E oil may be directly applied to a burn or other injury to help prevent scarring.

- Honey applied directly to the wound can greatly aid in healing, and raw honey is antibacterial.

- Some good clinical work has been done using chitosan (previously described in Lesson I-9 as a fat blocker) on wounds and burns. Open a chitosan capsule, pour the chitosan directly on the injury, and allow it to harden. This forms a sort of bandage that keeps the injury clean and aids in its repair; the chitosan will, over time, bond with the skin and minimize scarring. *Note:* If you have an allergy to shellfish, use chitosan with caution.

Any time the skin is injured, amino acids and the mineral zinc rush to the injured area to begin rebuilding the tissue and mending the wound. Other proteins such as enzymes and immunoglobulins come to assist. In the event of a burn or other skin injury, extra nutrition is essential during the healing period. Take the following steps:

- Increase protein in the diet, and consider using a supplemental free-form amino-acid complex.

- Increase your potassium by eating more fresh green vegetables and taking a potassium supplement.

- Vitamin A, zinc, and B-complex vitamins are critically important. Take 100,000 international units (IU) of vitamin A daily for one month, then reduce the amount to 50,000 IU daily for one month, and then take 10,000 IU daily. (*Caution:* If pregnancy is possible, do not use more than 7,500 IU of vitamin A per day.) Increase zinc supplementation to 30–50 mg per day, with meals, along with 100 milligrams (mg) of B-complex vitamins daily.

- Vitamin C is essential for burns. Take 75 percent of your flushing level (page 9) of vitamin C daily to promote the healing of the burn and the formation of collagen, which is the "glue" that holds the tissue together.

- Increase your intake of vitamin E to 600 IU per day.

- Drink plenty of fluids during the recovery time. As burns dehydrate the body, compensate by drinking extra water.

ADDITIONAL NOTES

Lesson IV-7. I Eat When I'm . . .

Lessons III-4 and III-8 dealt, to an extent, with emotional eating behavior. I suggested ways to provide comfort during stressful times that do not involve food, and I hope you are now putting those suggestions to use in your life; they may not, however, be enough. You may need to deal with emotional triggers on a different level. If emotional eating has become more than a habit, help may be needed to dig more deeply into the past and bring healing.

? TODAY'S QUESTION

When do you eat?

_____

_____

_____

_____

Make a list of all the occasions on which you eat. How many of these legitimately involve nutrition? Make a list of the different emotions that cause you to eat.

As previously noted, we eat for many reasons that have nothing to do with nutrition. We eat, for example, out of anger, depression, sadness, grief, or loneliness, and to participate in celebrations or grieving events. There is a lot of emotional baggage associated with food, isn't there? And eating occasions such as family meals and holiday festivities are often fraught with emotional connotations.

POTHOLES ON MEMORY LANE

We know that many people have been abused during childhood or even in adulthood. Some of these people have not faced their personal abuse issues, so these issues keep reappearing. They may encounter their past every time they get together with the extended family . . . when someone cuts them off in traffic . . . when a child drops a glass of milk on the floor . . . when their boss scolds them . . . when their spouse asks a "loaded" question. They may handle the encounter with something to eat.

Is this you? Do you recognize yourself in this picture? If so, I grieve with you. You have suffered great losses and unhappiness in your life. Life could have been easier (should have been easier), but life was hard, and you are still struggling with the consequences.

Important Questions

Now I am going to ask a series of questions regarding your eating behaviors. Please don't skip lightly over this section; spend some time with the questions, and think about your own eating cues. This information may prove invaluable to resolving your weight difficulty.

▪ What were meals like with your parents and siblings? Were they happy times? Nurturing times? Angry or disciplinary times? What about now: Have you carried these "traditions" into your current family? Are family meals a time of great anger or other stress? Do you get a knot in your stomach when you assemble the family for dinner? Is this knot a reaction to current circumstances, or is it a carryover from past experiences? Is one person in the family responsible for the majority of the mealtime tension?

✎ NOTES

_____

_____

_____

_____

_____

_____

▨ Are many of your eating occasions triggered by something other than true hunger? What is your anger response? Do you eat out of anger? Are you often depressed or discouraged? Do sad times trigger eating behaviors that are inappropriate to the occasion?

▨ Do you often feel lonely? If you live alone, you may find that you feel the most isolated at mealtimes. It isn't pleasant to decorate the table or to prepare a fabulous dinner for just one person to enjoy. Do you avoid preparing a "real meal" for this reason? Do you tend to graze rather than dine to compensate for loneliness?

▨ Do you celebrate the grand occasions in your life with a chocolate-chip cookie or a bowl of ice cream? Do festive events always mean eating "forbidden" foods? When you were a child, did your parents reward you with foods for good behavior? Do you now reward yourself with food?

ARE YOU CARRYING EMOTIONAL BAGGAGE?

Mealtimes and food can be laden with a huge emotional burden, to the point that you cannot even enjoy the preparation and participation in the meal. Seldom do we eat for purely nutritional reasons; we often eat to feed our emotions, not our bodies. If we occasionally indulge in comfort foods or celebratory foods, no harm is done; our bodies easily adapt to an occasional treat without adding extra pounds. Indulging once in a while is fun, and we should feel no guilt about enjoying dinner or parties with family and friends. The problem is not the occasional celebration: the problem is when eating for emotional reasons becomes a way of life, when it is more typical than occasional.

But if you tend to eat for emotional reasons, do not despair. Do not allow guilt to wash over you—it will send you back to the kitchen for another cookie! You can learn to overcome this pattern and get started on the right track again. What do you need to do to resolve your emotional triggers?

Unloading Your Baggage

If you have a hard time dealing with painful issues from the past, or with inappropriate or unhealthful eating behaviors brought on by emotional situations, do not be afraid to seek professional help. Ask your doctor to refer you to a licensed counselor. Talking these issues through with a professional can be very healing, and he/she can recommend ways to deal more proactively with the people who trigger unhealthful feelings and behaviors. A caring, competent counselor can become your most valuable ally!

Lesson IV-9 will discuss the types of people who purposely sabotage your efforts to be slim and healthy, and how to handle this problem. Even if you are dealing with very difficult people and situations, you have a choice in how to handle them. You may need to set clearer boundaries around yourself. You may even need to choose to avoid those people or situations. Whatever you need to do to bring yourself emotional strength, do it!

If You Eat Alone . . .

Eating alone can present real challenges for some people. Not everyone is like one of my friends who, as a single woman, always set her table with her best china and a vase of fresh flowers for dinner. She would say, "Why shouldn't I dress the table just for me? I'm worth it!" You are, too.

Here are some tips for "single eating" to help you stay focused on your health goals:

1. Do what my friend does: dress your table for dinner each night. Use your nice china and silverware and a placemat. Put a single flower or a vase full of flowers on the table, and decorate your table just as you would for guests. Make yourself feel special because you really are!

2. Prepare two meals at once, and set one portion aside for lunch the next day. Why mess up the kitchen twice?

3. Make your plate look pretty. Scout the aisles of your grocery store for specialty items that "dress up" the meal; dried cranberries, for example, look and taste wonderful on a salad. Buy seasonal fruits for a side dish or garnish.

4. Once or twice a week, share a meal with a friend. You are probably not the only "solitary eater" in your circle of friends. Trade meals, or host a cooking party once a week.

5. Do you know a single mom or dad? Single parents have the most difficult job in the world, and could use your help. Invite their children over for dinner, or get a sitter for the kids and invite the single parent to your home for a special dinner. What a blessing you will be to that tired person! Or, are *you* the single parent? Invite another single parent for dinner; hire a sitter for all the kids (share the cost),

cook dinner together, and eat in front of the fireplace or a movie. Do it often—life is too short to be alone.

6. Remember: a main purpose of any of these activities is to keep you on your program! Prepare a Wings meal. It's no fair comforting you (and your guest) with a gallon of ice cream!

And now, go to page 286 for your new recipes!

 TODAY'S ASSIGNMENT

EXPLORE YOUR CHILDHOOD

Write down some food-associated stories from your childhood. Do you remember how your relatives dealt with emotions? Were their emotional coping behaviors food related? How were you rewarded? Record these memories. Write down anything that will help you understand your own food triggers. Then, review your stories. Do these issues require further exploration? Work on a solution with a loved one, your counselor, or your accountability partner. Remember that you are not enslaved by your history!

LESSON IV-7 STUDY GUIDE

1. List some emotional triggers for eating behaviors.

2. What are some strategies for dealing with these emotional triggers?

3. How does eating alone often cause problems for people who want to control their weight?

4. If you are a single person, what strategies can you employ to make dining a pleasure?

 HEALTH TIP

PROSTATE CARE

About 50 percent of men over the age of fifty discover a problem with their prostate gland. Men, even if you are not yet fifty or are not yet experiencing symptoms (such as pressure in that area or frequent urination at night), now is the time to begin preventive care of this important organ. Several supplements, herbs, and natural therapies are especially helpful for preventing prostate problems, or (if you are already symptomatic) for reducing symptoms.

- On top of your daily multivitamin, take about 50–100 milligrams (mg) of the entire B-complex; vitamin B_6 is particularly important for lowering the risk of cancer.

- Take up to 80 mg of zinc daily, in divided doses with meals.

- Snack on pumpkin seeds, which are rich in zinc and other nutrients that benefit the prostate.

- Take at least 3 grams of fish oil (EPA/DHA) daily with meals to obtain the essential fatty acids that are very important to prostate function.

- Supplement your diet with the amino acids L-alanine, L-glutamic acid, and L-glycine, which are necessary for normal prostate function; Formula 600 by Nature's Life is a good supplement. Several other companies provide "prostate formulas" that combine these amino acids with pumpkin seeds, saw palmetto, and other herbs and nutrients (ask at the health food store).

- Make a tea from buchu, corn silk, juniper berries, parsley, slippery elm bark, or bearberry to use as a natural diuretic and urinary tract tonic.

- Chinese ginseng is beneficial for prostate health and sexual vitality.

- Eliminate tobacco, alcoholic beverages (especially beer and wine), caffeine, chlorinated and fluoridated water, spicy foods, junk foods, and tomato products.

- Drink 2–3 quarts of pure water every day.

- Get regular exercise. Do not, however, use a bicycle with a hard seat that puts pressure on the prostate.

- Dr. James Balch and Phyllis Balch, authors of *Prescription for Nutritional Healing* (New York, NY: Avery Publishing Group, 1997), recommend hydrotherapy to increase circulation in the prostate region. Sit in a bathtub of the hottest water tolerable for fifteen to thirty minutes once or twice per day; or, spray the lower abdomen and pelvis with water, alternating between three minutes of hot water and one minute of cold. Another method is sitting in hot water with the feet in cold water for three minutes, and then sitting in cold water with the feet in hot water for one minute.

ADDITIONAL NOTES

Lesson IV-8. The Other Side of the Coin: Eating Disorders and Activity Disorder

You might think it odd to talk about anorexia, bulimia, and other eating disorders in the context of a weight-loss curriculum. Don't these people do the opposite of what we do? They refuse to eat, or they vomit up what they ate. Many of them have lost too much weight, and are too thin already.

I present this material for a number of reasons. Some people's weight struggle begins with an eating disorder and progress, through poor health, to ongoing weight problems. Other people see their children beginning to struggle with weight as they do, and in an attempt to save them from the frustration they've endured, they become so strident that they actually induce eating disorders in their children. I want to prevent these situations from occurring, to help people develop healthful eating behaviors without going too far to the other extreme.

?   **TODAY'S QUESTION**

Have you ever had an eating disorder?

_____

_____

_____

_____

Did you struggle with any eating disorder like anorexia, bulimia, or uncontrolled eating before or after your weight problem began? Has anyone in your family struggled with an eating disorder?

As a nutritionist, I believe that there is a continuum of disordered eating. At one end are "picky eating" and consistent consumption of nutrient-poor foods; at the other end are diagnosed eating disorders like anorexia and bulimia, and even death.

WHERE DO EATING DISORDERS BEGIN?

Attitudes about weight are "caught" or taught very early in life. As the mother of four young daughters, I was amazed and dismayed at how early their body consciousness began. They became aware of their weight around the age of four or five, with no prompting from me. I never discussed overweight with them when they were little, but they began to make references to their own "overweight" when they started kindergarten and began associating with girls outside the home. Where did they pick it up? Possibly from other little girls, older girls, parents, the media—wherever this message about weight comes from, it is intensely harmful.

When researching the material for my first book, *Your Fat Is Not Your Fault* (New York, NY: Jeremy P. Tarcher/Penguin, 1998), I asked my daughters about their attitudes toward being overweight. Young as they were, they assured me they would rather be dead, or have a limb amputated, than be overweight. I was shocked! Unfortunately, their comments mirror research findings on the subject: children are terrified of being overweight and would rather suffer a disfiguring injury, or even die, than "be fat."

The incidence of eating disorders is rising rapidly among our very young, especially among young

✎   **NOTES**

_____

_____

_____

_____

_____

_____

girls. Eating disorders may begin as early as four or five years old, as little girls become aware of their bodies and aware that some children are heavy and some are slim. If they are a little heavy, or even if they just perceive they are a little heavier than their friends, they become incredibly self-conscious. If encouraged by the culture or by pressure from family and friends, they will lean more and more toward developing a full-blown eating disorder.

Is It a Control Issue?

Following is a list of "common states of being" for the eating-disordered individual:

- Low self-esteem

- Diminished self-worth

- Belief in the "thinness myth" (a notion that thinness is the "ultimate beauty," and that "good things" happen to thin people, or conversely, that "bad things" happen to overweight people)

- Need for distraction

- Dichotomous ("black or white") thinking

- Feelings of emptiness

- Quest for perfection

- Desire to be special/unique

- Need to be in control

- Need for power

- Desire for respect and admiration

- Difficulty expressing feelings

- Need for escape or a safe place to go

- Lack of coping skills

- Lack of trust in self and others

- Terror of not measuring up

Issues of control are part of the eating disorder syndrome. Children with eating disorders have an unusually strong need to control their bodies through food consumption as a means of establishing some form of control when the "uncontrollable" aspects of their lives cannot be changed. Most of the problem of anorexia is not loss of appetite but the desire to control it; many anorexics are extremely interested in food and dream about indulging their appetites, but they seem to have lost control over their lives—except in the area of food. The control issue becomes the driving force behind the disordered eating behavior.

However, once extreme malnutrition brought on by the eating disorder has robbed their bodies of the ability to digest food, and hypothyroidism and other health conditions have set in, anorexics may become unable to eat. Eating may actually make them sick. These children are very ill and desperately require the professional help of a doctor and a nutritionist. If you know someone is struggling with an eating disorder, seek help immediately, as his/her life is in danger.

Vegetarianism, Zinc Deficiency, and Disordered Eating

When I first heard of the increased popularity of vegetarianism, especially among young girls, I was pleased, thinking that these girls were becoming more conscious of the value of selecting healthful foods. I saw it as a trend toward health consciousness and good eating behaviors.

But as I interviewed many of these girls to learn what they ate, I became horrified. Most of these young vegetarians ate no vegetables at all! They ate pasta, cereal, and junk food. When I questioned the lack of vegetables in their "vegetarian" diet, raised the issue of protein deficiency, and talked about the likelihood of serious, chronic malnutrition, they laughed. They really had no concerns about a balanced diet or about meeting their nutritional needs. Most of them became vegetarian because they do not like the idea of killing animals for food, but they had little thought for their own welfare. I suspect, however, another reason that they chose vegetarianism: they are zinc deficient.

Zinc deficiency is becoming increasingly common, especially in young girls who do not eat balanced, healthful meals. One of the symptoms of zinc deficiency is distaste for protein foods, probably because enzymes (such as protease) that digest proteins are zinc dependent. A zinc-deficient body cannot produce the enzymes to digest meat, and therefore the body may choose to avoid eating a food that it cannot digest.

Perhaps a zinc deficiency leads to disordered eating, like the "vegetarianism" described above that is not based on healthful balance. A vegetarian diet is very low in zinc because high-zinc foods include red meats, whereas grains and vegetables do not provide adequate amounts of zinc. Do you see a vicious cycle here? Adolescents choose a predominantly grain-based diet, this zinc-deficient diet reduces their ability to digest animal and other proteins, they reject those proteins, and grains are the only foods they feel good about eating . . . leading to further decline in their zinc status. Interestingly, clinicians find that when zinc supplementation is given to patients with eating disorders, the disorders are resolved more easily and the patients gain weight.

Zinc deficiency has been causally linked to virtually every type of eating disorder. It is also linked to hyperactivity and to alterations in key hormones like thyroid, estrogen, and cortisol. Large amounts of zinc are present in areas of the brain that are involved in food seeking, weight regulation, and serotonin metabolism. Low levels of the calming neurotransmitter serotonin are linked to carbohydrate cravings. Also, people with eating disorders often have a problem with anger management that is thought to stem from serotonin dysregulation or inadequacy.

It is interesting to note that approximately one-half of women with anorexia nervosa are vegetarians. I have grave concerns about the long-term consequences of adolescent vegetarianism, and one of the reasons I do not endorse a vegetarian lifestyle is that the risk of nutritional deficiencies, leading to many health challenges, is virtually inevitable. Frankly, I have concerns about vegetarianism for adults as well, *unless* the adult is extremely knowledgeable about nutrition, eats a wide variety of foods including copious amounts of vegetables and vegetable sources of proteins, and supplements the diet with nutrients known to be undersupplied in a vegetarian diet. These nutrients include vitamin B_{12}, zinc, and several sulfur-bearing amino acids like L-cysteine and L-methionine.

ACTIVITY DISORDER

Hand-in-hand with eating disorders is a condition that health professionals have categorized as activity disorder. The achievement orientation, independence, self-control, perfectionism, persistence, and well-developed mental strategies of activity-disordered people can foster significant academic and vocational accomplishments in such a way that they appear to be healthy, high-functioning individuals. Their levels of activity, however, are beyond the "healthy zone." They are driven to excessive exercise as a way of maintaining control over their bodies. This obsession is as unhealthy as an eating disorder.

Activity disorder is characterized as follows:

▪ The person maintains a high level of activity and is uncomfortable with states of rest or relaxation.

▪ The individual depends on the activity for self-definition and mood stabilization.

▪ There is an intense, driven quality to the activity

that becomes self-perpetuating and resistant to change, compelling the person to continue the behavior while feeling unable to control it or stop it.

Although activity-disordered individuals may have coexisting personality disorders, there is no particular personality profile or psychological disorder that is known to underlie activity disorder. Activity-disordered persons will use rationalizations and other defense mechanisms to protect their involvement in the activity.

I encourage you to become an active person, but you must keep your eating and activity in balance. Eating and exercise should never become compulsive or have a driven quality about them. If you feel that you may be exercising to an extreme degree, or that your eating or exercise activities are dominating your life, please seek professional help to get your balance back.

PROMOTE HEALTHFUL EATING HABITS IN YOUR CHILDREN

Overweight moms and dads can trigger or encourage eating disorders by promoting dieting behaviors inappropriately. After all, children are easily influenced; when they see their parents struggling with weight, they become determined not to inherit that struggle. Being overweight can be a source of considerable shame, and peers are merciless in teasing overweight children. Were you teased as a child? Consider how that could have influenced your weight challenge. Teasing sets kids up for increased sensitivity to body shape and size and makes them self-conscious. Do not tease your children—or allow them to be teased.

My overweight clients have shared heartbreaking stories about parents who forbade them from enjoying the same foods that the rest of the family was eating, or parents who made huge issues of their child's weight in front of other people. One woman told of a mother who purposely overfed her daughter so she would gain weight and "be just like me." These insidious forms of abuse lead to emotional and physical problems that can last for a lifetime.

Moms and dads can also inadvertently encourage eating disorders, or at least disordered eating, by indulging childish whims about food selection. Young children can become very selective about what they will eat, and they seldom choose a healthful diet. In fact, several studies have shown that only 1 percent of children consistently receive the U.S. recommended daily allowance (RDA) for all vitamins and minerals. We know that chronic undernutrition is an issue in this country, even though we eat too many calories. And in Modules I and II of this book, you learned that chronic malnutrition or undernutrition plays a role in hypothyroidism and other conditions that directly lead to weight challenges.

I do not allow my children to consistently make their own food decisions because they lack the maturity and information to make those important choices. My girls have occasionally said, "I'm going to be a vegetarian," to which I've replied, "No, you are not. And here is why . . . . " Mom and Dad, you have the important job of building the foundation for your child's lifelong health. Don't abdicate your responsibility because of his/her whining or temperament: take a firm stand and make the right decisions for a healthful, well-balanced diet in your home. Your child's health, weight, and life depend on it!

If you struggle in the weight department, be especially sensitive to the emotional and physical needs of your children. Do not pressure them. Present the same marvelous food options you've been given in Wings, and teach your children to indulge in wonderful, natural foods that build health and vitality. Encourage them to live actively so they burn off excess calories by enjoying life. Don't let them plunk themselves down in front of a television and "vege out."

Better yet, work out with your children: join a club together, play tennis together, or go swimming. Biking is fun for the whole family, as are hiking and dancing. Be an active family! The weight issues children face are most often this simple: too many empty calories (junk food) and too little activity. Eliminate the junk, up the activity level, and most juvenile obesity problems are solved with no further involvement.

POST-DISORDER NUTRITION

If you have struggled with an eating disorder in the past, increase your supplemental nutrition to make up for years of gross malnutrition. Discuss your eating history with a nutritionist who can help you design a program to compensate for past malnutrition; your Wings nutritionist (at www.flywithwings. com/pnc.html, click on MyProConnect) can help make sure you are on track. Eating disorders damage the intestinal lining, so absorption of nutrients may be impaired, further increasing your need for adequate supplementation.

Remember that starvation is one of the driving forces behind hypothyroidism. If your thyroid gland is not working properly and you have struggled through an eating disorder, nourish your thyroid and work with your doctor to correct the endocrine problem and bring your whole body back into balance.

And now, go to page 286 for your new recipes!

 TODAY'S ASSIGNMENT

CHECKING AND BALANCING

How are you doing in the eating and activity departments? Are things getting out of control? Have you felt yourself becoming a little obsessive in your resolve to eat correctly and get adequate amounts of exercise? Talk to your spouse or a trusted friend and ask if your approach to health seems balanced. If he/she sends up some "red flags" of caution, take heed and evaluate your approach to the program as objectively as you can. Remember that the goal of Wings is to build vibrant health, not make you obsessive about your weight-management program!

LESSON IV-8 STUDY GUIDE

1. Why is information about eating disorders included in this weight-loss book?

2. List at least ten "common states of being" for the eating-disordered person.

3. What is an activity disorder?

4. Explain the link between zinc deficiency and eating disorders.

5. Discuss the "cons" of adolescent vegetarianism and how it can lead to eating disorders.

6. Explain some of the ways that parents can "encourage" eating disorders in their children.

HEALTH TIP

FIBROMYALGIA

Fibromyalgia is a condition of chronic tissue pain that ranges from mildly annoying to extremely painful. This pain may be in the lower back, neck, shoulders, back of the head, upper chest, and/or thighs; it is described by sufferers as burning, throbbing, shooting, and stabbing, with more pain in the morning. Among the other symptoms are headache, insomnia, depression, painful menstrual periods, anxiety, and dry eyes and mouth. Most individuals with this condition have some type of sleep disorder as well. Fibromyalgia's most distinctive feature, however, is the presence of "tender points" that are painful to the touch. One theorized cause of fibromyalgia is that reduced cellular energy production leads to a buildup of toxic waste materials in the cells.

Fibromyalgia is increasing in incidence. If you are experiencing symptoms of this painful disorder, try these natural tips to reduce or eliminate them:

- Take supplementary coenzyme Q_{10}, (CoQ_{10}) up to 240 milligrams (mg) per day, to improve the cells' oxygenation and energy production.

- Take up to 500 mg of magnesium malate per day, in a supplement that also provides about 1,200 mg of malic acid. Malic acid is involved in cellular energy production (a process called the Krebs cycle); supplemental malic acid may increase cell energy and aid in cell detoxification.

- Do the ascorbic acid flush frequently (pages 8–9), and maintain a daily vitamin C dosage of at least 75 percent of your flushing level. Vitamin C helps prevent the buildup of lactic acid, which is the energy-production byproduct that causes muscle pain after physical exertion.

- Take proteolytic enzymes to reduce inflammation. *Note:* Take these enzymes apart from food.

- Take 3,000–5,000 mg of fish oil per day to reduce inflammation.

- Take up to 25,000 international units (IU) of vitamin A per day, unless pregnancy is possible. *Caution:* If you are or may be pregnant, keep your vitamin A intake at no more than 7,500 IU per day.

- Consider getting B-complex vitamin shots to further increase your body's energy production.

- Reduce all potential dietary and environmental allergens; do the pulse test (pages 47–48; see also Appendix 5) on all of your commonly consumed foods, and remove every offending food from your diet.

- Do the Wings cleansing protocol (Lesson II-6) at least four times per year to aid in the body's detoxification.

- Take the amino acid L-cysteine to further detoxify the liver.

- Regularly drink teas of dandelion, red clover, and burdock root to promote liver function and cleanse the bloodstream.

- Get plenty of rest.

- Although exercise is important, let your body tell you when it is time to stop; don't push yourself beyond your abilities in the mistaken belief that you have to "push through the pain."

- For pain relief, try a topical cream that contains capsicum (an extract of cayenne pepper); this shuts down the transmission (via substance P) of pain signals to the brain, easing pain for several hours after the cream's application.

- Focus your diet on raw foods, with adequate amounts of protein and fresh fats.

- Drink plenty of fresh, pure water and herbal teas.

- Consider drinking freshly made vegetable juices and fruit juices, both a good source of energy.

- Avoid all caffeine, alcohol, sugar, wheat, and fermented products.

Lesson IV-9. Loving Saboteurs

Do you live in a nonsupportive environment? It is hard enough to make life-long changes in habits and customs, but when you face opposition from those you love most dearly, the challenge is even greater. It is like playing a constant game of tug-of-war, and that daily struggle can wear out the strongest person among us.

? TODAY'S QUESTION

Does your family encourage your efforts?

_____

_____

_____

_____

What does your spouse think of the Wings Program? Is he/she participating or cooperating with you? What do your children think of your program? Do they try to sneak things in behind your back? Do you feel that something—or someone—is holding you down, trying to thwart your progress? Is anyone sabotaging your best efforts to be healthy?

Maybe you are living with a "loving saboteur": someone who purposely tries to make you fail, who can make you feel incredibly guilty for simply working on your health goals, who can set up roadblocks at every juncture. Women especially struggle with guilt—it seems to be part of the female nature—and loving saboteurs can be masterful at manipulating that guilt.

A loving saboteur is someone who is purposely trying to defeat your plan to lose weight and become healthy. It could be a spouse, a child, or a parent; it could be your best friend or a favorite relative. A loving saboteur is someone who is influential in your life because of close familial or friendship ties, and who is trying to take control of you and your life through some sort of manipulation like guilt, intimidation, fear, anger, or more subtle forms of exploitation.

Why would people sabotage their loved ones' programs, especially goals like improved health and weight management? Following are some of the possible reasons:

- They are insecure, so any change, even positive change, is too difficult for them to handle. They are afraid that your weight loss will change your relationship with them—and it probably will! When you feel really good about yourself, you will change, and that will alter the relationship, which could be a positive thing; insecure people, however, see any change as negative.

- They may sincerely like to watch you enjoy foods that they can't enjoy for some reason, a type of vicarious eating pleasure. If they miss their favorite food, perhaps they get pleasure watching you eat it.

- Forcing others to eat may be a serious control or anger issue for some individuals. Compelling a loved one to remain unhealthy or heavy may be a way of keeping that person under close control, forcing him/her to remain in seclusion or "committed in the relationship," for example. They may

✒ NOTES

_____

_____

_____

_____

_____

_____

feel that if their loved one is more attractive, they may lose him/her to another lover—another form of insecurity.

- They may enjoy snuggling with a heavier, fuller figure. They simply don't like a thin spouse.

- They may simply want company as they indulge in their unhealthful foods. They want you to eat with them just for sociability. They don't want to eat alone.

- Tragically, some saboteurs even force-feed their partners to keep them obese, then use them as models for pornographic purposes. These women are trapped in a dangerous situation that requires professional (and possibly legal) assistance.

Relationships with food and people can be so complicated! How will they be resolved? If you are struggling to gain control over your eating and exercise habits because of a loving saboteur, how will you deal with it? You may have felt victimized by the person or situation for years. Marriage or relationship counseling may be necessary for deeply rooted issues. Be comforted to know that you always have options! You can choose to take control of your life and stop allowing the saboteur to control you. Remember that you are responsible for your own health, and you are responsible for what you eat. You can never hand this responsibility over to another person. The joy of becoming healthy is yours—alone.

Ask yourself the following questions:

- What do I really want for myself? Do I want to lose weight? Do I want to be healthy?

- Do I want to control my own health destiny? Who will decide how much I should weigh or how I should feel?

- What kind of opposition do I face? Who is my loving saboteur? How is that person sabotaging my goals? What is his/her method of manipulation: anger, guilt, shame, fear? Why is he/she trying to sabotage my goals? (You may not be able to discover the motives, but you can certainly realize the method of control.)

- What are my resources to deal with the sabotage? What are my options? How can I deal with the situation in a loving, strong way to take control of my life?

- Is my loving saboteur insecure? How can he/she get help for the insecurity? Am I trying to take the responsibility for my saboteur's problem? Am I preventing my saboteur from personal growth because I haven't forced him/her to take responsibility for the problem?

Healthy marriages are built on trust, companionship, and the mutual nurturing of two individuals who are free to pursue another course. A healthy marriage is not a trap, not a form of enslavement. True love always seeks the highest good of the loved one; as the Scriptures teach, love never seeks its own good. People in loving relationships truly seek the best for the loved one, even at the expense of their own unhappiness. Until self-sacrificing love is at the foundation of a marriage, the marriage cannot work, and the marriage partners will need to seek professional counseling to learn how to unconditionally love each other.

If love is not possible in a marriage or other relationship, the partner seeking health must choose to be healthy apart from the relationship. How is this to be accomplished? Set your personal goals around the obstacles put up by the noncompliant partner. Can you enforce your nutritional and emotional needs in the face of opposition? If your spouse is unwilling to eat your food, are you willing to prepare two meals, or will your spouse prepare his/her own meals? Are you willing to lose weight and push through to achieve your goals, even if your partner wants you to remain heavy?

Each marriage and situation is different. Here are some additional tips for dealing with a loving saboteur:

- Is your spouse willing to be taught good nutritional habits? Become the nutrition coach in your home. Prepare the wonderful meals in the Wings Program; the enticing aromas and flavors may be the best way to engage your partner's support.

- Although your spouse indulges in forbidden or unhealthful foods, you may still enjoy good, healthful foods. While your saboteur eats a slice of apple pie with ice cream, for example, you could have one of your homemade treats or a glass of wine, or nibble on a medley of fresh fruit. Going to the movies? Pack your own snack, and buy bottled water instead of a soft drink. Want something to munch while watching television with your loved one? Choose a fresh fruit platter, a nut mix, or a bowl of fresh popcorn (with a tiny bit of butter and salt). If your spouse is unhappy because you eat something different, that is his/her problem, not yours.

- Does your saboteur try to force you to eat a certain "forbidden food" just because he/she cannot have

My Loving Saboteur Story

I had a loving saboteur in my life for many years. When our relationship began, I weighed 135 pounds. He decided he wanted me to be heavier, so, without consulting me, he began "force-feeding" me. He didn't physically put food into my mouth, but he used guilt, badgering, and other ways to get me to eat more. He bought food I didn't want and badgered me to eat it. As I had never been heavy, I didn't even realize what was happening until four months later when I got on the scale—I had gained more than 35 pounds, and had to go shopping for new clothes.

As the relationship developed, the control issue never went away. In my childhood, I had been trained to submit to the men in my life, and that pattern of submission continued into my adulthood. He would put food on my plate—so I ate it. He chose the restaurants and selected the meals. If I complained or tried to insert my opinion, he used guilt, humor, trickery, and constant badgering to get me to eat what he wanted me to eat.

People with control issues tend to be involved with people with boundary issues. I had major boundary issues!

Years later, still heavier than I wanted to be, I finally grew up. I decided that I needed to establish firm boundaries and take charge of my health and weight. I learned to say no. I even stopped feeling guilty if I didn't eat something he wanted me to eat.

When he said, "I can't eat this, so it would give me pleasure if you ate it," I responded, "So I have to make myself sick and fat to give you pleasure?" When he put bread on my plate, I silently put it aside. When he put his unwanted food on my plate, I said, "Stop putting food on my plate," and put it back on his plate (sometimes that morsel got passed around several times before the waitress took it away). Eventually, he got the message, but it took several years of consistently reaffirming my boundaries before he realized that his control tactics would no longer work.

If I could do it, so can you! Reaffirming your boundaries will take consistency, patience, and probably a good dose of humor to make it stick, and may even take counseling, but you must do it!

---

it? This is a control issue that you must resolve. When the forbidden food is presented and persistently urged upon you, explain clearly that you do not care for that food. Say it lovingly but firmly. Each time the food is offered, smile and simply say, "No, thanks," and push it away; or, accept it but silently leave it on the plate. Just because someone gives you something to eat, you don't have to eat it. And there is no need to feel guilty.

- If your spouse likes you a little rounder than you prefer to be, you need to discuss your individual needs. Every person needs to be in control of his/her own body; a loving spouse will recognize the loved one's needs and allow him/her the privilege to choose personal weight and health goals.

- Is this a boundary issue? If you have trouble establishing boundaries in your life, I encourage you to read *Boundaries: When to Say Yes, When to Say No to Take Control of Your Life* by Dr. Henry Cloud and Dr. John Townsend (Grand Rapids, MI: Zondervan House, 1993). This book can help you establish healthful boundaries in your relationship. Just as "good fences make good neighbors," good boundaries help make a good marriage.

And now, go to page 287 for your new recipes!

 ## TODAY'S ASSIGNMENT

ERECT YOUR FENCES

Have a discussion with yourself this week about your health and weight goals. Is anyone hindering your progress? Do you have a loving saboteur in your life? If you do, brainstorm with yourself or talk with your accountability partner to discover your options. How will you handle the situation? Remember: you are not a victim of someone else's goals and desires, of someone else's insecurities or problems. You are in charge of your life and your body! It's time to take control.

LESSON IV-9 STUDY GUIDE

1. What is a loving saboteur?

_____

_____

_____

2. What are some reasons that people try to sabotage the health-improvement or weight-management programs of the people they love?

_____

_____

_____

_____

3. List some ways to reassert control over your body.

_____

_____

_____

_____

HEALTH TIP

PORTION CONTROL

If you have been on numerous diets in the past, you've been taught calorie counting and various other restrictions. You've tried to "push past the hunger" and to pretend that a bowl of lettuce is ultimately and gloriously satisfying. Then you came into the Wings Program—and I don't tell you how much food to eat. Why not? Because I don't know how much *you* should eat! How can I, when we are all different?

Even more confusing, your personal caloric needs can change on a daily basis. Some days, you feel particularly hungry; other days, you really don't feel like eating. But because you're used to being told how much to eat, you may be feeling uncertain when you sit down to your Wings meals. Here are some simple guidelines to help with portion control (some of these should be familiar by now):

- Eat slowly at each meal. Chew each bite thoroughly, at least twenty times, until the solid food is a liquid in your mouth.

- Relax when you eat. Never shove food into your mouth while you're hurrying to do something else. Don't get into an argument at mealtime. Make your dining a pleasurable experience and eat deliberately. Don't just gobble food mindlessly because you're distracted by something else. Get your whole body and mind involved in the enjoyment of your meal.

- Do I have to say it? Only eat *real* food. Junk food fills your stomach but doesn't satisfy your body, so you'll feel like you need to keep eating and eating to produce any satisfaction.

- Eat just until you are satisfied (not full), then stop. Is there still food on your plate? It is wasteful to eat it if you don't really need it! Your body is not a garbage can or a storage container for leftovers. Are you accustomed to filling your plate and then feeling obligated to eat everything on it? Use a smaller plate, put less food on it, and stop when you are barely satisfied. It takes twenty minutes from the time you have consumed enough food to the time your body tells your brain that it is satisfied; if you keep eating during those twenty minutes, you will have overeaten. You should never feel stuffed when you finish your meal. Be pleasantly satisfied—and that's it.

- Sometimes you will feel like you need more food. That is natural. If your activity levels are increased, if you are at a certain place in your menstrual cycle, if your immune system is fighting something, if you are under stress, or if you are healing an injury, you need more nutrition and your body will call for it. On the other hand, if your life is peaceful and calm and you are fairly sedentary, you will feel like you need less food.

- Above all, learn to listen to your body. It has great wisdom. Take heed!

Lesson IV-10. Making Health a Lifelong Journey

Here we are, at the end of the Wings curriculum. Hasn't it been a great year? Have you learned a great deal about your body? One of the main goals of Wings is to provide the information you need so that you can take responsibility for your own good health. I hope that goal has been fulfilled. Of course, there is still so much to learn. The human body is so marvelously complex that we will never feel like we've learned enough, but the tools provided in the Wings curriculum have given you a good start on knowing your body and exploring the world of natural health.

? TODAY'S QUESTION

Can you follow this program for the rest of your life?

_____

_____

_____

_____

Have you successfully put your new knowledge to work? What issues remain unresolved? How will you continue to maintain and improve your health for the rest of your life?

I encourage you to start again, at the very beginning, and go through this book a second time. You have probably forgotten some important information.

You may not have been able to complete all the work. It would certainly be beneficial to repeat the food sections (Module I). Food issues remain difficult for most of us, especially when we are asked to break habits that are several decades old—ditto for exercise issues.

If you are going to go through the material again, how about asking a friend or family member to do it with you? You may do better with someone to hold you accountable, and you will do that person a great favor as well. Plan to get together for lunch or dinner each week, for example. Creating a mutual support group is by far the best way to do the Wings Program.

Whether or not you intend to repeat the curriculum, I ask this question: "What are your health plans for the rest of your life?" There are several important points to remember:

■ As I have said, "If you are overweight now or have been overweight in the past, you are permanently potentially overweight. Period. You will never lose your tendency to be fat, no matter what you do."

What does this mean? Does it mean that you cannot lose weight? No, of course not: most of you have now achieved your weight goals and are looking forward to a life of health and vitality. It simply means that you have a permanent tendency to regain unwanted weight. It means that your body has stored too many fat cells and these fat cells want to get back up to their original (larger) size. It means that your metabolism may have slowed slightly if you are consuming fewer calories than you were before and have not yet sped it up again by following the suggestions in Lesson III-2.

So if you resume your former pattern of eating, you will regain your weight; if you wish to remain slender (or to lose more weight) and maintain your health, you must continue to follow the Wings

✒ NOTES

_____

_____

_____

_____

_____

_____

principles and enjoy healthful, delicious food forever. Do not be discouraged about this—you have been released from a life of "fat bondage"! You now know the secret of being healthy and slim, and you can enjoy your good health for the rest of your life.

- If you have lost your unwanted weight and reached your goal weight, you can maintain your goal simply by enjoying the rich abundance that nature provides. It is that simple—and that delicious. Avoid the temptation to sneak in many little "treats," or before you know it, you'll be hanging on to excess water, and fat tissue will accumulate as well.

- Encourage your own well-being through good health habits and by "going natural" as much as possible. You now know, for example, that prescription medications often cause weight gain through water retention or fat deposition, and that drugs can also interfere with your natural ability to maintain health by blocking your body's innate response mechanisms. Explore the world of natural health care; the more you use natural products to solve simple health problems, the healthier you will become.

- Avoid *at all costs* the temptation to read diet articles and books! They are generally wrong in their information and approach, and will only lead to confusion, frustration, and failure. The goal of magazine covers is to sell magazines, not to help you achieve maximum health; the goal of most weight-loss books is to sell books, not to inform. Very few weight-management books on the market today are worth anything, in fact, because they contain so much misinformation that they do more harm than good. Do not be tempted to chase a fad!

- Good health and a healthful weight are a lifelong journey, not a destination. If you have achieved your weight goal, great! Continue on your health journey and you'll continue to reap the benefits of good health. You really can keep feeling better and better! You really can stay on the Wings Program for the rest of your life—and enjoy it! I have lived my life on the Wings Program for more than fourteen years. I am healthier now, in middle age, than I was when I was "young and foolish." This is my life—and I love living (and eating) this way.

- The long and wonderful list of "side benefits" of eating correctly includes improved skin texture (soft, glowing skin), strong hair and nails, more energy, better sleep quality, normal cholesterol and triglyceride levels, normal blood sugar levels, improved digestion (less bloating, less intestinal gas, less undigested food in the stool) with regular bowel movements, better memory and mood, less depression or other mental and emotional conditions, and more . . . No wonder Wings students love this program so much. It is amazing how the body responds to natural, healthful food!

Measuring Up

Weigh yourself, and then take five girth measurements: bust at the largest point, waist at two inches above the navel, hips at the largest point, and right and left thigh circumference at the point where your extended fingertips reach with your arms hanging down at your sides. Record these figures, and your calculated BMI value, on your Progress Chart. What do you think of your progress?

And now, go to page 287 for your year-end recipe!

 TODAY'S ASSIGNMENT

WRITE IT DOWN AND MAKE IT STICK

This week, design and write down your personal strategy for lifelong health and weight management. How will you administer your own program? In formulating your strategy, consider the following:

1. How will you deal with the ever-enticing American junk-food culture?

2. How will you deal with boredom?

3. Who will hold you accountable each week? Accountability is an important part of success. If a trusted family member or spouse is unable to provide the support you need, work with a friend and be accountability partners for each other.

4. Are you keeping records of your food intake and exercise activities? Don't get so casual or overconfident that you abandon your daily Food Diary and your Exercise Diary. These are crucial tools of self-accountability.

5. If you cheat occasionally, do you put yourself back on track immediately?

6. Are you dealing with stress?

7. Do you get enough sleep at night?

8. Are you handling your loving saboteur(s)? Have you redefined your boundaries and made a plan for defending them if needed?

9. Have you taken care of any medical issues that have impeded your past health progress?

You may choose to "re-up" and repeat the Wings curriculum, and that would be wonderful. Whatever you decide, I wish you continued success and good health!

 HEALTH TIP

HYDROTHERAPY AND PAMPERING

Pampering is a good thing, and you should do it frequently (to yourself and someone else)! Is there anything quite as seductive as a warm bath? How about a foot bath? A hot-water massage? Water is very healing to the body and to the mind. Here are some lovely water-treatment ideas that will leave you breathless for more:

- Each week, prepare a mineral bath and give yourself at least one hour of uninterrupted pleasure in the tub. Bath minerals that originate from the Dead Sea or other natural mineral sources are available at health food stores. Make the water very warm so your muscles relax. If you feel overheated, apply a cool compress to your forehead while you bathe.

- For variety, instead of minerals, try using fragrant essential oils in the bath; some are specifically utilized as aromatherapy for their relaxing, calming, or stimulating effects, and you can experiment to find the ones you most enjoy.

- Fill a basin that is deep enough to bathe your feet with very warm water plus minerals or essential oils. Drape your favorite chair with a towel, dress comfortably with your lower legs exposed, sit back, and let the water caress your feet for as long as you wish. For added pleasure, ask your spouse to dry your feet and gently rub them with warm almond or coconut oil or another massage oil (health food stores carry a variety of these, some with essential oils for aromatherapy).

- If you have access to a water-massage device, take advantage of it as often as possible; one of the most relaxing devices has a fine-jet hose that emits very warm water at high pressure. Start your massage with the feet, and keep the parts of the body that are not being massaged covered as you go, so you don't feel a chill. It is fabulous!

- For information on many other water treatments, I encourage you to pick up a copy of *The Complete Book of Water Therapy* by Dian Dincin Buchman (New Canaan, CT: Keats Publishing, 1994).

ADDITIONAL NOTES

Menus and Recipes

Almost every diet has a food plan. Although Wings is a lifestyle to build health, and not a diet *per se*, we must discuss the foods and menus that are integral to this program. In the text of the lessons, the food picture is painted with a broad brush; in this section, I sketch in the details.

HOW TO USE THIS SECTION

As you read each lesson, turn to this section to learn what you'll eat for the next seven days. During the first three months of the program, I counsel you to follow the Wings food plan very carefully. Try not to deviate. The point of the menus in this section is to break very old habits, restore normal pH, balance blood sugar, increase energy, eliminate common allergens, and, in general, make you feel wonderful. You'll even start to lose weight.

Another goal is to reintroduce you to your kitchen as you enjoy these marvelous new foods. Get your pots and pans out of storage; pull out your knives and cutting board; rearrange your refrigerator to accommodate more vegetables; then tie your napkin around your neck and lay out the place mat, because I promise you will love the new flavors, aromas, and textures in real food!

As you would expect, the food plan follows the general principles of the Wings Program as described in the text. But being a purist is not always practical, so some of the recipes offer the option of using canned items like beans, broth, or other convenience foods to save time, or of using certain frozen vegetables because that is how they are generally available. Frozen fruits are also acceptable in moderation, particularly in the Wings Breakfast Drink. If you choose to use canned, jarred, or frozen items, please be sure to purchase low-sodium products that do not contain added sugars, MSG, or other artificial ingredients.

While I was writing this book, I was introduced to the concept of community sponsored agriculture (CSA), organic farms that allow customers who purchase a share of the crop in advance to receive farm-fresh produce weekly. If you have access to a CSA program, I urge you to check it out; your participation will support a local organic farmer, and you will also receive the most beautiful, fresh, and nutritious fruits and vegetables on the planet! Your local health food store can probably supply you with information on the nearest CSA farm.

THE WINGS BREAKFAST DRINK

I encourage you to use the Wings Breakfast Drink, or your chosen alternative (such as a rice-based protein mix from the health food store) for your first meal every day (see the Resource Guide for ordering information). You will, in time, design your own favorite variations, but meanwhile use the following Breakfast Drink recipes as a starting point.

The basic instructions are simple and the same for each Breakfast Drink recipe: combine all ingredients in a blender and whiz for a few seconds until the mixture is smooth and the desired texture (add more water if you want a thinner consistency). Each recipe is for one serving.

Purchase flaxseed oil at a health food store (if you cannot obtain flaxseed oil, use light olive oil, an excellent source of essential fatty acids that are good for the skin and metabolism, although the taste is slightly different). Almond milk is also available in health food stores and in many supermarkets; if you wish to make your own, it is simple, inexpensive, and delicious (see the recipe for Pure and Sweet Almond Milk on the next page). Rice milk can be substituted for almond milk, although the sugar content may be higher.

PEACHES AND CREAM

A rich and creamy breakfast.

4 scoops Wings Breakfast Drink
1 fresh ripe peach; or, 1 cup frozen peaches
1 cup vanilla almond milk
$1/4$ teaspoon vanilla extract
1 tablespoon flaxseed oil
$1/2$ cup ice-cold water

"MRS. REGULAR" BREAKFAST SHAKE

A delicious, rich blend.

4 scoops Wings Breakfast Drink
4 tablespoons prune juice (yes, really!)
1 cup vanilla almond milk
1 tablespoon flaxseed oil
$1/2$ cup ice-cold water

CARIBBEAN SUNRISE

You'll love the flavor and texture of ripe mango.

4 scoops Wings Breakfast Drink (vanilla)
$1/2$ fresh ripe mango, diced
1 cup vanilla almond milk
A splash of fresh orange juice
1 tablespoon flaxseed oil
$1/4$ cup ice-cold water

CHOCO-CHOCO LATTE

This variation is a little sweet for my taste,
but sometimes you just want chocolate!

4 scoops Wings Breakfast Drink
1 cup chocolate almond milk
$1/2$ teaspoon vanilla extract
1 tablespoon flaxseed oil
$1/2$ cup ice-cold water

BREAKFAST BANANA SPLIT

A very filling variation—prepare to be satisfied for hours.

4 scoops Wings Breakfast Drink
1 very ripe banana, cut into chunks
1 cup chocolate almond milk
$1/2$ cup ice-cold water

PEACH MELBA IN A GLASS

This one is even better if you can
get fresh raspberries and peaches.

4 scoops Wings Breakfast Drink
1 handful fresh or frozen raspberries
$1/2$ cup fresh or frozen peaches
1 cup vanilla almond milk
$1/4$ teaspoon vanilla extract
$1/2$ cup ice-cold water

PURE AND SWEET ALMOND MILK

This recipe is simple and the almond milk is delicious, particularly when served ice-cold. Adapted from the excellent book *Not Milk Nut Milks* by Candia Lea Cole (Santa Barbara, CA: Woodland Press, 1990).

Yield: about 3 cups

4 cups pure water
$1/3$ cup organic raw almonds
1 tablespoon fortified flaxseed
1 teaspoon lecithin granules
2 tablespoons honey
$1/4$ teaspoon almond extract

In a saucepan, heat the water until almost boiling, then turn the burner off and let the water cool slightly while you prepare the other ingredients. Process the almonds and flaxseed in a grinder, blender, or food processor until reduced to a fine powder. Add the lecithin granules, honey, almond extract, and $1/2$ to $3/4$ cup of the hot water to the mixture and process on medium speed to a smooth puddinglike purée. Add the remaining hot water to the purée, and process on high speed until creamy. If you wish, strain the almond milk before refrigerating; I like to leave it unstrained, however, to retain all the fibers and nutrients. Shake well before pouring.

Olive Oil or Macadamia Nut Oil?

Olive oil is a good source of heart-healthful monounsaturated fats, but only if you purchase a quality brand and use it within six months of its pressing. Olive oil's low smoke point can be troublesome when cooking above a light sauté, and a real problem in the oven. Macadamia nut oil, however, is an excellent substitute for olive oil in most recipes. Macadamia nut oil is 30 percent higher in monounsaturated fats; it also has a much higher smoke point, so there is no trans-fatty acid formation or oxidation when it is heated for cooking. Feel free to substitute this wonderful oil whenever you can. (Macadamia nut oil is available in health food stores.)

MODULE I

Module I emphasizes the body's acid/alkaline balance. The importance of this balance to your weight management and good health cannot be overestimated. But if you are like most Americans, you normally consume such a high proportion of acidic foods that your blood and urine remain acidic. Your stress level also contributes to your overall internal acidity.

The eating plan for the first eight weeks is directed toward restoring your pH balance, reducing your allergic potential, helping you drop water weight, and achieving other health goals. Don't skimp on this part of the program! Yes, the menus and recipes may differ substantially from what you've eaten in the past, but the results will be worth the effort.

WEEK I-1, DAY 1

- Breakfast: the Wings Breakfast Drink
- Lunch: a large salad including five different brightly colored raw vegetables, topped with 3–4 ounces of protein (such as tuna or chicken salad or leftover chicken) and dressed lightly with olive oil and balsamic vinegar
- Mid-afternoon snack: a handful of raw almonds or other raw nuts
- Dinner: a large salad (see Lunch above), Honey-Mustard Chicken (recipe below; 3–4 ounces, or enough to satisfy), ¼ baked potato with a pat of

butter and a dollop of sour cream, and Roasted Asparagus (recipe below)
- Evening snack: a handful of raw carrot and celery sticks or other raw veggies

Today's tip: Always prepare extra food so you can use the leftovers for lunch the next day.

HONEY-MUSTARD CHICKEN

Simple and tasty. The honey lends a little sweetness, and the mustard kicks up the flavor.

YIELD: 4 SERVINGS

¼ cup mayonnaise

2 tablespoons dijon-style mustard

1 tablespoon honey

*4 boneless, skinless chicken breast halves
(about 1 pound)*

In a small bowl, mix the mayonnaise, mustard, and honey. Place the chicken pieces on an oiled grill or on the rack of a broiler pan at 5–7 inches from the heat source. Brush the chicken with ½ of the sauce, and grill or broil 8–10 minutes. Turn the chicken, brush with the remaining sauce, and continue grilling or broiling until done—don't overcook.

ROASTED ASPARAGUS

NOT the mushy, slippery canned asparagus you may remember from childhood!

YIELD: 5 SERVINGS

1 bundle asparagus spears

A sprinkle of olive oil

Preheat oven to 375°F. Snap off and discard the tough ends of the asparagus spears (my daughters call this "cracking the knuckles" of the asparagus). Place the spears in a baking dish, sprinkle with olive oil, and roast until done but still a little crunchy (about 15–20 minutes).

WEEK I-1, DAY 2

- Breakfast: the Wings Breakfast Drink
- Lunch: a large tossed salad topped with leftover Honey-Mustard Chicken (3–4 ounces, or enough to satisfy) and dressed lightly with your favorite olive oil dressing

- Mid-afternoon snack: a handful of Roasted Toasted Pumpkin Seeds (recipe below)

- Dinner: Crab and Shrimp Casserole (recipe below), a large tossed salad dressed lightly with your favorite olive oil dressing, and a small baked sweet potato with a pat of butter

- Evening snack: a handful of raw carrot and celery sticks or other raw veggies

Today's tip: Prepare tomorrow's Black Bean Chili ahead of time by soaking the beans overnight tonight; then start cooking them tomorrow morning before work, and you can simply assemble the dish after work in time for your dinner.

CRAB AND SHRIMP CASSEROLE

The whole family will love the flavors of this casserole. Make sure your seafood does not originate in the South Pacific (for example, Indonesia), as those waters are extremely polluted with mercury and other heavy metals.

YIELD: 4 SERVINGS

2 cups cooked brown rice

1 cup mayonnaise

$\frac{1}{2}$ cup almond milk

$\frac{1}{2}$ cup chopped onion

$\frac{1}{4}$ cup chopped green pepper

1 cup fresh or canned crab

1 cup fresh or canned shrimp

1 cup tomato juice

$\frac{1}{4}$ cup slivered almonds

Combine all ingredients in a large bowl and place the mixture in a buttered 9x13-inch baking dish. Bake at 350°F for 1 hour and serve.

ROASTED TOASTED PUMPKIN SEEDS

A phenomenal snack: crunchy, salty, and healthful! Sprinkle some seeds on your salad, too.

YIELD: APPROXIMATELY 1 POUND

1 pound raw pumpkin seeds

A sprinkle of olive oil

A sprinkle of salt

Preheat oven to 325°F. Spread the pumpkin seeds in a baking pan, sprinkle lightly with the oil, toss to coat evenly, and roast until lightly browned (about 8–10 minutes)—be careful not to burn them! Remove from oven, sprinkle with salt, and cool before serving. Refrigerate leftovers in a covered dish.

WEEK I-1, DAY 3

- Breakfast: the Wings Breakfast Drink

- Lunch: lots of fresh veggies dipped in hummus, or leftovers from last night's dinner

- Mid-afternoon snack: a celery stalk stuffed with 1 tablespoon of almond or cashew butter

- Dinner: Black Bean Chili (recipe below) with a handful of baked tortilla chips

- Evening snack: a medium-sized salad of dark greens and sliced peppers and cucumbers, dressed lightly with olive oil and balsamic vinegar

Today's tip: Supermarkets usually carry various flavors of delicious, nutritious hummus, or you can easily make your own (see Homemade Hummus recipe on page 241).

BLACK BEAN CHILI

If you do not want to soak and cook dried black beans, substitute drained canned black beans. Add the optional chicken for more protein, or keep this a vegetarian meal if you prefer.

YIELD: 8–12 SERVINGS

2 cups dried black beans

4 cups water

1 tablespoon olive oil

1 tablespoon chopped garlic

$\frac{1}{4}$ cup peeled and diced carrots

$\frac{1}{2}$ cup peeled and diced onions

$\frac{1}{2}$ celery stalk, diced

$\frac{1}{2}$ cup seeded and diced red bell pepper

1 cup sun-dried tomatoes, sliced into $\frac{1}{4}$-inch pieces

2 cups chicken broth

2 tablespoons chili powder

$\frac{1}{2}$ teaspoon cayenne pepper

$1\frac{1}{2}$ tablespoons hot pepper sauce (optional)

1 pound boneless chicken breasts, cut into $\frac{1}{2}$-inch pieces (optional)

$\frac{1}{4}$ cup chopped scallions

1 cup diced fresh or canned tomatoes

Salt and pepper to taste

Soak the dried beans in water overnight; the next day, drain beans, put in a pot with enough water to cover by 1 inch, simmer gently until tender (approximately 1 hour), drain, and set aside. In a large pot, heat $\frac{1}{2}$ tablespoon of the olive oil and sauté the garlic over medium heat for 3 minutes, stirring constantly. Add the carrots, onions, celery, and peppers, and cook for 15 minutes. Add the cooked black beans, sun-dried tomatoes, and chicken broth, lower heat, cover, and let simmer for 20 minutes. Remove the lid, add the spices and hot pepper sauce, and simmer 20 minutes more. Meanwhile, in a sauté pan, heat the second $\frac{1}{2}$ tablespoon of olive oil and sauté the chicken pieces until done (approximately 15 minutes). Add the chicken to the chili along with the scallions and tomatoes, season with salt and pepper as desired, simmer 5 minutes more, and serve.

WEEK I-1, DAY 4

- Breakfast: the Wings Breakfast Drink
- Lunch: leftover Black Bean Chili and baked tortilla chips
- Mid-afternoon snack: a handful of raw sunflower seeds or an apple
- Dinner: Cobb Salad (recipe below)
- Evening snack: a sliced apple or other seasonal fruit dipped in almond or cashew butter

Today's tip: To save yourself some time, roast extra turkey breast when you are preparing tonight's Cobb Salad, and use the extra turkey in tomorrow's Chicken Enchilada Casserole.

COBB SALAD

Very satisfying! Traditionally, cobb salad toppings are arranged decoratively on the lettuce, not mixed throughout.

YIELD: 1–2 SERVINGS

Several cups chopped romaine lettuce

1 ripe tomato, seeded and chopped

1 hard-boiled egg, chopped

1 scallion, chopped

$\frac{1}{4}$ pound turkey bacon, fried crisp, drained, and chopped

3 ounces roasted turkey breast, chopped (leftovers are great for this purpose)

1 handful feta or blue cheese, crumbled

Olive oil to taste

Balsamic vinegar to taste

A sprinkle of kosher salt

Place the lettuce on dinner plates and arrange the toppings on the lettuce to suit your fancy. Sprinkle the salad with olive oil, balsamic vinegar, and kosher salt as desired, and enjoy.

WEEK I-1, DAY 5

- Breakfast: the Wings Breakfast Drink
- Lunch: leftover Black Bean Chili
- Mid-afternoon snack: a piece of fresh fruit, or a handful of homemade or purchased nut mix
- Dinner: Chicken Enchilada Casserole (recipe below) and a large salad of several brightly colored vegetables dressed lightly with olive oil and balsamic vinegar
- Evening snack: a handful of Roasted Toasted Pumpkin Seeds (recipe page 238)

Checking in: Do you love the food? Are you feeling "balanced"? I hope you are enjoying the dinner preparations! Food and kitchen time are to be savored.

CHICKEN ENCHILADA CASSEROLE

This is a "kid-friendly" recipe. To ramp up the flavor, add a little more spice. (You can substitute leftover turkey for the chicken breast if you like.)

YIELD: 2–4 SERVINGS

1 pound chicken breasts

$1\frac{3}{4}$ cups enchilada sauce

8 6-inch corn tortillas

1 cup canned green chilies

$\frac{1}{3}$ cup diced canned tomatoes

2 cups grated cheddar, goat, or almond cheese

Bake the chicken breasts at 350°F for 15 minutes, then shred or chop. Heat the enchilada sauce in a pan until it is just warm. In a 4-inch-deep casserole dish, layer (lasagna-style) the tortillas (1–2 per layer) dipped in enchilada sauce with some chicken, then some chilies, then some tomatoes, and then some cheese. Repeat the layer sequence two more times, pouring any remaining sauce over the top. Bake at 350°F for 45 minutes and serve.

WEEK I-1, DAY 6

■ Breakfast: the Wings Breakfast Drink

■ Lunch: leftover Chicken Enchilada Casserole

■ Mid-afternoon snack: a handful of raw almonds or other raw nuts

■ Dinner: Salmon Loaf (recipe below), a small baked sweet potato with a pat of butter, and a generous veggie tray of carrots, celery, cauliflower, broccoli, and grape or cherry tomatoes

■ Evening snack: more veggies from the veggie tray

Today's tip: To save time in making tomorrow night's soup, prepare the vegetables and store them in a plastic bag in the refrigerator.

SALMON LOAF

Delicious warm, or served cold with Lemon Mayonnaise (recipe follows). Try leftover loaf on a rice cake or atop a tossed green salad.

YIELD: 4 SERVINGS

1 pound cooked or canned salmon

1 egg, beaten

$1/4$ cup half-and-half (if you are intolerant to dairy products, substitute almond milk)

1 cup gluten-free cracker crumbs or bread crumbs

$1/2$ teaspoon salt

1 teaspoon pepper

2 teaspoons lemon juice

1 teaspoon Worcestershire sauce

1 tablespoon melted butter

3 tablespoons minced fresh parsley

$1/4$ cup chopped celery

$1/4$ cup chopped onions

Mix all ingredients together lightly, and spoon the mixture into a greased 5x9-inch loaf pan. Bake at 300°F for 30 minutes and serve warm.

LEMON MAYONNAISE

Serve over slices of cold Salmon Loaf (recipe above).

YIELD: ABOUT 1 CUP

1 cup mayonnaise

2 tablespoons fresh lemon juice

$1/2$ teaspoon grated lemon peel

$1/2$ teaspoon lemon-pepper seasoning

Blend all ingredients and refrigerate.

WEEK I-1, DAY 7

■ Breakfast: the Wings Breakfast Drink

■ Lunch: leftover Salmon Loaf

■ Mid-afternoon snack: a handful of rice crackers with nondairy cheese (almond, rice, or soy)

■ Dinner: Carol's Vegetable Soup (recipe on page 241) with nondairy cheese and a handful of crackers, and a handful of raw veggies dipped in store-bought hummus or Homemade Hummus (recipe on page 241)

■ Evening snack: a handful of rice crackers with nondairy cheese

HOMEMADE TURKEY BROTH

As part of Lesson I-7, make this delicious broth to use in soups, gravies, or casseroles.

YIELD: ABOUT 2 QUARTS

A splash of olive oil

6 pounds turkey parts (wings and such)

Several stalks celery, coarsely chopped (including the leaves)

2 large carrots, coarsely chopped

8–10 cloves garlic, crushed

1 large onion, coarsely chopped

3–4 small bay leaves

1 handful fresh basil; or, 1 tablespoon dried basil

1 sprig fresh thyme; or, 1 teaspoon dried thyme

3 quarts pure water

Any other seasonings you enjoy, to taste

In a large, heavy soup pot, heat the oil and sauté the turkey parts over medium heat, removing them to a plate once they are a nice brown color (make sure not to burn them). Put the vegetables in that same soup pot and stir until lightly browned. Return the turkey parts to the pot with the vegetables, add the herbs and the water, stir gently, cover loosely (to let a little steam evaporate), bring the pot to a simmer, turn the burner down so it barely simmers, and let it cook for 3–4 hours or until it is the desired strength, removing foam that floats to the top. Add any other seasonings as desired. When done, remove the turkey and cut any meat off the bones to use in other recipes. Strain the broth, pressing the juice out of the vegetables. Defat the broth when it cools, and store in the refrigerator.

Variation: If you would prefer not to spend so much time browning, you do not have to; it just gives the broth a richer flavor. You can simply place all the ingredients in the pot and cook the broth for several hours; it will be lighter in color and more delicate in flavor, but delicious nonetheless.

CAROL'S VEGETABLE SOUP

As you wander through the produce aisle, select what looks and feels good, and add it to this simple, flexible recipe for inexhaustible variety. Great with fresh CSA produce!

YIELD: *8–10 SERVINGS*

A splash of olive oil and a dab of butter

2–5 cloves of garlic, crushed or minced

1 large onion, chopped fine; or, 2–3 leeks, washed and chopped fine

2 large carrots, peeled and chopped

2 celery stalks, chopped fine

2 parsnips, peeled and chopped fine

1/2 rutabaga, peeled and chopped fine; or, 1–2 turnips, peeled and chopped fine

2 potatoes, peeled and chopped fine

1/4 head cabbage, shredded fine

1 large tomato, peeled and diced; or, 1 16-ounce can tomatoes, chopped with juice

4 quarts vegetable broth

2 bay leaves

1 8-ounce package frozen baby peas

1 8-ounce package frozen corn

Other fresh (or dried) herbs you enjoy (basil, oregano, parsley, and such), to taste

Salt and pepper to taste

In a large soup pot, heat the olive oil and butter and sauté the garlic until it softens. Add the onion or leeks, and cook for a few minutes, stirring frequently. Add the next six ingredients and continue sautéing, stirring frequently as it all cooks, until the vegetables are wilted (about 10 minutes). Add the tomato, broth, and bay leaves, put the lid on the pot, and allow the soup to simmer gently until the vegetables are done (about 20 minutes)—do not overcook, or they'll become soggy. Add the peas and corn, cooking just until they are heated through. Season with herbs and a little salt and pepper as desired, and serve immediately.

HOMEMADE HUMMUS

This simple recipe makes a delicious dip for raw veggies.

YIELD: *APPROXIMATELY 2 CUPS*

1 can garbanzo beans (chick peas) with their water

1 tablespoon olive oil

1 tablespoon lemon juice

1 tablespoon tahini

1–2 large roasted red bell peppers

1–2 small cloves garlic, peeled

Drain the garbanzo beans, reserving the water. In a food processor or blender, whirl the beans along with the rest of the ingredients until smooth and well blended, adding a little of the bean water as necessary to thin the hummus to the desired consistency. Serve at room temperature.

Variations: Try other "flavor accessories" instead of the roasted red peppers, such as a large dollop of pesto, or 1/4 cup roasted garlic, minced roasted onions, minced sun-dried tomatoes—you are only limited by your imagination, and every variety will be delicious and nutritious.

WEEK I-2, DAY 1

How do you feel after your first week on the Wings Program? You've broken some of your addictions, balanced your blood sugar, reduced your allergic load—and enjoyed some great food. This week, continue to focus on bringing your pH into alignment. Be encouraged to know that any withdrawal symptoms you may have struggled through last week should be dissipating. Each day that you enjoy the abundance from Mother Nature's table instead of eating nutrient-stripped processed foods, you take another giant step toward vibrant health!

▪ Breakfast: the Wings Breakfast Drink

- Lunch: a large mixed vegetable salad, topped with a slice of Salmon Loaf (page 240) or a scoop of tuna salad, and dressed lightly with olive oil and balsamic vinegar

- Mid-afternoon snack: a celery stalk stuffed with 1 tablespoon of almond or cashew butter

- Dinner: Crab-Stuffed Filet of Sole in Wine Sauce (recipe below), a small baked sweet potato or yam, 1/2 avocado sprinkled with olive oil and balsamic vinegar, and lightly steamed fresh green beans with a pat of butter and a sprinkling of sliced almonds

- Evening snack: a celery stalk stuffed with 1 tablespoon of almond or cashew butter

Checking in: Keep testing your first morning urine each day. If you have not yet achieved a pH of 6.5–7.5, revisit Lesson I-1. You may need to do the ascorbic acid flush (pages 8–9), increase your mineral intake, or cut back on acidic foods.

CRAB-STUFFED FILET OF SOLE IN WINE SAUCE

Even those who do not enjoy fish like this wonderful, simple dish. To avoid mercury contamination, be sure the crab does not originate in the South Pacific; or, use imitation crab—to most people, the difference in taste and texture is inconsequential.

YIELD: 8 SERVINGS

Crab Stuffing

1/4 cup chopped onion

1/4 cup butter

1/4 pound fresh mushrooms, cleaned and sliced

8 ounces real or imitation crab

1/2 cup coarse rice-cracker crumbs

2 tablespoons chopped parsley

1/2 teaspoon salt

A dash of pepper

Wine Sauce

3 tablespoons butter

3 tablespoons oat or spelt flour

1/4 teaspoon salt

1/2 cup rice milk

1/3 cup dry white wine

Sole

8 sole filets (about 2 pounds)

Paprika and chopped parsley for garnish

1. To make the stuffing, sauté the onion in the butter until it is tender but not browned, then stir in the mushrooms and cook until they are done. Add the remaining ingredients and mix well.

2. To make the sauce, melt the butter in a saucepan, stir in the flour and salt, and cook briefly. Add the milk and wine, whisking constantly, and continue cooking (keep stirring) until the sauce is thickened and smooth.

3. Spread the stuffing on the sole filets, roll the filets, and place them seam-side down in a buttered shallow baking dish. Pour the sauce over the fish (which may be refrigerated at this point). Bake at 400°F for 35 minutes, garnish with the paprika and more parsley, and serve.

WEEK I-2, DAY 2

- Breakfast: the Wings Breakfast Drink

- Lunch: leftover Crab-Stuffed Filet of Sole, a generous fresh veggie tray, and 1/2 cup steamed brown rice with a pat of butter

- Mid-afternoon snack: a piece of fresh fruit or a handful of nut mix

- Dinner: a large salad including at least five colorful vegetables dressed lightly with olive oil and balsamic vinegar and a three-salad plate with Mom's Cole Slaw, Carol's Potato Salad (recipes follow), and tuna or chicken salad or deviled eggs

- Evening snack: a piece of fresh fruit or a handful of nut mix

Today's tip: You will have leftovers from today's recipes tomorrow, so only dress the amount of salad that you will eat tonight and refrigerate the rest, dressing tomorrow's salad just before lunch so the vegetables do not get soggy.

MOM'S COLE SLAW

A recipe from my childhood. Slightly sweet and very crunchy—your kids will love it.

YIELD: 8 SERVINGS

1/2 head cabbage, shredded

1/4 head red cabbage, shredded

1 large carrot, peeled and shredded

1 can crushed unsweetened pineapple, with its own juice

1/2 cup mayonnaise, or enough to moisten

Prepare the vegetables and put them in a large mixing bowl. Drain the pineapple, reserving the juice, and add the pineapple to the vegetables. Thoroughly blend enough of the reserved juice with the mayonnaise to make a sauce with a fairly thin consistency. Pour the sauce onto the slaw, stir to blend, and serve immediately.

CAROL'S POTATO SALAD

A favorite at our house in the summer when it is too hot to cook. I take the leftovers to work for a satisfying lunch.

YIELD: 8 SERVINGS

6 large potatoes, washed but unpeeled

6 eggs

6 scallions, minced

1 can pimientos, chopped

3–4 kosher dill pickles, diced

Dill seed to taste

Mayonnaise to moisten

Enough pickle juice to thin the mayonnaise

Olives or tomato wedges for garnish

Salt and pepper to taste

Bake the potatoes at 425°F until they are done (about 30–40 minutes, depending on the size of the potatoes) and set them aside to cool. Meanwhile, hard-boil, cool, and peel the eggs. Peel and chop the potatoes, eggs, and scallions, and combine in a large bowl. Add the pimientos and pickles, and sprinkle with dill seed as desired. Blend the mayonnaise with enough pickle juice to make a creamy sauce, then mix enough sauce into the salad to moisten it. Taste the salad, correct the seasoning, and add the garnish. Serve at room temperature or chilled. If you anticipate leftovers, add the dressing only to the portion you will serve immediately, and add more dressing as you serve it.

WEEK 1-2, DAY 3

- Breakfast: the Wings Breakfast Drink

- Lunch: leftover salads from yesterday

- Mid-afternoon snack: a handful of Roasted Toasted Pumpkin Seeds (page 238)

- Dinner: Cuban Mojo Pork, Black Beans and Coconut Rice, and Unfried Plantains (recipes follow)

- Evening snack: a handful of Roasted Toasted Pumpkin Seeds

Today's tips: Today's meal takes 6–12 hours to marinate, so you may need to get up 10 minutes early and start it marinating in the morning. Also, you may want to roast the beets for tomorrow's dinner tonight to save time tomorrow night.

CUBAN MOJO PORK

Pork is not the most healthful meat, but eating it occasionally is okay, particularly if it's well cooked and roasted without fat. This marvelous dish in the Cuban tradition may become one of your family's favorite meals.

YIELD: PLAN ON 1/4 POUND OF PORK PER PERSON

1 large pork roast (3–6 pounds), trimmed of visible fat

1 bottle Mojo marinade (try the ethnic foods section of the supermarket)

You need to marinate the pork for at least 6 and up to 12 hours before cooking, so begin in the morning: stab holes throughout the pork on all sides with a sharp fork, place the meat in a refrigerator container, pour on enough of the Mojo sauce to nearly cover it, cover the container tightly, and place it in the refrigerator to marinate.

Preheat oven to 325°F. Place the roast and sauce in a roasting pan, cover tightly, and place it in the oven. Allow 40 minutes of cooking time per pound. Turn the meat occasionally as it cooks to keep it moist. Cook until the inner temperature reaches 180°F on a meat thermometer, then remove it from the oven and let it rest until the temperature goes to 185°F. Carve the roast into 1/2-inch slices, pour the sauce over them, and serve.

BLACK BEANS AND COCONUT RICE

A complete, light meal.

YIELD: 6–8 SERVINGS

3 1/2 cups water

2 cups uncooked white rice

1/2 to 1 cup unsweetened coconut milk

1–2 cans black beans

Bring the water to a boil, add the rice and coconut milk, and stir briefly. Reduce the heat to low, cover with a lid slightly ajar, and let the rice steam until done (about 10 minutes or so). Heat the black beans and serve them over the rice.

Variations: Add sautéed onions and garlic or chopped sun-dried tomatoes to the beans for more flavor.

UNFRIED PLANTAINS

There are two healthful ways to prepare plantains: baking and sautéing. For added sweetness and tenderness, let plantains ripen until the skins are almost black.

To bake, poke a couple of holes in the skin of the plantains and put them whole in a 325°F oven for about 45 minutes (you can do this while the Cuban Mojo Pork finishes roasting), then slice the skin open and scoop out the flesh to serve. Alternatively, to sauté, score the skin lengthwise and peel it off, cut each plantain into four chunks crosswise, and slice each chunk in half lengthwise; melt some butter in a skillet, sauté on each side until brown and crispy, and serve immediately. Fabulous!

WEEK I-2, DAY 4

- Breakfast: the Wings Breakfast Drink
- Lunch: leftover Cuban Mojo Pork, Black Beans and Rice, and Unfried Plantains
- Mid-afternoon snack: a piece of fresh fruit
- Dinner: Peas with Spinach and Shallots, Spinach, Beet, and Walnut Salad (recipes follow), and slices of nondairy cheese
- Evening snack: store-bought hummus or Homemade Hummus (page 241) with fresh veggies

Checking in: Because yesterday's dinner was a heavy meat meal, today's fare is lighter. The protein in these meals should be sufficient, but if you feel you need more, simply eat some more leftover pork from last night; just be careful not to overdo it.

PEAS WITH SPINACH AND SHALLOTS

Adapted from *Gourmet* magazine.

YIELD: 2 SERVINGS

2 medium shallots, thinly sliced

2 cloves garlic, thinly sliced

1 tablespoon olive oil

1 tablespoon unsalted butter

1 package frozen baby peas

1/4 cup water

5 ounces raw baby spinach

1/2 teaspoon salt

1/4 teaspoon black pepper

In a skillet, cook the shallots and garlic in the oil and butter over medium heat, stirring, until soft (about 6 minutes). Stir in the peas and water and cook, covered, until the peas are tender (about 5 minutes). Stir in the spinach, salt, and pepper, and cook, tossing, until the spinach is just wilted (about 1 minute).

SPINACH, BEET, AND WALNUT SALAD

Even if you are normally sensitive to dairy, you may be able to tolerate small amounts of goat cheese—if not, eliminate it. If you anticipate leftovers, hold the dressing on that portion until you are ready to serve it. This is a delightful salad! Enjoy it often. Adapted from *Bon Appetit*.

YIELD: 4 SERVINGS

1 1/2 pounds medium beets, ends trimmed

1/2 cup walnut oil or olive oil

1/4 cup sherry wine vinegar

2 large shallots, minced

2 6-ounce packages baby spinach

4 heads Belgian endive, thinly sliced crosswise

1 cup walnuts, toasted and coarsely chopped

6 ounces fresh soft goat cheese
(such as Montrachet), crumbled

Salt and pepper to taste

Preheat oven to 400°F, wrap beets in foil, and bake until tender when pierced with a knife (about 1 1/2 hours). Cool slightly, peel, cut each beet into eight wedges, and place in a covered medium-sized bowl. Whisk the oil and vinegar in a small bowl and then mix in the shallots. Pour 3 tablespoons of the dressing over the warm beets and toss. Combine the spinach, endive, and 3/4 of the nuts in a large bowl, pour the remaining dressing over them, and toss. Season with salt and pepper as desired. Divide the greens among plates, sprinkle the cheese over them, and top with the beets and remaining nuts.

WEEK I-2, DAY 5

- Breakfast: the Wings Breakfast Drink
- Lunch: a large salad including at least ten different brightly colored vegetables, topped with a scoop of

tuna salad or other protein and dressed lightly with olive oil and balsamic vinegar

- Mid-afternoon snack: a celery stalk stuffed with 1 tablespoon of almond or cashew butter

- Dinner: Chicken Breasts in Mushroom-Chive Sauce (recipe below), a small serving of steamed brown rice, and Roasted Asparagus (page 237) or steamed broccoli or another green vegetable

- Evening snack: a small-to-medium mixed vegetable salad tossed with your favorite dressing

CHICKEN BREASTS IN MUSHROOM-CHIVE SAUCE

Serve over steamed rice to savor the marvelous sauce.

YIELD: 4 SERVINGS

3 scallions, chopped

1 clove garlic, minced

1 pound mushrooms, sliced

4 tablespoons butter, divided

4 tablespoons olive oil

4 whole chicken breasts, boned, skinned, and halved

1 cup chicken broth

1 tablespoon lemon juice

1 cup almond or rice milk

2 tablespoons spelt flour

2 tablespoons finely chopped fresh chives

Salt and pepper to taste

Parsley for garnish

In a large saucepan on high heat, sauté the scallions, garlic, and mushrooms in 2 tablespoons of the butter until the mushrooms are lightly browned (about 5–10 minutes), and transfer the mushroom mixture to a plate. Add the oil to the pan, sauté the chicken in the oil until lightly browned (about 4–5 minutes per side), and transfer the chicken to another plate. Add the broth to the pan and boil until the liquid is reduced by half. Add the lemon juice and almond or rice milk to the pan and reduce heat to a simmer. In a separate small pan on medium heat, melt the remaining 2 tablespoons of butter, add the flour, and let it bubble for a minute or so to make a roux. Add the roux to the pan

of cream sauce, simmer until thickened, add the chicken, and simmer until done (about 10 minutes). Add the mushroom mixture and chives to the pan and heat through. Season with salt and pepper as desired, garnish with the parsley, and serve.

WEEK I-2, DAY 6

- Breakfast: the Wings Breakfast Drink

- Lunch: leftover chicken and vegetables from yesterday's dinner, and a mixed vegetable salad dressed lightly with your favorite dressing

- Mid-afternoon snack: a piece of fresh fruit or a handful of nut mix

- Dinner: chili (use your favorite chili recipe, or the Black Bean Chili recipe on page 238, or a healthful commercially made chili such as Health Valley's, which is organic and delicious) over baked tortilla chips with a sprinkling of grated nondairy cheese

- Evening snack: a handful of nut mix

WEEK I-2, DAY 7

- Breakfast: the Wings Breakfast Drink

- Remaining snacks and meals: throughout this day, enjoy your favorites from the past two weeks, or use up whatever leftovers you have on hand

Checking in: Is your pH restored yet to the normal range of 6.5–7.5? If not, reread Lesson I-1 and make the necessary adjustments to your diet and/or lifestyle.

WEEK I-3, DAY 1

- Breakfast: the Wings Breakfast Drink

- Lunch: a large mixed vegetable salad topped with a 3-ounce serving of protein and dressed lightly with your favorite dressing

- Mid-afternoon snack: a handful of raw almonds or cashews

- Dinner: Olive-Stuffed Chicken with Almonds (recipe follows), two green or orange vegetables of your choice, and a ½-cup serving of steamed brown rice

- Evening snack: a generous fresh veggie tray with your favorite dressing

OLIVE-STUFFED CHICKEN WITH ALMONDS

Really delicious! Adapted from *Gourmet* magazine.

YIELD: 4 SERVINGS

4 boneless chicken-breast halves with skin
(about 2 $\frac{1}{4}$ pounds total)

1 cup brine-cured green olives, pitted and chopped

Salt and pepper to taste

2 tablespoons unsalted butter

$\frac{1}{4}$ cup whole almonds with skins

3 tablespoons pure water

2 tablespoons chopped fresh flat-leaf parsley

Wash and dry the chicken breasts, cut a 2-inch long horizontal slit in the thickest part of each, stuff each with 1$\frac{1}{2}$ teaspoons olives, and season as desired with salt and pepper. Heat 1 tablespoon of the butter in a nonstick skillet over moderate heat until the foam subsides, and toast the almonds, stirring often, until they are a few shades darker (about 5–8 minutes). With a slotted spoon, transfer almonds to a plate to cool, leaving the remaining melted butter in the skillet. Increase heat to moderately high, place chicken breasts skin-side down in the skillet, sprinkle with the remaining olives, and sauté until the chicken skins are golden brown (about 8–10 minutes). Turn chicken over, cover skillet, and cook over moderate heat until done (about 5–7 minutes more), then transfer with tongs to plates; while the chicken cooks, chop the almonds. Add the remaining tablespoon of butter and the water to the skillet and heat, stirring, until the butter is melted, stir in the almonds and parsley, and sprinkle with pepper to taste. Spoon the sauce over the chicken and serve.

WEEK I-3, DAY 2

- Breakfast: the Wings Breakfast Drink
- Lunch: leftover Olive-Stuffed Chicken and a mixed vegetable salad
- Mid-afternoon snack: a piece of fresh fruit
- Dinner: Marinated Zesty Salmon with $\frac{1}{2}$ cup steamed brown rice, Sautéed Summer Squash (recipes follow), and a large mixed vegetable salad dressed lightly with your favorite dressing
- Evening snack: Banana "Ice Cream" (recipe follows)

Today's tip: Make plenty of salmon, because you'll need leftovers for tomorrow.

MARINATED ZESTY SALMON

A savory, slightly sweet preparation of one of the most healthful seafoods.

YIELD: 4 SERVINGS

$\frac{1}{3}$ cup Worcestershire sauce

2 tablespoons olive oil

1 tablespoon honey

$\frac{1}{4}$ teaspoon salt

$\frac{1}{4}$ teaspoon ground ginger

2 scallions, chopped

1 pound salmon filet

In a small bowl, combine all ingredients except the salmon. Place the salmon in a small baking dish and pour $\frac{1}{4}$ cup of the sauce over the fish, turning the pieces to coat them. Reserve the remaining sauce for basting. Cover and marinate the salmon in the refrigerator for 30 minutes, remove it from the marinade, and then grill or broil, turning it once and basting with the reserved sauce, until the fish is done (about 4 minutes per side).

SAUTÉED SUMMER SQUASH

This simple vegetable dish balances the richness of the Marinated Zesty Salmon, but you can spark up the flavor by adding herbs.

YIELD: 4 SERVINGS

2 summer squash (or zucchini)

A splash of olive oil

1 clove garlic, chopped

$\frac{1}{2}$ onion (preferably white onion), sliced

A dash of fresh or dried herbs (basil is good)

Wash the squash, cut into $\frac{1}{2}$-inch slices, and set aside. Heat the olive oil in a sauté pan until hot but not smoking, add the garlic, and sauté briefly. Add the squash and onion and cook, stirring, until the squash is still a little crisp but slightly tender (about 10 minutes). Remove from heat, sprinkle with herbs, and serve immediately.

BANANA "ICE CREAM"

What fruits work well with banana? Raspberries, blackberries, peaches—use your imagination!

YIELD: 4 SERVINGS

1 frozen banana, cut into 1-inch chunks

A handful of any other frozen fruit (unsweetened)

Process all ingredients briefly in a food processor or blender until just puréed (it should still be very cold). Scoop the purée into a container and freeze it until it's the texture of ice cream.

WEEK I-3, DAY 3

- Breakfast: the Wings Breakfast Drink
- Lunch: a large green salad topped with a protein serving of your choice and dressed lightly with olive oil and balsamic vinegar
- Mid-afternoon snack: a handful of Roasted Toasted Pumpkin Seeds (page 238)
- Dinner: Salmon Rice Salad, Confetti Cole Slaw (recipes follow), and Roasted Asparagus (page 237) or steamed broccoli topped with a pat of butter
- Evening snack: a piece of fresh fruit

SALMON RICE SALAD

Do not feel constrained by my ingredient suggestions; use your own and vary the salad each time you make it. Leftover Marinated Zesty Salmon works well here, as does regular poached salmon.

YIELD: 4 SERVINGS

2 cups cooked basmati or other good-quality rice, cooled

1 cup leftover cooked salmon, crumbled

1/2 cup prepared pesto

1 cup baby frozen peas, slightly heated, then cooled and drained

1/4 cup diced roasted red peppers

1 cup (more or less) mayonnaise, just enough to moisten

Salt and pepper to taste

Blend all ingredients together and serve on a lettuce leaf.

Note: If the entire salad will not be eaten at one meal,

only add mayonnaise to the portion that will be eaten immediately; don't add mayonnaise to the leftovers until just before serving.

CONFETTI COLE SLAW

Good for the tummy! You will definitely want leftovers for lunch tomorrow.

YIELD: 6–8 SERVINGS

1/4 head cabbage, shredded and chopped

1/8 head red cabbage, shredded and chopped

2 large carrots, peeled and shredded

1/4 cup peeled and shredded jicama

Enough mayonnaise to moisten

Combine all ingredients and serve immediately.

WEEK I-3, DAY 4

- Breakfast: the Wings Breakfast Drink
- Lunch: leftover Salmon Rice Salad and Confetti Cole Slaw
- Mid-afternoon snack: more Confetti Cole Slaw (if you still have leftovers; if you don't, a salad of mixed vegetables dressed lightly with your favorite dressing)
- Dinner: Tamale Pie, Great Guacamole (recipes follow) with baked tortilla chips, and a large green salad tossed with your favorite dressing
- Evening snack: leftover Great Guacamole and chips

TAMALE PIE

Adapted from *Round-the-World Cooking at the Natural Gourmet* by Debra Stark (New Canaan, CT: Keats Publishing, Inc., 1994).

YIELD: 4 SERVINGS

Filling

1 tablespoon olive oil

1 onion, chopped

2 cloves garlic, minced

4 cups diced tomatoes

1 green pepper, chopped

1 cup tomato purée

1 tablespoon chili powder

1 ¹/₂ teaspoons salt

¹/₄ cup sliced olives

4 cups cooked beans (kidney, lima, or black turtle)

Crust

3 cups water

¹/₂ cup corn grits

¹/₂ cup cornmeal

1 tablespoon olive oil

1 tablespoon grated pecorino Romano cheese

2 cups grated cheese (preferably almond or rice cheese)

1. To make the filling, warm the olive oil in a skillet and sauté the onion and garlic until soft (about 5 minutes). Add the tomatoes, pepper, tomato purée, chili powder, salt, and olives, and simmer 10 minutes. Add beans and simmer another 10 minutes.

2. To make the crust, boil the water and whisk in the corn grits and cornmeal until no lumps remain. Add the olive oil and Romano and simmer 10 minutes, stirring often to prevent sticking.

3. Spoon a layer of cornmeal crust into a greased 2-quart casserole dish, reserving 1¹/₂ cups for topping. Spread the filling over the bottom crust, the remaining batter over the top, and the grated cheese over all. Bake 30 minutes at 350°F. Let stand 10 minutes before serving.

GREAT GUACAMOLE

Nothing beats homemade guacamole. I have it often for a mid-afternoon or evening snack.

YIELD: 2–3 SERVINGS

1–2 medium-ripe avocados, sliced in half and pitted (Haas avocados have a better texture, but Florida avocados taste good too)

1–2 tablespoons salsa; or, 1 small tomato, diced fine

1 small clove garlic, mashed

A sprinkle of lime juice

Salt and pepper to taste

Scoop the flesh out of the avocado and mash, leaving a few lumps. Add all remaining ingredients, mix, and enjoy.

Variations: For more kick, throw in some minced onion and/or diced canned green chilies and/or chopped fresh cilantro; you may also wish to increase the amount of lime juice.

- Breakfast: the Wings Breakfast Drink
- Lunch: leftover Tamale Pie and a fresh veggie tray
- Mid-afternoon snack: baked tortilla chips and salsa
- Dinner: Forty-Cloves-of-Garlic Chicken, Roasted Vegetables (recipes follow), and your choice of salad
- Evening snack: Banana "Ice Cream" (page 247)

FORTY-CLOVES-OF-GARLIC CHICKEN

The aroma will bring the neighborhood to your door!
Adapted from *Round-the-World Cooking at the Natural Gourmet.*

YIELD: 8–10 SERVINGS

5 chicken thighs

5 chicken-breast halves

40 cloves garlic, unpeeled and whole

2 carrots, sliced

2 bulbs kohlrabi, diced

2 stalks celery, sliced

1 teaspoon dried or 2 teaspoons fresh thyme

1 teaspoon dried or 2 teaspoons fresh rosemary

1 teaspoon dried or 2 teaspoons fresh tarragon

1 teaspoon salt

1 teaspoon black pepper

Salt and pepper to taste

1. Wash and dry the chicken, and broil it until the skin is crisp and brown (about 10 minutes). Preheat oven to 325°F. Place the broiled chicken in a roasting pan with the garlic, vegetables, and seasonings, cover the pan with foil and the foil with a lid, and bake 1¹/₂ hours, uncovering during the last 15 minutes; the chicken is done when a fork inserted into the thigh comes out easily and the juice runs clear.

2. Transfer the chicken to a platter. Using a slotted spoon, scatter the garlic from the pan around the platter and spoon the vegetables over the chicken. Pour some of the cooking juices over all, sprinkle with salt and pepper as desired, and serve.

ROASTED VEGETABLES

Another recipe to get creative with—use seasonal, local vegetables when possible, and try a different vegetable blend each time. Turns "vegetable haters" into "vegetable lovers"!

YIELD: 6–8 SERVINGS

2 baking potatoes, scrubbed and cut into large chunks

1 white or yellow onion, peeled and cut into large chunks

Several whole cloves garlic, peeled

1 large butternut or other winter squash, peeled and cut into large chunks

1 parsnip, peeled and cut into chunks

A sprinkle of olive oil

Fresh or dried herbs to taste

Preheat oven to 425°F. Prepare all the vegetables, place in a shallow baking dish, and sprinkle generously with the olive oil and any desired herbs, stirring to coat all the pieces with oil. Roast uncovered in the oven, stirring occasionally but letting some get crisp on the bottom of the pan, until done and slightly browned (about 45 minutes)—do not overcook.

WEEK I-3, DAY 6

- Breakfast: Fruit Crisp or Brown Rice with Fruit (recipes follow)

- Lunch: your favorite salad topped with your favorite protein and dressed lightly with olive oil and balsamic vinegar

- Mid-afternoon snack: a piece of fresh fruit

- Dinner: leftover Forty-Cloves-of-Garlic Chicken, or your favorite bean soup

- Evening snack: fresh fruit dipped in almond butter

Today's tip: Today's recipes (and others you will see in future weeks) give you alternatives to the Wings Breakfast Drink, but you should only use these alternatives occasionally, such as for a family breakfast or brunch, or on days when you are going to be unusually active.

FRUIT CRISP

This sounds suspiciously like dessert, but I think it makes an excellent breakfast. Kids love it before heading off to school in the morning.

YIELD: 4 SERVINGS

5 cups sliced and peeled apples, peaches, or other fruit (or a mixture of fruits)

1/4 cup regular rolled oats

1/4 cup date sugar

1/4 cup oat flour or barley flour

1/4 teaspoon cinnamon

1/4 cup butter

1/4 chopped pecans or walnuts (optional)

Preheat oven to 375°F. Place the fruit in an 8x$^1/_2$-inch round baking dish. In a mixing bowl, combine the oats, sugar, flour, and cinnamon; then, using a pastry cutter or two knives, cut in the butter until the topping resembles coarse crumbs. Sprinkle the topping over the fruit and sprinkle the nuts over the topping. Bake until the fruit is tender and the topping is golden brown (about 30–35 minutes). Serve warm.

Variation: Especially delicious with fresh pie cherries mixed in with the apples, or even fresh rhubarb, although rhubarb may require a little more sweetening.

BROWN RICE WITH FRUIT

Absolutely delicious for breakfast on a cool fall or winter morning. Especially attractive with blueberries, which turn the whole dish an appetizing purple color— kids love purple rice!

YIELD: 4 SERVINGS

2 cups hot water

A sprinkle of salt (optional)

1 cup uncooked brown rice (preferably short-grain, but long-grain also works well)

1 teaspoon butter

1–2 cups fresh fruit (blueberries, strawberries, raspberries, or sliced peaches)

Bring the water to a boil, sprinkle in a little salt as desired, add the brown rice and butter, stir once or twice, set the lid slightly ajar, turn heat down, and let simmer slowly until tender (about 45 minutes). Remove from heat and gently stir in the fruit, being careful not to over-stir and make the rice sticky. Serve immediately.

Note: As this dish takes a while to cook, you may want to start early. Or, the night before, bring the water to a boil, add the rice, stir a couple times, replace the lid, turn off heat, and let the rice sit on the stove all night to soften; in the morning, you'll only need to cook it for about 10 minutes before it is tender.

WEEK I-3, DAY 7

- Breakfast: the Wings Breakfast Drink
- Lunch: a mixed vegetable salad topped with leftover Forty-Cloves-of-Garlic Chicken and dressed lightly with your favorite dressing, plus leftover Roasted Vegetables if you're still hungry
- Mid-afternoon snack: a small or medium green salad dressed lightly with olive oil and balsamic vinegar
- Dinner: your choice from a previous menu or another favorite dinner of your own, including at least three different vegetables (make sure your dinner is balanced among proteins, carbohydrates, and fats, and is prepared from whole, real foods with no artificial ingredients)
- Evening snack: a piece of fresh fruit

Checking in: Keep testing your first morning urine and keep its pH steady at 6.5–7.5; remember, pH is a key factor in your body's ability to heal and to prevent premature aging.

WEEK I-4, DAY 1

Feeling great? Losing weight? Hopefully, you've lost some of your allergies and other symptoms are disappearing. Isn't it wonderful to feel and look good? Continue on your program and stay faithful to the food plan.

- Breakfast: the Wings Breakfast Drink
- Lunch: a large green salad dressed lightly with olive oil and balsamic vinegar, and any leftovers you have in the refrigerator
- Mid-afternoon snack: a piece of fresh fruit
- Dinner: Shrimp Curried Rice (recipe follows), Roasted Asparagus (page 237) or another green vegetable, and sliced tomatoes topped with fresh basil and olive oil

- Evening snack: a handful of raw almonds

Today's tip: Start soaking the beans for tomorrow's soup before you go to bed tonight.

SHRIMP CURRIED RICE

This simple dish is lovely for a quick family dinner. Try it for brunch too!

YIELD: 4 SERVINGS

3 cups water
1 1/2 cups uncooked white rice
1 teaspoon olive oil
1 pound large shrimp, peeled
2 cloves garlic, minced
2 cups frozen green peas, thawed
1 tablespoon curry powder
1/2 teaspoon salt
2 tablespoons chopped fresh cilantro
2 teaspoons dark sesame oil
Soy sauce to taste

Bring the water to a boil, add the rice, cover lightly, turn heat down, and simmer until barely tender (about 10 minutes). Meanwhile, heat the olive oil in a nonstick skillet or wok over medium-high heat, add the shrimp and garlic, and sauté for 2 minutes. Add the peas, curry powder, and salt, and stir-fry for 1 minute. Stir in the cooked rice and stir-fry until thoroughly blended and warm (about 1 minute). Serve on individual plates, sprinkled with the cilantro, sesame oil, and soy sauce to taste.

WEEK I-4, DAY 2

- Breakfast: the Wings Breakfast Drink
- Lunch: leftover Shrimp Curried Rice and a small green salad tossed with your favorite dressing
- Mid-afternoon snack: rice or other non-wheat crackers with nondairy cheese (soy or almond)
- Dinner: Bean Soup with Ham Chunks (recipe follows), several slices of nondairy cheese, and two slices of Kamut, spelt, or brown rice bread (this may be a new type of bread for you; do not substitute, as you do not want to introduce wheat or other highly allergenic grains into your diet)

- Evening snack: one slice of Kamut, spelt, or brown rice bread with your favorite nut butter

Today's tip: Before work this morning, place the pre-soaked beans for tonight's soup in the 2¹/₂ quarts of water, bring to a boil, simmer gently for 5 minutes, and then turn off heat, cover tightly, and let them sit on the stove for quicker cooking this evening.

BEAN SOUP WITH HAM CHUNKS

Ham isn't a great food, but it makes a wonderful flavoring agent for this satisfying dish. By the time the longer-cooking beans in the mixture are done, the others will have turned to mush, producing a creamy, thick soup.

YIELD: 8–12 SERVINGS

2 cups natural bean-soup mix

1 package (2 or 4) smoked ham hocks

2 ¹/₂ quarts water

1 cup chopped onion

2–3 large ripe tomatoes, chopped and seeded

1¹/₂ teaspoon chili powder

2 teaspoons garlic powder

2 cloves garlic, minced

Soak the beans overnight, drain, and rinse. In a soup pot, bring the beans and ham hocks and water to a boil, reduce heat, and simmer for 3 to 3¹/₂ hours. Remove the ham hocks, allow them to cool a bit, and chop the meat finely. Add the remaining ingredients and the chopped ham to the pot, simmer for 30 minutes, and serve.

WEEK 1-4, DAY 3

- Breakfast: the Wings Breakfast Drink

- Lunch: leftover Bean Soup and a small or medium mixed green salad tossed with your favorite dressing

- Mid-afternoon snack: store-bought hummus or Homemade Hummus (page 241) with a handful of rice crackers or other non-wheat crackers

- Dinner: Barbecued Salmon Filets, Vegetable Rice Pilaf, and Colorful Vegetables (recipes below)

- Evening snack: a piece of fresh fruit

Today's tip: Make extra rice and salmon, and before you close the kitchen for the night, assemble the ingredients for Salmon Rice Salad (page 247), but reserve the dressing so it doesn't dry out before tomorrow's lunch.

BARBECUED SALMON FILETS

This recipe is ridiculously simple and the result is deeply satisfying. Enjoy it often!

YIELD: 4 SERVINGS

4 salmon filets (about 2 pounds)

A splash of olive oil

¹/₂ cup barbecue sauce
(my favorite is Original Masterpiece)

Preheat oven to 325°F. Wash the salmon filets and dry thoroughly. Heat a little olive oil in a heavy skillet and brown the salmon for a couple of minutes on the non-skin side. Remove from the skillet and place skin-side down in a baking dish, spread the barbecue sauce over the non-skin side, and roast in the oven until the inside of the salmon has barely turned color (about 5–10 minutes)—be sure not to overcook, or it will be dry and flavorless. Remove carefully, cut into 3-ounce portions, and serve immediately.

VEGETABLE RICE PILAF

This pilaf blends nicely with the salmon or any other meat dish.

YIELD: 4–6 SERVINGS

2 tablespoons butter

¹/₄ cup minced carrots

¹/₄ cup minced onions

¹/₄ cup minced celery

2–3 cloves garlic, minced

2 cups chicken broth

1 cup cooked basmati rice

1 teaspoon minced fresh basil

Melt the butter in a heavy saucepan, add the vegetables and garlic, and stir until lightly browned. Add the broth, stir in the rice, cover tightly, and let it simmer slowly until done *al denté* (about 5–8 minutes). Stir in the basil and serve immediately.

Variation: If you are not dairy intolerant, add 2–4 tablespoons grated Parmesan cheese for extra flavor.

COLORFUL VEGETABLES

Beautiful as well as delicious. Serve leftovers in an omelet.

YIELD: 4–6 SERVINGS

2–4 tablespoons olive oil

1 bunch fresh broccoli, cut into bite-sized pieces

2 carrots, peeled and sliced thin

1 medium red bell pepper, seeded and sliced

1 medium orange, green, or yellow bell pepper, seeded and sliced

$1/2$ white or yellow onion, peeled and sliced

4 cloves garlic, sliced

A sprinkle of soy sauce

A sprinkle of sesame oil

Heat the olive oil in a wok or heavy skillet. Making sure the vegetables are dry, add them to the oil, and stir with a wooden spoon until they are crisp yet tender—do not overcook. Sprinkle with the soy sauce and sesame oil and serve immediately.

WEEK I-4, DAY 4

- Breakfast: the Wings Breakfast Drink

- Lunch: Salmon Rice Salad (page 247) and a generous veggie platter with your favorite dressing

- Mid-afternoon snack: an apple or other raw seasonal fruit, sliced and dipped in nut butter

- Dinner: Buffalo Burgers (yes, really!) and Oven-Baked "Fries" (recipes below)

- Evening snack: a piece of fresh fruit

Today's tip: Are you wary of buffalo? It is very much like beef, except leaner. If you can't find ground buffalo (available at some health food stores), substitute *very lean* ground beef.

BUFFALO BURGERS

And you thought you knew burgers . . .

YIELD: 4 BURGERS

1 pound ground buffalo

1 tablespoon Worcestershire sauce

2 tablespoons minced onion

Salt and pepper to taste

Lettuce leaves

4 tomato slices

Several pickle slices

1–4 tablespoons mayonnaise

1–4 tablespoons catsup

8 slices non-wheat bread such as Kamut, spelt, or brown rice bread

Mix the Worcestershire sauce and minced onion into the ground buffalo, along with salt and pepper as desired, and form into 4 patties about 1-inch thick. Grill, broil, or sauté a few minutes on each side to the desired "done-ness." Be sure, for safety's sake, not to undercook, but don't overcook either, as buffalo is very lean and can get dried out; you may need to add a little oil to the grill or pan. Then, assemble your burgers with the remaining ingredients.

OVEN-BAKED "FRIES"

"Fries" don't have to be unhealthful.
These are terrific and kids love them.

YIELD: 4 SERVINGS

3–4 large russet or other baking potatoes, scrubbed but unpeeled

2 tablespoons olive oil

Salt and pepper or other seasonings to taste (see "Flavors for Your Fries" below)

Preheat oven to 425°F. Cut the potatoes into French-fry sticks, place them in a bowl of ice water for a few minutes, then remove and dry thoroughly. Sprinkle them with the oil, stir to coat all the pieces evenly, sprinkle with the salt and pepper or other seasonings as desired, and spread them one layer deep in baking pans. Bake, stirring and turning them frequently with a spatula, until done and golden (about 20–30 minutes)—do not stir for the last few minutes, so they get a bit crispy on the bottom. Remove from the oven and serve immediately.

Flavors for Your "Fries"

CHILI SEASONING

$1/2$ teaspoon sugar

$1/4$ teaspoon chili powder

$1/4$ teaspoon cayenne

$1/8$ teaspoon paprika

HERB SEASONING

1 tablespoon minced fresh thyme

1 tablespoon minced fresh rosemary

1 tablespoon minced fresh oregano

CHEESE SEASONING

¼ cup finely grated Parmesan cheese

1 tablespoon Italian seasoning

WEEK I-4, DAY 5

- Breakfast: the Wings Breakfast Drink
- Lunch: leftover Bean Soup with Ham Chunks if you still have it; otherwise, a large green salad topped with a scoop of your favorite protein or leftover Buffalo Burger and dressed lightly
- Mid-afternoon snack: a piece of fresh fruit
- Dinner: Mesclun Salad (recipe follows)
- Evening snack: a piece of fresh fruit

Checking in: Was last night's burger a little heavy for you? Don't worry, you're eating lightly today.

MESCLUN SALAD

Very light yet very satisfying.

YIELD: 4 SERVINGS

1 package mesclun mix (available at supermarkets or health food stores)

Other raw vegetables of your choice, cut and prepared for the salad

1 handful dried cranberries or cherries

1 handful Roasted Pecans or Walnuts (recipe follows)

1 handful feta cheese (sheep, goat, camel— but not the cow's milk variety)

Olive oil and vinegar dressing to taste

Assemble the greens and vegetables on dinner plates. Sprinkle with the cranberries or cherries, roasted nuts, and cheese. Dress the salad as desired and enjoy immediately.

ROASTED PECANS OR WALNUTS

These are an excellent snack and a wonderful salad topping.

YIELD: 1 CUP

A splash of olive oil or macadamia nut oil

1 cup raw pecans or walnuts

In a heavy skillet, heat the oil on medium heat, then add the nuts, and stir constantly for a few minutes until lightly browned—they burn easily, so be careful not to overcook.

WEEK I-4, DAY 6

- Breakfast: the Wings Breakfast Drink
- Lunch: two deviled eggs and a fresh veggie tray with your favorite dressing
- Mid-afternoon snack: a handful of raw almonds or other raw nuts
- Dinner: Sautéed Halibut or Salmon Medallions (page 255), a large mixed green salad tossed with your favorite dressing, and a small baked sweet potato with a pat of butter
- Evening snack: a handful of Roasted Toasted Pumpkin Seeds (page 238)

WEEK I-4, DAY 7

You've been doing so well that tonight you get a real treat for dinner. Brace yourself . . .

- Breakfast: the Wings Breakfast Drink
- Lunch: leftover Sautéed Halibut or Salmon Medallions and a salad of your choice
- Mid-afternoon snack: fresh veggies with your favorite dressing
- Dinner: a small filet mignon or other steak, a small baked potato with a pat of butter and a dollop of sour cream, a small green salad tossed with your favorite dressing, and Roasted Asparagus (page 237)
- Evening snack: although you probably won't feel that you need a snack, drink a cup of miso soup to balance your pH, because steak can be highly acidic

Today's tip: Prepare the steak according to your favorite method. Do not overeat! Three to four ounces of beef is plenty to fulfill your protein requirement; share with your spouse or a friend.

WEEK I-5

This week, change the pace and give your body a new perspective by trying the Two-Hour Diet. (Don't worry; we'll go back to normal next week.) Ready? The concept is very easy to understand and the diet is easy to follow.

Thermogenesis, which is the production of heat (in this case, body heat from calories), is important to the dieter and non-dieter alike, as you will learn in later lessons. Calories are used to maintain a body temperature of 98.6°F, at which enzymes and other proteins work at optimum levels. When enzymes function properly, cellular activity is increased, so the body "runs" more efficiently and loses weight or maintains a healthful weight more easily.

The simple act of eating increases the body's energy expenditure, and eating certain types of food raises body temperature; scientists call this "diet-induced thermogenesis." Studies show that eating frequent, highly nutritious, smaller meals increases diet-induced thermogenesis and burns more calories than eating larger, less frequent meals; even if the total calorie content is the same, the body tends to burn the calories rather than store them as fat. The benefit of eating frequent small meals lies in the way the body uses short "bursts" of food to raise body temperature and increase the number of calories burned—without hunger, dieting, or cravings!

The key to losing weight on the Two-Hour Diet is to eat regularly and frequently, and to eat nutrient-dense foods only. No junk foods allowed! Converting food into ATP for cellular energy is an extremely complex task: the body utilizes a great deal of metabolic energy, many micronutrients, and several thousand biochemical steps toward this goal. Junk food does not contain adequate amounts of the critical nutrients, so the building blocks of cellular energy are missing, and the body has no choice but to convert such nutrient-poor "delectables" into body fat rather than into useable energy.

The Two-Hour Diet is one of the easiest weight-management protocols to follow—*if* you plan ahead. Follow this protocol for one week. Expect both your body temperature and your energy level to increase slightly. You will not lose tons of weight, but you should drop a little water weight and fat weight. *And* you should feel terrific! I recommend doing this Two-Hour Diet every few weeks, just to give your body a change of pace. Most people find that it really does help with weight loss.

Suggested Two-Hour Diet Schedule, Meals, and Menu

The first challenge is disciplining yourself to eat a small meal every two to three hours; this amounts to six to eight small meals per day. Here is a sample schedule:

- Meal #1: 7:00 A.M.
- Meal #2: 10:00 A.M.
- Meal #3: 1:00 P.M.
- Meal #4: 4:00 P.M.
- Meal #5: 7:00 P.M.
- Meal #6: 10:00 P.M.

The second challenge is rethinking your idea of a meal. This involves careful planning to minimize meal preparation and prevent overeating. The secret to portion control is to eat slowly, chew thoroughly, and stop eating when you feel slightly satisfied, *before* you feel full. If you eat too much at one meal, your body spends too much energy in digestion, hindering its ability to turn the food into cellular energy instead of fat.

Here is a list of typical Two-Hour Diet meals:

- Half a serving of the Wings Breakfast Drink (highly recommended as the first daily meal, because it provides an optimal balance of proteins, carbohydrates, and fats that keeps blood sugar steady throughout the day; it is also quickly and easily prepared, as well as delicious and satisfying)

- A celery stalk stuffed with 1 tablespoon of almond or cashew butter

- A small green salad topped with 1 ounce of chicken and dressed lightly

- Bean salad with black or pinto beans

- 1 cup of Two-Hour-Diet Vegetable Soup (recipe follows)

- 1 ounce tuna fish moistened with 1 teaspoon mayonnaise

- One baked or broiled chicken leg with a small romaine salad

- 1/2 cup cottage cheese with 1/2 apple

- 4 tablespoons Great Guacamole (page 248) with baked tortilla chips

- 1/4 cup store-bought hummus or Homemade Hummus (page 241) with fresh vegetables (like carrots, broccoli, and cauliflower)

- 2 ounces baked or broiled tilapia, halibut, or other white fish, with a small salad

- Two hard-boiled eggs or deviled eggs

- 2 tablespoons Roasted Toasted Pumpkin Seeds (page 238)

- 2 tablespoons raw almonds or other nuts

- Half an avocado with 2 tablespoons cottage cheese

Here is a sample menu to get you started. Follow this model first, and then you should be able to design your own Two-Hour Diet menus for the rest of the week.

- Meal #1: half a serving of the Wings Breakfast Drink

- Meal #2: a celery stalk stuffed with 1 tablespoon of almond or cashew butter

- Meal #3: a small romaine salad topped with 2 ounces of baked or broiled tilapia, halibut, or other white fish, and dressed lightly

- Meal #4: bean salad with black beans or pinto beans dressed with olive oil

- Meal #5: half a serving of the Wings Breakfast Drink

- Meal #6: a large green salad topped with 2 ounces of protein and dressed lightly

- Meal #7: 1 cup of Two-Hour-Diet Vegetable Soup (recipe follows), to finish the day by alkalinizing the body

Be cautious in your Two-Hour Diet menu design: (1) only include nutrient-dense food (whole, real food), and (2) keep the calories per meal at no more than 200–250 so your total calorie count per day will be 1,200–1,400. Pack each calorie full of good nutrition!

SAUTÉED HALIBUT OR SALMON MEDALLIONS

This recipe is so simple, you'll want to use it frequently.

YIELD: 8–10 SERVINGS (SERVING SIZE IS 1 CUP)

1 tablespoon butter
1 tablespoon olive oil
4 halibut or salmon filets

Heat the butter and oil in a heavy frying pan. When it is slightly bubbly, add the filets and brown quickly on one side, then turn to brown the other side. Cover the pan with a lid, lower the temperature, and allow the filets to cook on the inside. Do not overcook.

TWO-HOUR-DIET VEGETABLE SOUP

A good, basic vegetable soup recipe that works well in this (or any other) context.

YIELD: 8–10 SERVINGS (SERVING SIZE IS 1 CUP)

1 tablespoon olive oil

½ cup chopped onion
½ cup chopped celery
½ cup chopped carrots
1 cup shredded cabbage
½ cup canned kidney beans
½ cup canned garbanzo beans
2 cups vegetable broth

In a heavy saucepan, heat the oil and add the onions, celery, carrots, and cabbage. Cook over low heat, stirring, until the vegetables begin to soften (about 20 minutes). Add the beans and broth, bring the soup to a slow simmer, and let it simmer until the vegetables are done (about 20 minutes).

WEEKS I-6 TO I-10

Repeat the original Wings menus for weeks I-1 to I-5, which includes last week's Two-Hour Diet. If you have some favorites out of this selection, enjoy them more frequently. Remember that one of the purposes of these menus is to remove common allergens from your diet.

The focus of Lesson I-10 is food allergies, so now is a good time to schedule your ELISA/Act LRA test (see page 47). If you find that you are allergic to foods in the Wings recipes, eliminate those foods completely for at least six weeks. You may then try to reintroduce them, but if you still get a reaction or gain a few pounds, you will have to eliminate them permanently. Don't worry: you'll still have lots of wonderful foods to enjoy! If you have a number of allergies and are having difficulty putting a food plan together, go to the website www.flywithwings.com/pnc.html and click on MyProConnect for a consultation with your Wings nutritionist.

WEEK I-11

Starting now, the concept for the rest of the Wings Program eating plan is to use the menus and recipes provided in the first four weeks as your base. From here forward, I will provide new recipes each week that you can rotate into these "core menus." If you have any uncertainty about what to include on your day's menu, just go back to one of the core menus and follow its format. Remember to include protein, carbohydrates, and fats with each meal, and to eat natural food only (as much as possible). It's simple, really, and you've been doing it for several weeks now. You're a pro!

This week's new recipes feature breakfasts, or, if you like, desserts.

OAT COTTAGE-CHEESE PANCAKES

If you can handle cottage cheese (some people with dairy intolerance can tolerate cottage cheese or yogurt), you'll love these high-protein pancakes for an occasional special breakfast. Serve with warm Homemade Applesauce (recipe follows) instead of syrup.

YIELD: 4 SERVINGS

1/2 cup oat flour (if oats bother you, use barley, Kamut, or spelt flour)

1/2 teaspoon nonaluminum baking powder

2 teaspoons honey

1/2 teaspoon salt

2 eggs, beaten

1 cup creamed cottage cheese

Mix the dry ingredients and add the beaten eggs and honey. Sieve the cottage cheese and add to the flour-egg mixture. Fry on a well-greased medium-hot griddle, spreading the pancakes out as you place them (they don't spread themselves) and watching carefully so the cottage cheese doesn't burn, and serve immediately.

HOMEMADE APPLESAUCE

I'm almost embarrassed to include such a simple recipe, but if you've never made homemade applesauce, you'll love it. No added sugar: a little cinnamon tricks your mouth into thinking it is sweeter than it is. Especially good on warm pancakes, but an excellent snack or dessert by itself.

YIELD: 6–8 SERVINGS

6 Rome or Granny Smith apples
(these are best, but you can use other varieties)

1 tablespoon cinnamon,
or more or less to taste

Peel, core, and slice the apples, place in a large saucepan, and *almost* cover with water. Bring to a boil, lower the temperature, simmer until soft (about 10 minutes), and remove from heat. With a potato masher, mash the apples into a sauce texture, and then stir in the cinnamon. Serve warm or cold.

Variation: If you are really adventurous, add some fresh rhubarb to lend tartness.

REALLY GOOD MIXED-GRAIN PANCAKES

Fluffy, tender, and so delicious that you will never be tempted by restaurant pancakes again! Top with warm applesauce or fresh fruit. As an alternative to oat or barley flours, I sometimes use Kamut or quinoa flours, which are more appropriate for gluten-sensitive individuals.

YIELD: 4 SERVINGS

1 cup oat or barley flour

3/4 cup spelt flour

2 tablespoons date sugar

1 tablespoon non aluminum baking powder

1/2 teaspoon salt

2 eggs, beaten

13/4 cups almond, rice, or soy milk

1/3 cup butter, melted

In a large bowl, combine the flour, sugar, baking powder, and salt. In a medium-sized bowl, combine the eggs, milk, and butter. Stir the egg mixture into the flour mixture until just blended, but do not over-stir (only break up big lumps, leaving the batter slightly lumpy). Heat a large skillet over medium heat until a few drops of water sprinkled in bounce before evaporating. Brush skillet lightly with butter, pour 1/4 cup batter for each pancake onto skillet, cook until bubbles break on top of pancakes, turn with a spatula, cook until browned, and serve immediately.

WEEK I-12

How is it going designing your own menus? Remember to balance your proteins, carbohydrates, and fats with each meal, and to eat natural food.

Also, remember to start your day with the Wings Breakfast Drink most of the time, saving last week's pancakes for an occasional treat.

This week's first new recipe takes a little preparation time, but the payoff is that one batch is the base for at least three well-balanced meals (recipes follow), each of which can be ready to go within minutes.

TRIPLE-BATCH BEEF

My family really enjoys this recipe, which was designed by the Oregon Beef Council. This beef makes the best chili and stew my kids have ever eaten. Once the meat is cooked, divide it into three portions and freeze or refrigerate for later.

YIELD: 6 CUPS COOKED BEEF TO USE IN OTHER RECIPES

3 $1/2$ pounds beef (chuck or blade roast)

1 tablespoon olive oil

Salt to taste

$1/2$ teaspoon black pepper

2 cups chopped onions

4 cloves garlic, crushed

1 $1/2$ cups water

Trim the fat from the beef and cut the meat into $3/4$-inch pieces. In a Dutch oven or similarly heavy pot, heat the olive oil over medium heat until hot. Add a quarter of the beef at a time and brown evenly, stirring occasionally. Remove the beef to a plate and season with the salt and pepper. Add the onions and garlic to the same pot and cook, stirring occasionally, until onions are lightly browned. Return the beef to the pot, add the water, bring to a boil, reduce heat to low, cover tightly, and simmer until tender (about 1$1/2$–2 hours). Place about 2 cups of beef into each of 3 freezer containers, cover tightly, and freeze or refrigerate.

TWENTY-MINUTE BEEF CHILI

My kids like to pile this chili on baked corn chips, sprinkle it with a little cheese (almond cheese is good), and eat it with their fingers. It is also excellent on an omelet, or right out of a bowl on a cool evening.

YIELD: 4 SERVINGS

$1/3$ portion Triple-Batch Beef (recipe above)

8 ounces salsa (commercial or homemade)

1 tablespoon chili powder

1 15-ounce can red kidney beans, undrained

2 scallions, chopped, for garnish

In a medium saucepan, combine the beef, salsa, and chili powder, bring to a boil, reduce heat to low, cover tightly, and simmer for 10 minutes. Stir in the beans and heat through (about 5 minutes). Garnish with the scallions and serve.

WEEKNIGHT BEEF STEW

I've suggested my favorite root vegetables for this stew, but you can use any seasonal fresh vegetables you like and make the stew different each time.

YIELD: 4 SERVINGS

2 medium potatoes

1 large carrot

1 medium parsnip

1 medium turnip

$1/3$ portion Triple-Batch Beef (recipe above)

1 teaspoon dried oregano

1 $1/2$ cups water

$1/4$ teaspoon salt

1 cup petite frozen or fresh peas

Peel the vegetables and cut into uniform pieces. In a medium saucepan, combine them with the beef, oregano, water, and salt, bring to a boil, reduce heat, and simmer until the vegetables are barely done (about 20 minutes)—do not overcook, and add more water if necessary. Stir in the peas, turn off heat, let peas heat through (about 5 minutes), and serve immediately.

QUICK-AND-EASY BEEF-BARLEY SOUP

Barley is "comfort food" for the intestinal tract, and this nourishing, delicious soup goes down easy, especially on cool fall and winter evenings.

YIELD: 4 SERVINGS

1 cup fresh green beans

1 small carrot

$1/3$ portion Triple-Batch Beef (recipe above)

3 cups water

$1/4$ cup quick-cooking Scotch barley, dry

1 cup beef broth

1 teaspoon dried thyme

Cut the beans into 1-inch pieces and remove the stem ends. Peel and cut the carrot into 1-inch pieces. Combine all ingredients in a large saucepan, bring to a boil, reduce heat to low, cover tightly, simmer until the barley is tender (about 12 minutes), and serve.

MODULE II

I know you are staying on track—because you feel so good! Remember to balance your proteins, carbohydrates, and fats with each meal. Begin each day with the Wings Breakfast Drink to balance your blood sugar and energy level. Ready for a whole new module and more great food? Here we go . . .

WEEK II-1

Welcome to "Vegetable Week"! Too many of us were raised on limp, soggy, canned vegetables and never really learned to enjoy the marvelous textures, colors, and flavors of well-prepared fresh vegetables. I am going to change that with three new vegetable dishes that will make your taste buds stand up and cheer! As a bonus, these delicious dishes are simple to prepare.

PIKE STREET CAFÉ'S WILD FOREST MUSHROOM SOUP

Soup is light yet warm and filling, and can be prepared ahead of time for a quick meal-on-the-run; serve with a salad. This dish is a favorite at the Sheraton Hotelin Seattle.

YIELD: 4 SERVINGS

1 bulb garlic, peeled
4 tablespoons olive oil
$\frac{1}{2}$ cup chopped onion
1 medium carrot, peeled and chopped
2 cups button mushrooms
$\frac{1}{2}$ pound dried shiitake mushrooms
1 teaspoon dried thyme
8 ounces dry white wine
2 quarts vegetable broth

Roast the garlic cloves (sprinkled with a little olive oil) at 375°F until tender (about 30 minutes), then set aside. Meanwhile, dice the onion and carrot, and clean and slice the mushrooms, reserving 9 shiitake mushrooms whole for garnish. In a saucepan, heat the oil and sauté the onion for 5 minutes, add the carrot and thyme and sauté for 3–4 minutes; then add the wine, roasted garlic, and mushrooms, and sauté for 3 minutes. Add the vegetable broth, bring to a boil, then reduce heat and simmer until the liquid is reduced by a quarter. Remove from heat and purée in a blender or food processor. Garnish with the 9 reserved mushrooms and serve.

RATATOUILLE

Serve hot or cold as a vegetable side dish.

YIELD: 10 SERVINGS

1 cup olive oil
2 large onions, sliced
3 cloves garlic, chopped very fine
2 large eggplants, peeled and cut into small cubes
2 large zucchini squash, washed and sliced
2 large green bell peppers, seeded and sliced
6 ripe red tomatoes (preferably in season), peeled, seeded, and chopped
Salt and pepper to taste
1 bouquet garni (a parsley sprig, celery top, bay leaf, and pinch of thyme tied in cheesecloth)

Heat the olive oil until sizzling, sauté the onions until limp, then add the garlic and cook 5 minutes. Add the eggplant, zucchini, green peppers, and tomatoes, season with salt and pepper as desired, add the *bouquet garni*, cover the pot, and simmer 1 hour; if the ratatouille is too liquid, remove the lid for the last half hour to reduce.

ROASTED GARLIC

Roasting mellows the flavors of garlic deliciously for spreading on rice crackers, enjoying as a side dish, mixing with hummus, or adding to vegetable soups. To make it even easier, purchase whole, fresh cloves of garlic that are already peeled and ready to cook.

YIELD: APPROXIMATELY 1 CUP

1 cup fresh, peeled garlic cloves
A sprinkle of olive oil

Place the garlic in a small roasting pan, sprinkle with the oil, bake at 375°F until soft (about 30–35 minutes), and serve immediately.

WEEK II-2

Drink lots of water this week: at least 1 ounce of water for every 2 pounds of your body weight, daily, spaced out between meals.

VEGETABLE SAUTÉ

Delicious and beautiful—make a little extra to put on top of a breakfast eggs treat.

1 bunch broccoli, divided into florets (stalk ends removed) and cut into thin slices

4 large bell peppers (red, green, orange, and yellow), washed, seeded, and cut into 1-inch squares

Several cloves fresh garlic, minced

1/2 large white onion, cut in to 1/4-inch slices

1–2 tablespoons olive oil

1–2 tablespoons soy sauce

1/2 teaspoon sesame oil

In a large sauté pan, heat the olive oil until it is hot, add all the vegetables and cook, stirring frequently until tender but still crunchy (about 10–15 minutes). Add the soy sauce and stir to coat all pieces. Just before serving, sprinkle the sesame oil over the vegetables.

FRIJOLES NEGROS

Fabulous with a small salad or a grilled chicken breast, or over brown rice for a complete meal. (*Note:* Before you begin, sort through the dried beans to discard any small stones or other debris, then rinse the beans under running water and soak them overnight, or for at least 4 hours.) Adapted from *Gourmet* magazine.

1 1/2 pounds dried black beans, rinsed and pre-soaked (see note above)

1 bay leaf

1 sprig fresh oregano

4 tablespoons olive oil

1 tablespoon cumin powder

12 scallions, trimmed and finely chopped

8 cloves garlic, finely chopped

1 small green bell pepper, cored, seeded, and finely chopped

Salt and pepper to taste

Put the pre-soaked beans, bay leaf, oregano, and 1 tablespoon of the oil into a large pot, cover with cold water by 3 inches, bring to a boil over high heat, reduce heat to medium-low, and simmer until beans are tender (about 2 hours), adding more water as needed to keep beans covered. Heat the remaining oil in a small skillet over medium heat, add the cumin, scallions, garlic, and green pepper, and sauté, stirring often, until peppers are soft and scallions are golden (about 10 minutes). Add to bean pot and continue cooking, stir-

ring occasionally, for 10–15 minutes. Remove bay leaf, season as desired with salt and pepper, and serve.

This week, in preparation for the upcoming cleansing week, plan to enjoy several high-fiber meals (the following two recipes feature beans, a great source of fiber). Also, try a new twist on your Wings Breakfast Drink: add 1–2 tablespoons of ground flaxseed to the drink, mix thoroughly, and drink immediately before the fiber gels. Flaxseed is a good source of essential fatty acids, is wonderfully soothing to the delicate gastrointestinal lining, and provides a form of fiber that softens the stool and adds bulk.

SQUASH AND WHITE BEAN SOUP

Butternut squash makes a fabulous soup; the beans add a bit of flavor, protein, and fiber.

1 large clove garlic, minced

2 tablespoons olive oil

1/2 small butternut squash, cut into 1/2-inch pieces

2 cups chicken broth

2 cups water

1 can white beans, rinsed and drained

2 cups canned whole tomatoes, chopped

1 teaspoon finely chopped fresh sage

1/4 cup Roasted Toasted Pumpkin Seeds for garnish (optional; page 238)

In a heavy saucepan, cook the garlic in 1 tablespoon of the oil for about 1 minute, stirring frequently. Add the squash, broth, water, beans, tomatoes, and sage, and simmer, covered, stirring occasionally, until squash is tender (about 20 minutes). Using a potato masher, mash some of the squash to thicken the soup. Remove from heat, correct seasoning to taste, garnish with the pumpkin seeds, and serve.

BABY LIMA BEANS AND CORN IN A CHIVE SAUCE

Bacon isn't a great food, but it sure is a good seasoning agent, used sparingly and occasionally.

4 slices bacon, cut into 1/2-inch pieces

1 medium onion, chopped

1 green bell pepper, diced

1 10-ounce package frozen baby lima beans

1 10-ounce package frozen corn

1 cup water

$1/2$ teaspoon salt

$1/4$ teaspoon pepper

$1/4$ cup tahini

2 tablespoons chopped fresh chives;
or, 1 teaspoon dried chives

1 tablespoon chopped fresh parsley;
or, 1 teaspoon dried parsley

Cook the bacon in a skillet over moderate heat, stirring, until crisp, then transfer bacon to paper towels to drain. Cook the onion and bell pepper in the skillet with the bacon fat over moderate heat, stirring frequently, until softened (about 5–6 minutes). Add the lima beans, corn, water, salt, and pepper, and simmer, covered, until tender (about 8 minutes). Add the tahini and cook, uncovered, until the soup thickens. Stir in the herbs, correct the seasoning as desired, and serve sprinkled with bacon bits.

WEEK II-4

Have you always relied on canned soups? Lesson II-4 about "nonfoods" points out the problems of eating from cans. Why not prepare a delicious homemade soup instead? It's simple, and your family will love it.

BASIC VEGETABLE SOUP

A large bowl of this light, satisfying soup counts as two servings of vegetables! Use whatever vegetables are in season—hopefully, organic produce from your local CSA farm—to vary the flavor from pot to pot.

YIELD: 6–8 SERVINGS

2 tablespoons butter

2 cups diced leeks or onions

2 cloves garlic, chopped

1 28-ounce can tomatoes (dice the tomatoes)

1 large carrot, diced

4 celery stalks, diced

1 large turnip, peeled and diced

$1/4$ cup uncooked long-grain brown rice

8 cups beef broth

1 cup fresh string beans cut into 1-inch pieces

1 large zucchini, diced

2 cups shredded Chinese cabbage

1 tablespoon chopped fresh parsley

$1/2$ teaspoon oregano

Salt and pepper to taste

In a large saucepan, heat the butter and cook the leeks or onions until wilted (about 5–10 minutes), add the garlic, cook for 30 seconds, and add the tomatoes, carrot, celery, turnip, rice, and broth. Bring to a boil, reduce heat, and cook gently for 5–8 minutes. Add the string beans, zucchini, and cabbage, and cook until tender (about 30 minutes). Stir in the herbs, season with salt and pepper as desired, and serve.

AUTUMN CAULIFLOWER SOUP

Creamy, rich, and absolutely delightful as a main course. Serve with a slab of piping hot Carol's Cornbread (recipe follows).

YIELD: 6 SERVINGS

1 head cauliflower

3 tablespoons butter

1 large onion, chopped

1–2 slices fresh ginger root

$1/2$ cup uncooked long-grain white rice

3 celery stalks, chopped

Salt to taste

Cayenne pepper to taste

2 teaspoons dried chives

2 teaspoons chopped fresh parsley

$1/2$ teaspoon curry powder

2 cups chicken stock

$1/4$ cup tahini

In a large pot, cover the cauliflower with water, bring to a boil, and simmer until tender (about 15 minutes)—do not overcook! Reserving the water, remove the cauliflower and set it aside. In a large pot, melt the butter and sauté the onion and ginger for 5 minutes. Add the rice, celery, and reserved liquid from the cauliflower, season with salt and cayenne as desired, and simmer until rice is tender (about 10 minutes). In a blender or food processor, blend 2 cups of the soup at a time until smooth (be careful that the hot mixture does not burst up and burn your hands), and return to the pot. Add the chives, parsley, curry, and chicken stock. Chop the cooked cauliflower fine and add to soup, stir in the tahini, and heat thoroughly, but do not boil. Serve hot.

CAROL'S CORNBREAD

A moist, wheat-free cornbread. My kids love it hot from the oven, with a dab of butter melted on top and slathered with fruit-only jam. Slice any leftover pieces in half lengthwise, and toast on both sides for breakfast the next day.

YIELD: 6 SLICES

1 1/3 *cups stone-ground cornmeal*

1 1/3 *cups spelt flour*

1 tablespoon nonaluminum baking powder

1 teaspoon salt

3 eggs, beaten

1/4 *cup honey or maple syrup*

1 can cream-style corn

1 cup soy or almond milk

1/3 *cup melted butter*

Preheat oven to 400°F, placing an iron skillet in it to heat while you prepare the batter. In a mixing bowl, stir together all the dry ingredients. In another mixing bowl, stir together the remaining ingredients until blended, then combine the two mixtures and stir just until smooth. Remove the skillet from the oven, butter the bottom and sides, pour the batter into the skillet, and quickly place it back into the hot oven. Bake for 40–50 minutes or until the top is golden and a toothpick inserted in the center comes out clean. Let it sit for a couple of minutes, then slice into wedges and serve.

WEEK II-5

SNAPPER ALMONDINE

Snapper is a delightful fish, slightly sweet with a soft texture; if it is unavailable or too expensive, substitute another soft white fish. Serve with a little brown rice (pilaf, perhaps?), a vegetable, and a salad.

YIELD: 4 SERVINGS

16 ounces red snapper

Salt and pepper to taste

1 tablespoon lemon juice

4 ounces sliced almonds

1/2 *cup oat flour or barley flour*

2 tablespoons olive oil

4 ounces white wine

1 tablespoon chopped fresh parsley for garnish

Cut the snapper into four equal pieces, sprinkle with the salt, pepper, and lemon juice, and coat both sides of the filets with the flour. Heat the oil and sauté the fish about 4–5 minutes on each side (actual cooking time depends on the thickness of the fish and the temperature of the oil)—don't overcook! Remove to a heated serving dish. Add the almonds to the remaining oil and sauté until golden, add the wine, and reduce until the mixture is thickened. Pour the gravy over the filets, garnish with the parsley, and serve.

WEEK II-6

This week, set aside the usual Wings meal plan to do the cleansing program described in Lesson II-6. Please follow the protocol in the text carefully. You'll continue to have the Wings Breakfast Drink for breakfast each day (are you still adding extra flaxseed?). For your lunch and dinner from Day 1 through Day 7 of the cleanse, your menus are as follows (recipes except where noted can be found over the next few pages):

Day 1

- Savory Black Beans and Rice
- Raw veggies with Tofu and Red Pepper Spread

Day 2

- Chalupas
- Raw veggies (choose a wide variety: broccoli, cauliflower florets, carrots, celery sticks, radishes, red onion, and any others you like) with Tahini Sauce

Day 3

- Lima Bean Soup over brown rice
- Babaganoush

Day 4

- Rice Topped with Sautéed Veggies
- Roasted Garlic and Baked Onion

Day 5

- Gardener's Pie
- Mixed green salad dressed lightly with olive oil and balsamic vinegar

Day 6

- ▨ Soup of Many Beans

- ▨ Store-bought hummus or Homemade Hummus (page 241) with raw veggies

Day 7

- ▨ Baked Winter Squash with a sprinkle of black pepper (if desired) and a dollop of hummus

- ▨ Avocado with Olive-Oil Dressing

- ▨ Mixed green salad dressed lightly with Tahini Sauce

SAVORY BLACK BEANS AND RICE

Here's another delicious variation of a versatile dish. Makes a light but satisfying dinner for the entire family.

YIELD: 4 SERVINGS

1 cup water

¹/₂ cup uncooked brown rice

2 cups cooked black beans

1 clove garlic, minced

1 bay leaf

¹/₂ teaspoon cumin powder

¹/₂ teaspoon salt

¹/₄ teaspoon dried oregano

¹/₈ teaspoon red pepper

¹/₂ cup chopped onion

¹/₂ cup chopped sun-dried tomatoes

¹/₄ cup chopped parsley

In a 2-quart saucepan, bring the water to a boil, stir in the rice, reduce heat to simmering, cover, and simmer for 30 minutes. Stir in the beans and the remaining ingredients (except the parsley), cover, and simmer until most of the liquid is absorbed (about 20 minutes). Remove the bay leaf, stir in the parsley, and serve immediately.

TOFU AND RED PEPPER SPREAD

A great dip with raw veggies. Adapted from *Cooking with the Right Side of the Brain* by Vicki Rae Chelf (New York, NY: Avery Publishing Group, 1991).

YIELD: 2 SERVINGS

1 cup mashed tofu

¹/₂ large red pepper

¹/₂ cup cashews

¹/₄ cup chopped onion

1 tablespoon yellow miso

1 tablespoon dijon mustard

In a blender or food processor, mix all ingredients until smooth and creamy. The spread will thicken slightly when chilled. If too thick, add about 1 tablespoon water (as needed); if not thick enough, add more tofu or cashews.

CHALUPAS

My kids love these simple, flat tacos; you may want to add this recipe to your list of favorites. Adapted from *Cooking with the Right Side of the Brain.*

YIELD: 6 SERVINGS

6 corn tortillas

Olive oil as needed

3 cups cooked pinto or red kidney beans

¹/₄ cup water reserved from cooking the beans

1 teaspoon dried basil

¹/₂ teaspoon dried oregano

1 teaspoon cumin powder

1 teaspoon chili powder

Cayenne pepper to taste

¹/₄ cup tomato paste

2 tablespoons shoyu sauce or tamari

¹/₂ cup grated almond cheese

Topping

1 medium avocado, pitted and peeled

2 tablespoons lemon juice

2–3 cloves garlic, pressed

2 handfuls shredded lettuce

2 ripe tomatoes, chopped

Brush the tortillas with a small amount of oil, and toast them in a toaster oven or under the broiler until crispy—be careful not to burn them. In a bowl, mash the beans with enough of the water reserved from cooking them to obtain a spreadable consistency, and mix in the herbs, spices, tomato paste, and shoyu sauce or tamari. Spread the toasted tortillas generously with the bean mixture, sprinkle with the cheese, place on a cookie sheet, and bake at 400°F until thoroughly heated and cheese melts (about 10–15 minutes; almond cheese does not spread and glaze over like dairy cheese). Meanwhile, mash together the avocado, lemon juice, and garlic. Top the hot chalupas with the lettuce and tomato, garnish each with a big spoonful of the avocado mixture, and serve.

BABAGANOUSH

Adapted from *Round-the-World Cooking at the Natural Gourmet* by Debra Stark (New Canaan, CT: Kents Publishing, Inc., 1994).

YIELD: 4 SERVINGS

2 large eggplants

4 cloves garlic, peeled

$1/2$ teaspoon salt

$1/4$ teaspoon cumin powder

$2/3$ cup sesame tahini

$1/4$ cup lemon juice

A pinch of cayenne pepper

Paprika to garnish

Prick the eggplants with a knife (so they won't explode in the oven), bake them on a cookie sheet at 350°F until the flesh feels soft, cool them slightly, and then scrape the flesh out of the skin into a food processor. Using the processor's steel blade, blend the eggplant with the garlic, salt, cumin, tahini, and lemon juice to the desired smoothness. Spoon the babaganoush into a bowl, garnish with the paprika, and serve at room temperature. (Can be refrigerated for up to 2 weeks.)

TAHINI SAUCE

Lovely on a salad, as a dip for rice crackers or vegetables, or as a flavoring for soups. Adapted from *Round-the-World Cooking at the Natural Gourmet.*

YIELD: APPROXIMATELY 1 CUP

$1/4$ cup tahini

$1/4$ cup lemon juice

$1/2$ cup water

2 cloves garlic, peeled

1 teaspoon salt

Using the steel blade of the food processor or a blender, blend all ingredients until sauce is smooth and no garlic pieces remain. Add more water if necessary to reach pouring consistency.

LIMA BEAN SOUP

This smooth, creamy soup is the ultimate comfort food, and I make it often, even when I'm not cleansing. Serve it over brown rice for a rich, delicious flavor. Adapted from *Cooking with the Right Side of the Brain.*

YIELD: 4 SERVINGS

1 cup dried baby lima beans, washed well and soaked in water overnight

3 cups water

3 bay leaves

2 tablespoons tahini

2 tablespoons arrowroot

1 teaspoon tarragon

3 tablespoons tamari

1 tablespoon cider vinegar or rice vinegar

Cayenne pepper to taste

Finely chopped scallions and parsley for garnish

Drain the pre-soaked beans, place them in a large kettle with the water and bay leaves, cover, bring to a boil, reduce heat, and simmer until very tender (about $1\frac{1}{2}$ hours). In a small bowl, combine the tahini and arrowroot, and stir it well into the kettle of beans. Add the tarragon, tamari, vinegar, and cayenne, and simmer, stirring constantly, until the soup thickens (if it becomes too thick, add some water). Garnish with the scallions and parsley and serve.

RICE TOPPED WITH SAUTÉED VEGETABLES

This is the outline for a "do-as-you-please" recipe . . .

YIELD: 4 SERVINGS

2 cups water

1 cup uncooked brown rice

Salt to taste

2 tablespoons olive oil

4 cups mixed vegetables (as many different colors as you like)

Soy sauce or Tahini Sauce (recipe above) to taste (optional)

Bring the water to a boil, add the rice and salt, stir briefly, cover lightly, reduce heat, and let simmer until the rice is done and the water is gone (about 45 minutes). During the last 20 minutes of the rice's cooking time, heat the oil in a skillet, add the vegetables, sauté until they are tender but still crunchy, cover, and let them steam until they are a little more done. Season with soy sauce or Tahini Sauce as desired, spoon the vegetables over the rice, and serve.

ROASTED GARLIC AND BAKED ONION

Roasted garlic is one of life's great culinary treats—and don't forget the sweet and delicious onion! You can use this simple recipe often as a wonderful side dish.

YIELD: 2–4 SERVINGS

1 large Vidalia or other white onion, with top cut off
Olive oil as needed
1 bulb garlic, separated into cloves and peeled

Place the onion, root-side down, in a baking dish, sprinkle with a little oil, and bake at 375°F (about 40 minutes). Push the onion a little to the side in the dish, add the garlic, sprinkle with a little oil, and continue baking until both vegetables are soft and done (about 20–25 minutes). Remove and serve immediately.

GARDENER'S PIE

This delicious version of shepherd's pie isn't from the animal kingdom. I've suggested my favorite vegetables, but you and your family may prefer to use others—just be sure to include root vegetables, as they are so good for the liver; and according to Oriental philosophy, shiitake mushrooms are an anti-aging food.

YIELD: 6 SERVINGS

1 large rutabaga, peeled and diced
1 small-to-medium butternut squash, peeled and diced
2 tablespoons olive oil
Sprinkle of fresh herbs to taste
1 large red bell pepper, diced
1 large yellow bell pepper, diced
1 large onion, peeled and diced
4–6 large cloves garlic, chopped
3–4 cups mashed potatoes, seasoned to taste
1–1 1/2 cups soy milk or almond milk
Salt and pepper to taste
8–10 Brussels sprouts, quartered
1 package (2 ounces or so) shiitake mushrooms, cleaned and diced
1 tomato, sliced

Preheat oven to 375°F. Place the rutabaga and squash on a baking sheet, drizzle with 1 tablespoon of the oil and sprinkle with the herbs, and bake until slightly browned and tender (about 20–25 minutes). Meanwhile, place the peppers, onions, and garlic on a separate baking sheet and bake until slightly browned and tender (about 20–25 minutes). Prepare the mashed potatoes, using the soy or almond milk and salt and pepper, and set aside. In a skillet, brown the Brussels sprouts in the second tablespoon of oil until done.

To assemble the pie, strew the pepper mixture over the bottom of a casserole dish, sprinkle with the mushrooms, arrange the rutabaga and squash over the mushrooms, spread the Brussels sprouts over that, spread the mashed potatoes over the top, then place the tomato slices on the potatoes. Bake at 375°F for about 25 minutes and serve. (You may wish to brown the topping under the broiler for a few minutes, but be careful not to dry out the potatoes.)

SOUP OF MANY BEANS

Adapted from *Boutique Bean Pot* by Kathleen Mayes and Sandra Gottfried (Santa Barbara, CA: Woodbridge Press, 1992).

YIELD: 6–8 SERVINGS

1/4 pound dried white kidney beans,
soaked overnight and rinsed
1/2 pound dried fava beans,
soaked overnight and rinsed
1/4 pound dried garbanzo beans (chick peas),
soaked overnight and rinsed
1/4 pound dried lentils, any color
1/4 pound dried split yellow peas
9–10 cups water
1 5-ounce can water chestnuts, drained and sliced
3 stalks celery, chopped
1 medium onion, diced
1 medium carrot, peeled and chopped
6 sun-dried tomatoes, chopped small
2 cloves garlic, mashed
3 teaspoons ground fennel seed
Salt and freshly ground black pepper to taste

Drain and rinse the legumes, put them in a soup pot with the water, bring to a boil, and simmer until tender (about 3 hours). Halfway through cooking (1 1/2 hours), add the water chestnuts, celery, onion, carrot, tomatoes, garlic, and fennel seed. When cooked, season with salt and pepper as desired and serve.

BAKED WINTER SQUASH

How easy is this?

YIELD: 2–4 SERVINGS

1 winter squash, such as butternut or acorn

A sprinkle of olive oil

Freshly ground black pepper to taste

Cut open the squash, remove the seeds, coat lightly with a little oil, and bake at 375°F until soft (about 1 hour). Serve with a little black pepper.

AVOCADO WITH OLIVE OIL DRESSING

This one doesn't really need a recipe . . .

Cut a ripe avocado in half, remove the pit, peel gently, sprinkle with your favorite olive oil and vinegar dressing, and enjoy immediately.

WEEK II-7

This is the healing week after your cleanse! Focus on restoring your body's pH and getting your intestinal tract back to vibrant health. Return to modeling your daily menus on the core Wings menus while you follow the rest of the healing protocol in Lesson II-7. This protocol includes the four recipes below, adapted from an excellent book that I highly recommend, *Nourishing Traditions* by Sally Fallon (San Diego, CA: ProMotion Publishing, 1995).

BIELER BROTH

Maverick physician Henry Bieler recommended this broth for fasting, energy, and overall health. He felt this combination of vegetables was ideal for restoring acid/alkaline and sodium potassium balance to organs and glands (especially the sodium-loving adrenals). Bieler broth is highly recommended for people under stress or suffering from stress-related conditions.

YIELD: 4–6 SERVINGS

4 medium summer squash, washed and sliced, ends removed

1 pound wax beans, ends removed

2 stalks celery, chopped

2 bunches parsley, stems removed

Fresh herbs such as thyme or tarragon, tied together with a string (optional)

1 quart filtered (clean) water (not tap water)

Place all ingredients in a pot, bring to a boil, skim, reduce heat, cover, and simmer for about $1/2$ hour. Remove the bundle of herbs. Purée the soup in a blender to a thick consistency.

VEGETABLE JUICE COCKTAIL

Alkalinizing vegetable juice is good for correcting an acidic condition of the blood.

YIELD: 2–4 SERVINGS

1 green pepper

2 carrots, peeled

2 stalks celery

1 bunch parsley

$1/2$ zucchini or yellow squash

Handful string beans

Run all vegetables through a juicer, and thin the beverage with a little filtered (clean) water if desired.

BEET KVASS

This medicinal drink is an excellent blood tonic; it promotes regularity, aids digestion, alkalizes the blood, cleanses the liver, and, according to author Sally Fallon, is a good treatment for kidney stones and other ailments. (Whey is extremely hard to find, so check with your local health food store. Do not confuse whey and whey proteins, which are different altogether. If you cannot find whey, leave it out.)

YIELD: 1–2 SERVINGS

3 small or 2 medium organic beets, peeled and chopped coarsely

2 tablespoons whey

1 teaspoon sea salt

Filtered water as needed

Place the beets, whey, and salt in a 2-quart jug, and add enough filtered water to fill the container. Stir well, cover securely, and keep at room temperature for 2 days before refrigerating. Drink $1/2$ cup of the broth once or twice per day, as desired. When most of the liquid has been drunk, you may fill the container with water and keep at room temperature another 2 days (the second brew will not be as strong).

Note: Sally Fallon warns not to grate the beets in the preparation, as they will exude too much juice, resulting in rapid fermentation that favors the production of alcohol rather than lactic acid. (One doesn't want to get drunk on one's tonic!)

BARLEY JUICE

Barley is very healing to the intestinal lining.

YIELD: 1–2 SERVINGS

4 tablespoons pearl barley (dried)

Water

Wash the barley, cover with cold water in a saucepan, heat to boiling, and strain. Place the barley and 1 quart of water in top of a double boiler, simmer for 2 hours, and strain the mixture. Drink the barley juice warm or cold.

WEEK II-8

I hope you feel wonderful after your cleansing and healing weeks! Here are some high-fiber recipes to keep your intestinal tract scrubbed clean.

GRANOLA WITH FRUIT AND NUTS

If you are completely intolerant of grains, you can't use this recipe, but most people can handle eating this granola for breakfast once a week. One serving provides about 537 calories, more than 5 grams (g) of fiber, more than 15 g of protein, 43 g of carbohydrate, 34 g of fat, and an excellent balance of vitamins and minerals.

YIELD: 6–8 SERVINGS

4 cups rolled oats

2 cups oat bran

1 cup raw sesame seeds

2 cups raw sunflower seeds

1 cup unsweetened coconut flakes

1 cup chopped almonds

1 cup chopped walnuts

1/3 cup olive oil

1/4 cup honey

1 cup raisins

1 cup diced dried apricots

1 cup diced dried papaya or figs

In a large roasting pan, mix the oats, oat bran, seeds, coconut, and nuts. Over a low flame, heat the oil and honey until very thin and easily poured, then drizzle it over the dry ingredients, mixing constantly, until evenly coated. Bake at 325°F, stirring thoroughly every 15 minutes or so, until lightly browned (about 45–60 minutes). When the granola cools slightly, stir the fruit in thoroughly. Once it cools completely, refrigerate in food-storage bags or plastic containers.

ORIENTAL ASPARAGUS

Remember canned asparagus? This delicious dish is nothing like that! Very simple and flavorful, it makes an excellent accompaniment to a seafood meal.

YIELD: 4 SERVINGS

1 1/2 pounds fresh asparagus

1 tablespoon light soy sauce

1 teaspoon sesame oil

2 drops red hot chili oil (optional)

1/2 teaspoon toasted sesame seeds for garnish

Trim the hard ends off the asparagus and slice the stalks diagonally into 1-inch pieces. Bring a medium pot of water to a boil over high heat and cook the asparagus until tender-crisp and bright green (about 1 1/2–2 minutes)—do not overcook. Drain, plunge it immediately into a bowl of ice water, and set aside to cool (2–3 minutes). In a medium bowl, whisk together the soy sauce, sesame oil, and chili oil, add the asparagus, and toss. Garnish with the sesame seeds and serve.

SAUTÉED SHRIMP WITH SNOW PEAS

One of my kids' favorite dishes, and so easily prepared that it's one of my favorites, too. Serve with steamed rice. Adapted from *Secrets of Fat-Free Chinese Cooking* by my friend Ying Compestine (Garden City Park, NY: Avery Publishing Group, 1998).

YIELD: 5 SERVINGS

1 pound raw shrimp, peeled and deveined

1 tablespoon cooking wine

1 teaspoon lemon juice

1/4 teaspoon Mrs. Dash seasoning (available in health food stores and supermarkets)

2 teaspoons cornstarch

2 cups fresh snow peas

1 scallion, chopped

1 tablespoon minced fresh ginger

2 teaspoons soy sauce

$\frac{1}{4}$ teaspoon sesame oil

Rinse the shrimp with cold water and pat dry. In a bowl, combine the wine, lemon juice, Mrs. Dash, and cornstarch, add the shrimp, and marinate in the refrigerator for 30 minutes. Lightly coat a nonstick wok or frying pan with cooking spray (or 1 teaspoon olive oil) and place over medium heat. Reserving the marinade, sauté the shrimp until just pink (about 2–3 minutes), then transfer to a bowl. Add the snow peas, scallion, and ginger to the wok or pan, stir-fry for 1–2 minutes, add the reserved marinade, soy sauce, and cooked shrimp, mix well, and cook until most of the sauce is absorbed (about 1–2 minutes). Transfer to a serving bowl, sprinkle with the sesame oil, and serve hot.

WEEK II-9

We have more Chinese cooking this week, and you will *love* these easy vegetable recipes.

DRY-COOKED GREEN BEANS IN SZECHUAN SAUCE

Excellent as a side dish to the Sautéed Shrimp with Snow Peas—lots of vegetables! Adapted from *Secrets of Fat-Free Chinese Cooking.*

YIELD: 4 SERVINGS

3 cups green beans, tips removed

$\frac{1}{4}$ cup water

1$\frac{1}{2}$ teaspoons soy sauce

1$\frac{1}{2}$ teaspoons chili paste

$\frac{1}{2}$ teaspoon sugar

2 teaspoons minced fresh garlic

1 teaspoon canola or other oil

1 teaspoon Eden Foods Sesame Shake
(available at health food stores or supermarkets)
or chopped sesame seeds

2 scallions, minced, for garnish

If the green beans are long, break them into 3-inch pieces. In a small bowl, mix together the water, soy sauce, chili paste, and sugar, and set aside. Lightly coat a nonstick wok or frying pan with cooking spray and sauté the garlic on medium-low heat until it begins to brown (about 1–2 minutes). Increase heat to medium, add the canola oil and green beans, and stir-fry until wrinkled (about

10–12 minutes). Mix the Sesame Shake or seeds in thoroughly, add the bowl of sauce, reduce heat to medium-low, and stir frequently to prevent burning. Allow the dish to cook down (about 4 minutes), remove from heat, garnish with the scallions, and serve.

TOFU AND SPINACH MISO SOUP

A meal that is "light to the touch," this delicate broth features flecks of green spinach and cubes of soft tofu (if your family says they don't like tofu, call it soy cheese). Adapted from Ying Compestine's book, *Cooking with Green Tea* (Garden City Park, NY: Avery Publishing Group, 1999). Green tea is an excellent antioxidant and helps speed metabolism!

YIELD: 4 SERVINGS

2 cups brewed green tea (see below)

2 cups vegetable stock

4 slices ginger root, each the size of a quarter

1 12-ounce package firm silken tofu
(cut tofu into $\frac{1}{4}$-inch cubes)

2 tablespoons miso

2 cups packed spinach leaves, large stems removed

2 teaspoons sesame oil

$\frac{1}{4}$ cup chopped scallions

Soy sauce to taste

In a large saucepan, bring the green tea, stock, and ginger to a boil, add the tofu, return to a boil, reduce heat, cover, and simmer until tofu is heated through (about 2–3 minutes). In a bowl, combine the miso with about $\frac{1}{2}$ cup of broth from the pan and stir into a smooth, thin paste, then pour the paste back into the soup. Add the spinach, return to a boil, stir in the sesame oil, and remove from heat. Ladle into bowls, garnish with the scallions and another drop or two of sesame oil, and serve hot. Soy sauce may be passed at the table if desired.

Brewed Green Tea

For the best flavor and the most infusion, brew green tea at 160–170°F, when the water first begins to stir (it's restless but not simmering). It is better to steep green tea at this lower temperature for a little longer than to force the leaves to give up their essence at higher temperatures, which ends up making a bitter brew. According to research, all the health benefits of green tea are yielded by 3–4 minutes of brewing time.

WEEK II-10

You can purchase beef and chicken broth from your grocery store, but in some parts of the country, it is difficult to find a good broth that doesn't contain MSG or huge amounts of salt. So this week and next, you are "going to cooking school" to learn the art of making some more broths and sauces. Although it is not difficult, it takes a lot of time, so I enjoy making broth while I'm doing something else; after the initial preparation, it simmers on the back burner of the stove, sending a beautiful essence throughout the house.

Homemade broth is not as strong as commercial broth, unless you reduce it substantially when cooking. Use your own taste to govern how rich you make your broth. It can then be used as base for gravies or soups. Pour into freezer containers and mark the date on the container; it will keep frozen for 2–3 weeks or more without losing taste.

RICH BROWN CHICKEN BROTH

Adapted from my book *The Crazy Makers: How the Food Industry Is Destroying Our Minds and Harming Our Children* (New York, NY: Jeremy P. Tarcher/Penguin, 2000).

YIELD: APPROXIMATELY 2 QUARTS

A splash of olive oil

1 medium-sized stewing hen

1 cup chopped onions

1 cup chopped celery

1 cup chopped carrots

8–10 cloves garlic, chopped

3–4 small bay leaves

1 teaspoon dried basil; or, 1 large stalk fresh basil

1 teaspoon dried thyme; or, 3 teaspoons fresh thyme

Any other seasonings you may enjoy

3 quarts hot water

Heat the oil in a large, heavy soup pot. Remove the giblets from the chicken (set aside for another use), cut the hen into manageable pieces, and sauté in the oil on medium heat, making sure the pieces don't burn, and removing them when they are nicely browned on both sides. Add the vegetables to the same oil, stir until lightly browned, add the chicken, herbs, and any other seasoning, and gently stir in the hot water. Bring the broth to a boil, turn heat down so it barely simmers, cover loosely (to let a little of the steam evaporate), and let it cook for 3–4 hours or until it is the desired strength. Remove foam as it floats to the top, remove the chicken pieces for use in another recipe when finished cooking, and strain the broth, pressing the juice out of the vegetables. Defat the broth and refrigerate.

HOMEMADE BEEF BROTH

Adapted from *The Way to Cook* by Julia Child (New York, NY: Knopf, 1989).

YIELD: APPROXIMATELY 3–4 QUARTS

3–4 pounds meaty raw beef bones, in small pieces

2 each: large carrots, onions, and celery stalks, chopped

6 quarts cold water

1 tablespoon dried basil; or, 2 tablespoons fresh basil

1 tablespoon dried parsley; or, 2 tablespoons fresh parsley

1 tablespoon dried oregano; or, 2 tablespoons fresh oregano

2 large cloves unpeeled garlic, smashed

Salt and pepper to taste

1 large unpeeled tomato, cored and roughly chopped; or, 1/3 cup chopped canned tomatoes

Preheat oven to 450°F. In a roasting pan, arrange the bones and 1/2 cup each of the chopped vegetables and brown in the upper third of the oven, turning and basting with accumulated fat several times until they are a good walnut-brown color (about 15–20 minutes). Pour out and discard fat, and scoop bones and vegetables into a large soup pot. Pour 2 cups of the water into the roasting pan, bring to a boil over moderately high heat, scrape the browning juices into the liquid with a wooden spoon, then pour the liquid over the browned bones in the soup pot. Add the herbs, the rest of the vegetables, garlic, and tomato, with enough water to cover by 2 inches, and bring to a simmer. Skim off and discard the gray scum that will collect on the surface for several minutes. Cover loosely and maintain at a slow simmer, skimming off fat and scum occasionally, and adding a little boiling water if the liquid evaporates below the surface of the ingredients. Simmer until you feel the bones have given their all. Strain the stock through a colander into a large bowl, pressing juices out of the vegetables. Degrease the stock, season lightly to taste, and strain again, this time through a fine-mesh sieve into a clean pan or container. The broth can be kept covered in the refrigerator for 2 days, or frozen for 2 weeks.

WEEK II-11

You are continuing cooking school this week, with more of my favorite sauces.

BEEF WINE SAUCE

This rich, versatile sauce (one of my children eats it like soup) is fabulous with grilled or broiled steaks or with pork or beef roasts; substitute chicken broth for beef broth, and it's great with grilled chicken or turkey. Using Madeira in the final step makes the sauce very rich (you may prefer it without). Adapted from Julia Child's *The Way to Cook.*

YIELD: APPROXIMATELY 2 CUPS OF FRAGRANT,
BEAUTIFULLY FLAVORED BROWN LIQUID

2 tablespoons olive oil

3 tablespoons each finely chopped onion and celery

2 tablespoons chopped carrot

1 small clove garlic, chopped

1 bay leaf

1 pinch dried thyme; or,
2 teaspoons fresh thyme

8 fresh stems parsley; or,
1 teaspoon dried parsley

1 allspice berry

$1/3$ cup dry white French vermouth or white wine

3 cups beef stock and/or chicken stock

1 small ripe tomato, chopped;
or, 1 teaspoon tomato paste

$1 1/2$ tablespoons cornstarch, blended with $1/4$ cup dry
Madeira or port wine; or, blended with a few
tablespoons of the broth

In a small, heavy-bottomed saucepan, heat the oil and sauté the onion, celery, carrot, and garlic over moderately low heat until tender (about 7–8 minutes), then increase heat slightly and brown lightly, stirring, for several minutes. Stir in the herbs, white wine, stock, and tomato, cover loosely, and simmer 1 hour. Correct seasoning and strain into a clean pan, pressing juices out of the vegetables with a spoon. Skim off surface fat. When ready to serve, beat $1/2$ cup of the broth into the cornstarch-wine or cornstarch-broth mixture, pour back into the base, and bring to a slow simmer for 2 minutes. The sauce should be lightly thickened; if too thick, stir in dribbles of additional stock.

Variation: For really rich gravy over a beef, lamb, or pork roast, deglaze the saucepan with the broth and add the glaze to the sauce.

MADEIRA WINE SAUCE WITH PRUNES

No, this is not a strange recipe—it is absolutely wonderful with any roast beef or pork! My kids always ask for extra prunes; substitute other fruits, if you wish, for a delicious variation.

YIELD: APPROXIMATELY 2 CUPS

The entire quantity of Beef Wine Sauce (recipe above)

1 cup whole, pitted prunes

When the Beef Wine sauce is finished, stir the prunes into the warm sauce and heat thoroughly (about 10–15 minutes). Pour over roast and serve immediately.

WEEK II-12

This week's recipe for Chicken Pot Pie takes a *lot* of time, but the results are well worth the extra trouble; fortunately, it makes a lot of pie and is easily frozen for several subsequent meals. And in keeping with our cooking-school theme, you will learn to make a white stock, velouté sauce, and pastry-crust topping that can be used in other recipes. Use your imagination! If you are allergic to even small amounts of wheat, I've provided an alternative wheat-free crust recipe that will work beautifully also, or you can simply cover the pie with a thin layer of mashed potatoes (sweet potato mash would be terrific).

WHITE STOCK

This easily prepared, lightly colored and flavored chicken broth is excellent in the Velouté Sauce recipe that follows, or as a base for other gravies or soups. For variety or convenience, you can substitute any vegetables you desire or have on hand. Adapted from *Cuisine* magazine.

YIELD: APPROXIMATELY 2 QUARTS

3 pounds chicken wings or other chicken parts

4 carrots, peeled and chopped

2 parsnips, peeled and chopped

2 onions, peeled and chopped

2 leeks, cleaned and chopped

2 whole cloves garlic, peeled

3 quarts water

8 sprigs fresh thyme

6 sprigs fresh parsley

3 bay leaves

1 teaspoon whole black peppercorns

Place the chicken pieces in an 8-quart stockpot, add the chopped vegetables and the garlic, and add water to cover. Bring to a simmer over high heat, reduce heat to medium, and simmer the stock (don't let it boil) for 2 hours, skimming off any foam that rises to the top. After 2 hours, add the herbs and peppercorns, and simmer for 1 hour more. Pour finished stock through a fine-mesh strainer (don't press the solids to release more liquid, as it will make the stock cloudy). Refrigerate until cold, preferably overnight, and skim off the layer of fat that solidifies on top.

VELOUTÉ SAUCE

An excellent base for soups, pot pies, or gravies, and used in the Chicken Pot Pie recipe that follows. I suggest preparing this sauce ahead of time while something else is cooking. Adapted from *Cuisine* magazine.

YIELD: APPROXIMATELY 8 CUPS

1/4 cup unsalted butter or olive oil

1/2 cup peeled, diced carrots

1/2 cup diced celery

2 tablespoons peeled, minced shallots or onion

1/2 cup dry white wine

6 cups White Stock (recipe above) or chicken broth

6 sprigs fresh thyme

4 sprigs fresh parsley

2 bay leaves

2 teaspoons whole black peppercorns

Roux

6 tablespoons unsalted butter

1/2 cup all-purpose gluten-free flour
(Bob's Red Mill makes a great gluten-free flour)

Salt and pepper to taste

1. Melt the butter (or heat the oil) in a large saucepan over medium heat and sauté vegetables until soft (about 8 minutes). Deglaze the pan with the wine, reduce until liquid is almost gone (about 8–10 minutes), add the White Stock or broth, herbs, and peppercorns, and simmer uncovered for 1 hour.

2. To make the roux, melt the butter in a small pan over medium heat, whisk in the flour, cook and stir until thickened and very light brown (about 2–3 minutes), and remove from heat.

3. Strain the simmered stock (from step 1) into a clean pan, return to a simmer, whisk in the hot roux, and continue to whisk until the velouté coats the back of a spoon (about 2–3 minutes). Simmer 10 more minutes and season with salt and pepper as desired.

CHICKEN POT PIE

I'll make no apologies: this takes a lot of time to prepare and makes a *big* mess in the kitchen—but it has become such a favorite of my children that they beg me to make it, even if they have to help clean up. You will get several meals from this recipe, and that saves time, doesn't it? Choose any vegetables you like for the filling; I use whatever is seasonal and suits my mood, and I love changing the taste each time.
Adapted from *Cuisine* magazine.

YIELD: 12–14 SERVINGS

Crust

4 cups all-purpose gluten-free flour (The Gluten-Free Pantry, www.glutenfree.com, makes an excellent gluten-free pastry mix that would also be suitable)

2 teaspoons minced, each: fresh parsley, thyme, and rosemary

1 teaspoon salt

1 teaspoon black pepper

1 1/2 cups cold unsalted butter, in cubes

8–12 tablespoons ice water

Filling

1 5–7 pound whole roasting chicken, rinsed and trimmed of excess fat

2 cups 1-inch cubes peeled butternut squash (approximately 1 small squash)

2 cups 1-inch cubes peeled parsnips (approximately 2–3 parsnips)

2 cups quartered, unpeeled red potatoes (approximately 5–6 potatoes)

8 ounces shiitake mushrooms, stemmed

1 package fresh peeled pearl onions; or, 1 large white onion, cut into large chunks

1 package fresh asparagus or green beans (cut vegetables into 1-inch pieces)

1/4 cup olive oil

2 teaspoons salt (preferably kosher salt)

1 teaspoon black pepper

4 cups Velouté Sauce (recipe above)

1 tablespoon chopped fresh flat-leaf parsley

1 tablespoon chopped fresh thyme

1. To prepare the crust, combine the flour, herbs, salt, and pepper in a food processor and pulse a few times to mix, add the butter, and pulse processor 10–12 times, until the mixture looks like coarse cornmeal. Add 6–8 tablespoons of the ice water and pulse until the dough clumps. To test, press a little bit of dough together: if it is too crumbly, add 2–3 tablespoons more water, 1 tablespoon at a time, until it is the right texture and holds together. Wrap dough in plastic, flatten into a disk, wrap in plastic, and chill for ½ hour.

2. To prepare the filling, preheat oven to 425°F, place the chicken breast-side up on a roasting pan and roast, uncovered, for 45–55 minutes. Meanwhile, toss the vegetables with the olive oil, sprinkle with the salt and pepper, spread on two baking sheets, and roast at 425°F for 15–20 minutes (stir after 10 minutes to prevent sticking to the pan), then remove from oven. When chicken is done, remove the skin and meat from the bones and tear into bite-sized pieces (any uncooked meat will finish cooking in the pies). In a large mixing bowl, combine the chicken and vegetables, and stir in the Velouté Sauce and herbs.

3. To finish the pies, preheat oven to 400°F. Divide the dough in half, refrigerate half, and roll other half to ¼-inch thickness on a floured surface. Using an empty pie pan as a guide, cut out rounds of dough 1 inch larger than pan all the way around. Fill pie pans with the chicken-vegetable mixture, place a dough round over each without stretching it, turn the edge under around the pie, and crimp the edges. Place the pans on a baking dish and bake until crust is golden and filling is bubbly (about 25–30 minutes)—some may leak. Cool 5–10 minutes before serving.

ALTERNATIVE POTATO-SPELT PIE CRUST

This wheat-free recipe makes a 9- or 10-inch crust that is easy to roll out, tender, and delicious.

YIELD: 1 PIE CRUST

1 cup unseasoned mashed potatoes,
at room temperature

¼ cup oil (preferably olive oil)

1 cup spelt flour (available at natural food stores)

2 teaspoons minced, each: fresh parsley,
thyme, and rosemary

1 teaspoon nonaluminum baking powder

¼ teaspoon sea salt

1 tablespoon ice water (or more, if needed)

Using a whisk or fork, whip together the mashed potatoes and oil. Mix together the flour, herbs, baking powder, and salt, add to the potato mixture, and blend using a fork or your hands—do not overwork the dough. If it is too dry to hold together, gradually add a little ice water until it is moist enough (you may not need to do this if the mashed potatoes are fairly moist already). Sprinkle a counter or tabletop with a few drops of water to keep a piece of waxed paper secure, sprinkle the dough with flour to keep the rolling pin from sticking, roll out the dough onto the paper, cover with another piece of waxed paper, roll it out further, and follow the sizing instructions in the Chicken Pot Pie recipe above. Pick up dough by edges of paper, place dough (paper-side up) over filled pie pan, crimp crust edges, and bake as in the recipe above.

WEEK II-13

This delicious Mexican recipe will make your taste buds sparkle with delight.

ENCHILADAS DE POLLO Y QUESO

My family loves this dish, served with a salad. If you need to substitute soy yogurt for the sour cream and almond cheese for the Monterey Jack, you'll find little difference in taste and texture.

YIELD: 6 SERVINGS

1 cup chopped onion

½ cup chopped green bell pepper

5 tablespoons butter

2 cups chopped cooked chicken or turkey

1 4-ounce can green chili peppers
(rinsed, seeded, and chopped)

¼ cup oat flour

1 teaspoon ground coriander seed

¾ teaspoon salt (optional)

2 ½ cups chicken broth

1 cup dairy sour cream or soy yogurt

1 ½ cups shredded Monterey Jack or nondairy cheese

12 6-inch corn tortillas

In large saucepan, cook the onion and green pepper in 2 tablespoons of the butter until tender, combine in a bowl with the chopped chicken or turkey and chili peppers, and set aside. In the same saucepan, melt the remaining 3 tablespoons of butter, blend in the flour, coriander, and salt, stir in the broth all at once, and cook, stirring, until thickened and bubbly. Remove from heat, stir in the sour cream or yogurt and ¹/₂ cup of the cheese, and then stir ¹/₂ cup of the sauce into the chicken mixture. Dip each tortilla into the remaining warm sauce to soften it, fill each with about ¹/₄ cup of the chicken mixture, roll up, and arrange in a 13x9x2-inch baking dish. Pour the remaining sauce over the dish, sprinkle with the remaining cheese, bake uncovered at 350°F until bubbly (about 25 minutes), and serve.

MODULE III

I hope you are excited about the new territory you will be entering. Don't forget about your food plan while you explore this module's medical information. Food is an important healer! Are you staying on track? Remember to balance your proteins, carbohydrates, and fats at each meal. Begin each day with the Wings Breakfast Drink to balance your blood sugar and energy level.

WEEK III-1

Week III-1 is actually two weeks for one lesson: Lesson III-1 instructs you to repeat the cleansing and healing weeks before you go on to Lesson III-2 and Week III-2's recipes. See page 261 for the cleansing week and page 265 for the healing week.

WEEK III-2

Sometimes you just want a piece of bread like everyone else. When you're allergic to wheat, however, it is hard to get a piece of bread that won't kick off your allergies and make you gain water or fat weight. Thanks to the generosity of Pat Cassady Redjou's son, the following three recipes for biscuits, scones, and bread are adapted from her book, *The No-Gluten Solution: The Cooking Guide for People Who Are Sick and Tired of Being Sick and Tired* (unfortunately, it is out of print). Unusual baking ingredients can be purchased at natural food stores.

POTATO-FLOUR BISCUITS

A simple, satisfying substitution for "regular" biscuits.

YIELD: 6 BISCUITS

1 egg, well beaten
¹/₃ cup polyunsaturated oil

1 ¹/₂ cups potato-starch flour
¹/₂ teaspoon salt

Combine all ingredients and mix well, pat out dough on a floured board, cut into biscuit shapes, bake at 350°F for 12–15 minutes, and serve immediately. Store in an airtight container.

SCONES

Scones, the British version of biscuits, are best served hot with butter and a little fruit-only jam.

YIELD: 6 SCONES

3 tablespoons cornmeal
3 tablespoons soy flour
2 tablespoons potato flour
¹/₈ teaspoon salt
1 tablespoon brown sugar
1 teaspoon dry pectin
1 teaspoon nonaluminum baking powder
2 ¹/₂ tablespoons butter
3 tablespoons plus 1 teaspoon cold water

In a bowl, combine the cornmeal, flours, salt, sugar, pectin, and baking powder. Cut the butter finely into this mixture, then mix in the cold water. Knead the dough into a ball, divide into 6 portions, pat to flatten, brush each with a dab of butter, bake at 350°F for 15–18 minutes, and serve immediately.

WEEK III-3

Keep in mind that this week's recipes are for occasional treats! Stick with the Wings Breakfast Drink and then give yourself a "goodie" on Sunday morning. Keep balancing your proteins, carbohydrates, and fats, just like you did in the first four weeks of the Wings Program.

COTTAGE-CHEESE BREAD

If you can tolerate some dairy, this bread satisfies the occasional hankering for a morning piece of toast.

YIELD: 3 SMALL LOAVES

1 cup milk
2 tablespoons yeast
¹/₂ cup warm water
2¹/₄ cups brown rice flour

1 1/2 cups potato-starch flour

2/3 cup powdered milk; or, 2/3 cup soy flour

2 teaspoons nonaluminum baking powder

2 teaspoons sugar

2/3 cup cottage cheese

2 tablespoons safflower oil

2 eggs

Scald the milk and cool it to lukewarm. Dissolve the yeast in the warm water and let it froth until doubled. In a bowl, combine the flours, powdered milk, baking powder, and sugar. Stir in the cottage cheese, oil, and eggs. Add the warm milk and the yeast mixture to the bowl, beat with a mixer at high speed for 4 minutes, pour into 3 small greased bread pans, and let rise 30–45 minutes. Bake 10 minutes at 400°F, lower temperature to 325°F, and bake another 20 minutes.

WHEAT-FREE GRANOLA BARS

Delicious and fun for breakfast "on the run."

YIELD: 12 BARS

1 cup homemade granola (recipe page 266)

1 cup quick-cooking rolled oats
(those from a health food store have better texture)

1 cup chopped walnuts or sunflower seeds

1 tablespoon sesame seeds

1/2 cup less 1 teaspoon spelt flour

1/2 cup raisins

1 egg, beaten

1/3 cup honey or maple syrup

1/3 cup cooking oil or butter

2 tablespoons brown sugar

1/2 teaspoon cinnamon

Line an 8x8-inch baking pan with waxed paper, grease the paper with butter, and set aside. In a mixing bowl, combine the dry ingredients except for the cinnamon. In a separate bowl, stir together the moist ingredients and the cinnamon. Mix the two combinations together thoroughly. You may need to use your fingers. Press the mixture evenly into the baking pan and bake at 325°F until lightly browned (about 30–35 minutes). Cool, lift the paper out of the pan to remove the contents, discard the paper, and cut the granola into bars.

Note: For easier handling, you can press the mixture into the lightly buttered cups of a muffin tin and bake.

Like last week's Wheat-Free Granola Bars, this week's Breakfast Brownies are fairly high in carbohydrates, so if you feel better with more protein in your morning meal, add some eggs or other protein food to balance the carbs.

BREAKFAST BROWNIES

Only for mornings when you feel particularly festive—and a little decadent. These are, however, wheat- and dairy-free.

YIELD: 16 BARS

2 eggs, beaten

1/4 cup maple syrup or honey

1/4 cup soy milk

1/4 cup carob powder

1/4 cup spelt flour

1/4 cup oat bran

2 tablespoons soy flour

1 tablespoon nonaluminum baking powder

3/4 cup unhulled sesame seeds

1 cup chopped dates

1/2 cup raisins

1/2 cup sunflower seeds or chopped walnuts

Beat together the eggs, syrup or honey, and soy milk until smooth and creamy. In a separate bowl, combine the dry ingredients and the sesame seeds, then add to the moist mixture, stir until well blended, and fold in the fruits and nuts. Pour the batter into an 8x8-inch baking pan. Bake at 325°F for about 30 minutes, let cool slightly, and cut into bars.

MINESTRONE SOUP

Delicious and chock full of vegetables—a bowl of this soup is a meal by itself. Adapted from *Cuisine* magazine.

YIELD: 8 SERVINGS

1 cup dried cranberry beans (or kidney, cannelloni, pinto, or any medium-sized bean)

1/2 teaspoon salt

2 ounces diced pancetta or bacon

2 tablespoons olive oil

1 cup chopped yellow onion

1 tablespoon minced garlic

3 cups chopped cabbage

2 cups trimmed green beans

1 cup diced celery

1 cup sliced carrots

1 cup diced fennel

1 cup diced zucchini

1 cup peeled, diced russet potatoes

4–5 cups beef broth

1 14-1/2-ounce can diced tomatoes

1/4 cup dry red wine

1 2-ounce Parmesan rind

2 tablespoons Italian seasoning

2 cups chopped red Swiss chard (stalks removed)

In a small pot, combine the cranberry beans and salt, add water to 2 inches above, cover, bring to a boil, turn off heat, and allow to sit 30 minutes (the beans will finish cooking in the soup). In a large pot, sauté the pancetta in the oil (pancetta is not as greasy as bacon and will stick to the pot otherwise) over medium-high heat until crisp (about 10 minutes). Add the onion and garlic to the pot and cook 2 minutes. Add the cabbage, sauté a little, add the green beans, sauté a little, and continue with the celery, carrots, fennel, zucchini, and potatoes in this way, sautéing each a little before adding the next. They will begin steaming and the juices will begin flowing. Once all the vegetables have been added, let them steam about 10 minutes. Add 4 cups of the broth, the diced tomatoes, and the wine, stir well, then add the cranberry beans, Parmesan rind, and Italian seasoning. Simmer over medium heat for 1½ hours, stirring occasionally until the vegetables and beans are soft; if necessary, add the remaining 1 cup of broth. When the cranberry beans are soft, add the Swiss chard and stir until wilted. The soup will have reduced considerably at this point. Remove and discard any visible chunks of rind before serving.

WEEK III-5

Can you be trusted with more dessert recipes? Desserts are not to be eaten every day or as comfort food when you're depressed. Nor are they for stashing away and sneaking a bite of in the afternoon or evening when no one can see! Desserts are to be enjoyed once in a while (one evening per week?) at the end of a meal. These nutrition-rich recipes are low in sugar and grains, and they taste good too. You and your family will enjoy these special treats.

DEEP, DARK, DELICIOUS CHOCOLATE PUDDING

Very creamy and decadent, and no one will believe it is "diet food." Don't tell your kids it contains tofu, or they will not allow themselves to enjoy it! And be sure to use this exact kind of tofu, as others will make the pudding slightly bitter. Adapted from one of my favorite cookbooks, *Secrets of Cooking for Long Life* by Sandra Woodruff (Garden City Park, NY: Avery Publishing Group, 1998).

YIELD: 5 SERVINGS

2 12.3-ounce packages light silken extra-firm tofu

3/4 cup plus 2 tablespoons dark brown sugar

1/3 cup plus 1 tablespoon Dutch-processed cocoa powder

2 teaspoons vanilla extract

2 tablespoons coffee liqueur (optional)

Combine all ingredients in a food processor and process until smooth and creamy (about 3 minutes), scraping down the sides as needed. Divide the pudding among 5 serving dishes or wine glasses, cover with plastic wrap, and chill for at least 2 hours before serving.

Note: I also whip up some heavy cream with a tiny bit of sugar and 1/2 teaspoon of vanilla, and dob some on each portion—I know it is high in fat, but sometimes life should be rich, shouldn't it?

CAROL'S OATMEAL COOKIES

Wheat-free cookies can be a little more crumbly, but they taste great (you can also try Kamut or spelt flour instead of oat flour, for better handling).

YIELD: ABOUT 36 COOKIES

3/4 cup butter

1 1/4 cups oat flour

1 cup date sugar

1 egg

1 teaspoon nonaluminum baking powder

1 teaspoon vanilla

1/4 teaspoon baking soda

1/2 teaspoon cinnamon

1/4 teaspoon ground cloves

2 cups quick-cooking rolled oats (available at health food stores)

1/2 cup chopped walnuts or pecans

In a mixing bowl, beat the butter with a mixer on medium-to-high speed for 30 seconds, stir in about ¹/₂ of the flour and all of the sugar, egg, baking powder, vanilla, baking soda, cinnamon, and cloves, and beat until thoroughly combined. Beat in the remaining flour and stir in the oats and nuts. Drop by rounded teaspoons, 2 inches apart, onto an ungreased cookie sheet, bake at 375°F until edges are golden (about 10–12 minutes), and cool on a wire rack.

FRUITY OATMEAL BARS

These are a little crumbly too—thanks to the oat flour—but they taste buttery delicious.

YIELD: ABOUT 25 SMALL BARS

Crust

1 cup oat flour

1 cup quick-cooking rolled oats
(available at health food stores)

²/₃ cup date sugar

¹/₄ teaspoon baking soda

¹/₂ cup butter

Filling

2 medium apples, peeled, cored, and chopped

2 tablespoons sugar

2 tablespoons water

1 tablespoon lemon juice

¹/₂ teaspoon ground cinnamon

1. To make the crust, combine the flour, oats, date sugar, and baking soda in a mixing bowl, and cut in the butter until the mixture resembles coarse crumbs. Feel free to add a little more butter if it seems too dry and doesn't stick together. Reserve ¹/₂ cup of the mixture, and press the remaining mixture into the bottom of an ungreased 9x9x2-inch baking pan.

2. To make the filling, combine the apples, sugar, water, lemon juice, and cinnamon in a medium saucepan, bring to a boil, reduce heat, and simmer until tender (about 8–10 minutes).

3. To finish the cookies, spread the filling over the crust base in the baking pan, sprinkle the reserved crust mixture over the top, bake at 350°F until the top is golden (about 30–35 minutes), cool in the pan on a wire rack, and cut into bars.

Let's try some more main entrée recipes. Remember: if you are having trouble staying on the Wings food plan, go back to the first four weeks of Module I and follow those menus and recipes all over again. Repetition resets the concepts in your mind.

HONEY CHICKEN

Delicious served over steamed rice.

YIELD: 4 SERVINGS

¹/₂ cup honey

¹/₃ cup lemon juice

2 tablespoons butter

1¹/₂ tablespoons soy sauce

4 chicken breasts

A dash of spelt flour

Salt and pepper to taste

Combine the honey, lemon juice, butter, and soy sauce in a saucepan, bring just to a boil, and set aside. Toss the chicken breasts in just enough spelt flour to lightly coat, sprinkle with salt and pepper as desired, and place in a baking dish. Pour the sauce over the chicken and bake at 350°F for 30 minutes, turning once while cooking.

ALMOND CHICKEN

Another simple dish with lots of flavor and nutrition.

YIELD: 4 SERVINGS

1 cup slivered almonds

A splash of olive oil

1 bunch celery, trimmed and diced

1 green pepper, seeded and diced

1 medium or large onion, diced

1 cup chicken broth

1¹/₂ tablespoons light soy sauce

2 tablespoons cornstarch or arrowroot powder

4 chicken breasts, cooked and diced

Salt and pepper or soy sauce to taste

Toast the almonds at 350°F for 10 minutes and set aside. In a skillet, heat the oil and sauté the vegetables until the onions turn glassy. In a small dish, mix the broth, soy sauce, and cornstarch until there are no lumps. Add the diced chicken and sauce to the vegetables, stir until sauce thickens, add almonds, season as desired with salt and pepper or more soy sauce, and serve.

GRILLED RED SNAPPER

Red snapper is one of my favorite fish: mild and flaky, with just a hint of the ocean.

YIELD: 4 SERVINGS

4 red snapper filets (about 1 1/4 pounds)
3 tablespoons olive oil
1 tablespoon lemon juice
1 teaspoon dried thyme
2/3 cup red wine
1 tablespoon soy sauce
1 teaspoon honey
4 scallions, julienned (cut into long thin strips)

Rinse the fish, pat dry, and place in a deep dish. Combine the oil, lemon juice, and thyme, pour over the fish, and marinate at room temperature for 1–2 hours. In a saucepan, heat the wine, soy sauce, and honey for a few minutes, add the scallions, and cook for another 2 minutes. Brush the filets with oil so the fish don't stick, grill or broil them for 2 minutes, turn them over, and grill or broil the other side for 2 minutes. Place the filets on hot plates, top with a little of the wine sauce, and serve immediately with the rest of the sauce on the side.

WEEK III-7

Like the Triple-Batch Beef (page 257), the Mexican Meat Mix recipe below makes a large quantity to use in many delicious dishes. Keep some frozen to thaw for a quick meal on a busy evening.

MEXICAN MEAT MIX

The first step is cooking a 5-pound beef roast ahead of time, either overnight in a crock-pot (without adding salt or water) or for about 12 hours in a 200°F oven in a large roasting pan or Dutch oven covered with a tight lid (also without adding salt or water). Don't forget to reserve the juices from the roast . . .

YIELD: ABOUT 9 CUPS OF MEAT MIX

5 pounds beef roast
3 onions, chopped

1 4-ounce can chopped green chilies
3 tablespoons olive oil
2 7-ounce cans green chili salsa
1/4 teaspoon garlic powder
4 tablespoons white spelt flour
4 teaspoons salt
1 teaspoon cumin powder
Reserved juices from roast

Remove the bones from the roast, shred the meat, and set aside. In a large skillet, sauté the onions and green chilies in the oil for 1 minute, add the salsa, garlic powder, flour, salt, and cumin, cook over medium-low heat for 1 minute, stir in the reserved meat juices and shredded meat, and cook over medium-low heat until thick (about 5 minutes). When cooled, divide into thirds (about 3 cups each) and put into 1-quart freezer containers, leaving about 1/2-inch space at the top. Seal and label containers, freeze, and use within 6 months.

MEXICAN MEAT-MIX TACOS

All you have to do for this recipe is fill the tortillas as desired and enjoy.

YIELD: 8 SERVINGS

1 quart Mexican Meat Mix (recipe above), heated
Lettuce, shredded
Tomatoes, chopped
Scallions, chopped
Soy or almond cheese, shredded
8 corn tortillas, soft or fried crisp in olive oil

MEXICAN MEAT-MIX TOQUITOS

Delicious with Great Guacamole (page 248).

YIELD: AS MANY AS YOU WOULD LIKE

Olive oil
Corn tortillas
Mexican Meat Mix (recipe above)

In a deep frying pan, heat about 1 inch of oil to medium-high. Using tongs, dip the tortillas in the hot oil for a few seconds until soft, and drain on paper towels. Put a small amount of Mexican Meat Mix in a line down the center of each tortilla, roll it up, hold it with the tongs for a minute or so in the hot oil until crisp on the edges, then drain again on paper towels , and serve.

BRAISED LAMB SHANK SHEPHERD'S PIE

I adore this version of an old favorite . . . Preparing it involves a few steps, but the end result is an exquisite comfort food. Serve with a salad. Adapted from *Gourmet* magazine.

YIELD: 8 SERVINGS

5 1/2 pounds lamb shanks or lamb roast

2 tablespoons olive oil

Salt and pepper to taste

2 small onions, trimmed and quartered

1/2 cup fresh thyme sprigs

1/2 cup fresh rosemary sprigs

1/2 cup dry white wine

1 1/4 cups beef broth

1 1/2 cups water

3 pounds potatoes (preferably baking potatoes)

3/4 cup soy or other nondairy milk

5 medium carrots, sliced 1/4-inch thick

1 package fresh baby spinach

2 tablespoons cornstarch or potato starch

1 tablespoon butter, melted

1. To prepare the lamb, preheat oven to 450°F. Put the shanks or roast in a large metal roasting pan, rub with the oil, season with salt and pepper as desired, place onions around lamb, and roast in the middle of the oven for 40 minutes. Turn lamb over, scatter with the herbs, and roast another 40 minutes. Pour the wine, broth, and water into the roasting pan, cover tightly, and braise until tender (about 45 minutes to 1 hour). Transfer the lamb to a plate, remove the meat and discard the bones, and pour the cooking liquid (including onions) into a large glass measuring cup. Do not clean the roasting pan.

2. To prepare the vegetables while the lamb roasts, pierce each potato once with a fork and bake on rack in lower third of oven until cooked through (about 45–50 minutes), cool 10 minutes, halve lengthwise, scoop out warm flesh and force through a ricer into a bowl, then stir in the soy milk and salt and pepper as desired (or,

peel potatoes, cut into small pieces, cook in water until just soft, mash, and stir in the soy milk and salt and pepper as desired). Cook the carrots in boiling water until barely tender (about 10 minutes), then rinse under cool running water. Rinse the spinach thoroughly to remove any grit, place in a large pot (do not add more water), cover tightly, cook over moderate heat until just limp (about 1–2 minutes), drain in a colander, rinse until cool, squeeze to remove as much moisture as possible, then coarsely chop.

3. To make the gravy, skim and discard the fat from the cooking liquid (or use a defatting cup); you should have about 2 1/2 cups of broth. In a large bowl, whisk 1 cup broth and the cornstarch or potato starch into a thin paste, then whisk in the remaining broth (including onions). Set the lamb's roasting pan across two burners, pour in the broth mixture, and boil over moderate heat, whisking, until thickened (about 5 minutes). Remove from heat and season with salt and pepper as desired.

4. To assemble and bake the pie, reduce oven to 350°F. Cut the lamb into bite-sized pieces, stir it into the gravy, and spoon the mixture evenly into a casserole baking dish. Scatter the carrots evenly over the lamb, then the spinach evenly over the carrots, and spread the mashed potatoes on top to cover the filling completely to the edges. Make some swirls in the potatoes with the back of a spoon, drizzle with the melted butter, and bake until the top is golden and the filling is bubbling (about 30 minutes). Serve immediately.

Main-course salads are so easy to prepare and so satisfying . . .

GARDEN CRAB SALAD

I enjoy this delicious salad two or three times per week—for variety, you can change the vegetables to make it seasonal, or dress it up with a beautiful salsa.
(Be certain not to use crab from the South Pacific, which is dangerously polluted with mercury and other toxins.)

YIELD: 2 SERVINGS

1 8-ounce container fresh crab

1/4 cup minced red onion

1/4 cup minced celery

1/4 cup minced red or yellow bell pepper

¹/₄ cup (or to taste) mayonnaise

Salt and pepper to taste

1 package mesclun or other salad mix

Olive oil and balsamic vinegar to taste

In a mixing bowl, combine the crab, onion, celery, and bell pepper, mix in the mayonnaise, and season with salt and pepper as desired. Arrange the salad greens on two salad plates, sprinkle with olive oil and balsamic vinegar, top with the crab mixture, and serve immediately.

SHRIMP AND AVOCADO SALAD

Another dish you'll want to enjoy often—simple, cooling, and tasty. Note that the recipe calls for marinating part of the salad 1–2 days before serving.

YIELD: 4 SERVINGS

2 pounds medium-sized shrimp, peeled and deveined

³/₄ cup white-wine balsamic vinegar

1 cup olive oil

¹/₄ cup capers

¹/₂ teaspoon kosher salt (or to taste)

1 teaspoon freshly ground black pepper

1 teaspoon celery seed

¹/₂ teaspoon Tabasco sauce

1 cup thinly sliced red or white onion

¹/₂ cup chopped celery

7 bay leaves

2 firm-ripe Haas avocados

Soft lettuce such as Boston lettuce

In a 5-quart pot of boiling salted water, cook the shrimp until just barely done and turned pink (about 2–3 minutes). In a large bowl, whisk together the vinegar, oil, capers, salt, pepper, celery seed, and Tabasco sauce, add the warm shrimp, onion, celery, and bay leaves, and toss to combine. Cover and marinate in the refrigerator for 24 hours to 2 days, then discard bay leaves. Just before serving, cut the avocados into cubes, stir gently into the shrimp mixture, and spoon the salad onto a bed of lettuce.

WEEK III-10

You will see from the following recipes that Wings students become creative cooks . . .

SIMPLY DELICIOUS CHICKEN MADE SIMPLY

This fabulous recipe comes from a Wings student in Florida—thanks, Vicki! Serve with a salad and a vegetable dish.

YIELD: 4 SERVINGS

1 cup uncooked brown rice

¹/₂ or 1 whole chicken, cut into serving pieces

1 teaspoon coarse kosher salt

1 teaspoon freshly ground pepper

1³/₄ cups water

2 whole cloves garlic, peeled

1 stem fresh cilantro with leaves

10 pimiento-stuffed olives

1 28-ounce can tomatoes (dice tomatoes and retain liquid)

Preheat oven to 350°F. Use a casserole dish that will fit the chicken pieces without crowding. Place the rice in the bottom of the casserole, wash and dry the chicken, place it skin-side down on the rice, and sprinkle with the salt and pepper. Add the water, garlic, cilantro, and olives to the casserole, and top with the tomatoes and their juice, making sure some of the tomato flows to the rice. Cover, bake for 1 hour, reduce temperature to 325°F, bake for 1 more hour, and serve.

CABBAGE-AND-CARROT SALAD

This fresh, healthful substitute for "normal" cole slaw was provided by another generous Wings student, Suzanne—thanks, friend!

YIELD: 4 SERVINGS

¹/₂ cabbage, chopped to fit into the food-processor bowl

1 carrot, grated

2 tablespoons olive oil

1 tablespoon lemon juice

Sea salt to taste

A sprinkle of fresh herbs of your choice (optional)

Process the cabbage and carrots in a food processor until fine but not mushy. In a large serving bowl, stir the oil and lemon juice together, add the vegetables, mix well, and season as desired with the sea salt and herbs. Chill for the flavors to blend before serving.

SUZANNE'S KISS* BEAN SALAD (*KEEP IT SIMPLE, SWEETIE)

Another recipe from our "sweetie" Suzanne.

YIELD: 4–6 SERVINGS

1 1/2 cups (1 16-ounce can) drained
and rinsed black beans

1 1/2 cups (1 16-ounce can) drained and
rinsed red or pinto beans

1/2 cup diced celery

1/2 cup diced red onion

1 cup diced fresh tomato

1/4 cup chopped fresh parsley

Dressing

1/4 teaspoon cumin powder

1/2 teaspoon sea salt

1/4–1 teaspoon chili powder, to taste (optional)

1 clove garlic, crushed

2 tablespoons lemon or lime juice

2 tablespoons olive oil

In a large serving bowl, combine the beans, celery, onion, tomato, and parsley. In a small bowl, combine all dressing ingredients and mix, pour over the bean salad, and stir well. Serve at room temperature or chilled.

WEEK III-11

GARLIC-AND-GINGER PORK

Pork isn't a great meat to eat often, but you can enjoy it occasionally for variety. Overcooking makes pork dry and tasteless, so use a meat thermometer to assure a properly cooked tenderloin. This recipe comes from another Wings student in Florida—thanks, Jill! Serve over steamed rice and sautéed baby bok choy, with the cooking juices poured over all.

YIELD: 4–6 SERVINGS

1 tablespoon sesame oil

1 tablespoon chopped fresh ginger root

2 cloves garlic, crushed

1 cup Chinese cooking wine or dry sherry

1/4 cup soy sauce

1/4 cup hoisin sauce

2 tablespoons honey

2 pork tenderloins, cut in half;
or, 4–6 boneless chicken breasts

In a bowl, combine all ingredients except the meat and mix well. Place the meat in a shallow casserole dish, pour the sauce over it, cover, and marinate for 2 hours in the refrigerator. Preheat oven to 400°F. Cook covered dish about 25–30 minutes, reduce temperature to 350°F, and continue to roast until done (about 15 more minutes). Remove the meat to dinner plates and serve with the cooking juices poured on top.

SHRIMP ETOUFFÉE

(pronounced "eay-too-fay")

Do you enjoy spicy food? You'll enjoy preparing this easy meal-in-a-pot for your family. Serve over steamed rice. (If you can eat butter without triggering allergies, you should be able to tolerate the small amount of heavy cream in this recipe; if not, leave it out.) Thanks again, Jill!

YIELD: 4 SERVINGS

1/2 cup butter

1 1/2 cups finely chopped onion

1/2 cup finely chopped green bell pepper

1/2 cup finely chopped celery

3 cloves garlic, minced or crushed

2 tablespoons rice flour or white spelt flour

1 1/2 cups good (nonalcoholic) Bloody Mary mix

3 tablespoons heavy cream

1 teaspoon salt, or to taste

1 1/2 pounds raw shrimp, cleaned
and deveined

1/2 teaspoon cayenne pepper, or to taste

1/8 teaspoon Tabasco sauce

Lemon juice to taste

In a heavy saucepan, melt the butter, add the vegetables and garlic, and sauté until just tender. Stir in the flour, then the Bloody Mary mix, and cook lightly as you stir in the cream. Continue stirring so the cream does not curdle, add the shrimp, cayenne, and Tabasco sauce, cook until the shrimp just turns pink (about 2–3 minutes), and serve with a squeeze of lemon juice.

OATMEAL COCONUT CHEWS

Sometimes you just need a cookie (can you be trusted not to eat the whole batch?).

YIELD: 4 DOZEN COOKIES

1 cup butter, softened

1/2 cup brown-rice syrup

1/2 cup date sugar

1 teaspoon vanilla

2 eggs, beaten

1 1/2 cup Kamut flour

1 teaspoon salt

1 teaspoon baking soda

3 cups rolled oats

3/4 cup flaked coconut

1/2 cup chopped walnuts

Preheat oven to 350°F. Cream the butter, syrup, and sugar together until fluffy, stir in the vanilla, and add the eggs one at a time, beating after each. Sift together the flour, salt, and baking soda, and add to the creamed mixture, then stir in the oats, coconut, and nuts. Drop by tablespoons, about 2 inches apart, onto well-buttered baking sheets and bake for 12–15 minutes.

CHICKEN RISOTTO WITH ROASTED PEPPERS

Excellent for the entire family, and the splashes of green, red, and white make this a very festive dish. Saffron is frightfully expensive; you may substitute turmeric for its bright color and richer flavor. Serve with two side vegetables or a salad.

YIELD: ABOUT 6 SERVINGS

7 cups chicken broth

1/2 teaspoon saffron or turmeric powder

1 1/2 pounds boneless, skinless chicken breasts, cut into 1/2-inch-wide strips

Kosher salt and freshly ground pepper to taste

Several tablespoons olive oil

1 onion, chopped

3 cloves garlic, minced

1/4 teaspoon red pepper flakes

2 1/2 cups uncooked arborio rice

1 cup dry white wine

1 1/2 teaspoons dried rosemary

1 red bell pepper, roasted, skinned, and cut into strips

1 1/2 cups thawed frozen peas

In a saucepan, bring the broth to simmer, cover, and adjust heat to keep it warm. Sprinkle the chicken with the kosher salt and pepper as desired. In a heavy saucepan, heat a couple tablespoons of the oil, and sauté about half of the chicken pieces at a time, stirring frequently, to a light golden brown (about 3–4 minutes). Transfer each batch to a plate and set aside. In the same pan over medium heat, add more olive oil and sauté the onion and garlic, stirring, until they begin to color slightly (about 3–4 minutes). Stir in the pepper flakes, sauté for about 1 minute longer, add the rice, and stir until white spots appear in the center of the grains (about 1 minute). Add the wine and rosemary, stir until wine is absorbed (about 2 minutes), add a ladleful (about 1/2 cup) of the warm broth, adjust heat to maintain a simmer, and cook, stirring constantly, until the liquid is absorbed. Continue adding broth a ladleful at a time, stirring each time until the liquid is absorbed. Add the chicken, bell pepper, and peas at the final ladleful of broth. Continue stirring, and cook until rice is just tender but slightly firm in the center and mixture is creamy (about 20–25 minutes). Adjust the seasoning with salt and pepper as desired, and serve.

WINE-POACHED SALMON

For a simple, quick dinner, arrange these filets over a garden-fresh mixed vegetable salad sprinkled with a splash of olive oil and balsamic vinegar and a pinch of kosher salt.

YIELD: 4 SERVINGS

1 tablespoon olive oil

2 tablespoons minced onion

1 clove garlic, minced

4 salmon filets (3–4 ounces each)

1/2 cup dry white wine

1/2 cup chicken broth

2 fresh basil leaves, minced

In a skillet, heat the oil on medium heat, add the onion and garlic, and sauté until soft but not browned (about 1–2 minutes). Add the salmon, sauté briefly (3–4 minutes), and turn the filets. Add the wine and broth, cover, lower heat, and let simmer until filets are done (about 3–4 minutes) but still a little pink in the center. Remove salmon with a slotted spoon to a serving plate, raise heat to high, and continue to cook, stirring occasionally, until the liquid is reduced by half. Pour the sauce over the salmon, sprinkle with the basil, and serve immediately.

WEEK III-14

CREAMY POLENTA

You won't miss pasta after you try this Italian side dish. Feel free to "dress it up" by adding minced sun-dried tomatoes, roasted garlic cloves, or other favorites while it cooks, and serve topped with your favorite marinara sauce or Italian Peppers and Onions (recipe follows).

YIELD: 8 SERVINGS

6 cups water

½ teaspoon salt

2 cups Bob's Red Mill Polenta
(available at health food stores)

Grated cheese (Parmesan, Romano, or Fontina)
to taste (optional)

In a deep pot over high heat, bring the water and salt to a boil, lower heat, and *very* gradually stir in the polenta, continuing to stir with a long-handled wooden spoon as it cooks (be careful, polenta bubbles and pops vigorously). Continue stirring and cooking until very thick. Stir in the cheese as desired and serve.

Note: Press leftover polenta into a buttered baking dish, cover, and refrigerate. The next evening, tip it out onto a cutting board, cut into ½-inch slices, and sauté in a little butter for another delicious side dish.

ITALIAN PEPPERS AND ONIONS

This "little taste of Italy" is a good side dish and also a beautiful topping for Creamy Polenta (recipe above) or scrambled eggs.

YIELD: 6–8 SERVINGS

1 tablespoon olive oil

3 large bell peppers (red, green, and yellow),
seeded and cut into 1-inch pieces

1 large white onion, peeled and cut into large pieces

Several cloves garlic, peeled

3 cups chopped canned tomatoes, with juice

1 teaspoon chopped fresh oregano

1 teaspoon chopped fresh basil

In a large skillet, heat the oil on medium heat, add the peppers, onion, and garlic, and cook, stirring frequently. When the peppers are nearly cooked through (about 10 minutes), add the tomatoes and herbs, cover, lower heat, allow to cook slowly until vegetables are done (about 10 more minutes), and serve.

MODULE IV

You are headed into new territory again! But do not forget the Wings food emphasis: fresh, natural, and delicious. And remember, every morsel of natural food invites healing into your body.

WEEK IV-1

You get to try some new vegetables this week . . .

CAROL'S ASPARAGUS SOUP

I love soup . . . Asparagus soup is particularly delicious and a real comfort food.

YIELD: 6 SERVINGS

A splash of olive oil

1 medium white onion, diced

2 stalks celery, diced

3–4 cloves garlic, minced

1 bunch of asparagus, tough ends removed,
cut into 1-inch pieces, with the heads set aside

6 cups vegetable broth

4 tablespoons tahini

In a heavy soup kettle or saucepan, heat the oil, add the onion, celery, and garlic, and cook over medium heat until nearly soft. Add the asparagus stalks (reserving the heads), stir for a few minutes, add the broth, reduce heat to simmer, cover tightly, and simmer until asparagus is done (about 20 minutes). Meanwhile, in a separate saucepan, cook the asparagus tips in a little water until they are bright green and still crisp (about 5 minutes maximum), remove from heat, drain, and set aside. When the asparagus stalks are done, transfer all the vegetables from the broth with a slotted spoon to a blender or food processor, and process until puréed.

Return the purée to the broth, add the tahini, and bring to a slow simmer, stirring until mixed and heated through. Ladle the soup into bowls, garnish with the asparagus heads, and serve immediately.

PROSCIUTTO-WRAPPED SALMON

Serve this delicious fish over Herbed Bean Ragout (recipe follows). Adapted from one of my favorite cooking magazines, *Gourmet*. (I encourage you to get a subscription to *Gourmet* because it features marvelous seafood and vegetable recipes.)

YIELD: 6 SERVINGS

6 6-ounce center-cut salmon filets, skinned

12 very thin slices (¹/₄ pound) prosciutto

Pepper to taste

2 tablespoons olive oil

Preheat oven to 425°F. Wrap each salmon piece in a slice of prosciutto, leaving the ends of the salmon exposed. Transfer the wrapped salmon, seam-side down, to an oiled, large, shallow baking pan. Season with pepper as desired and drizzle each piece with ¹/₂ teaspoon of the olive oil. Bake in the middle of the oven until just cooked through (about 8–9 minutes) , and serve.

HERBED BEAN RAGOUT

If you cannot find *haricots verts*, use regular green beans. You can find *edamame* at the supermarket or health food store.

YIELD: 6 SERVINGS

6 ounces haricots verts (thin French green beans), trimmed and halved crosswise

1 1-pound bag frozen edamame (soybeans) in the pod, not thawed; or, 1¹/₄ cups frozen shelled edamame, not thawed

²/₃ cup finely chopped onion

2 cloves garlic, minced

1 bay leaf

2 3-inch fresh rosemary sprigs

¹/₂ teaspoon salt

¹/₄ teaspoon pepper

1 tablespoon olive oil

1 medium carrot, diced into ¹/₈-inch pieces

2 stalks celery, with strings removed, diced

1 15-ounce can small white beans, rinsed and drained

1¹/₂ cups chicken stock or broth

2 tablespoons unsalted butter

2 tablespoons finely chopped fresh flat-leaf parsley

1 tablespoon finely chopped fresh chervil

In a large pot of boiling salted water, cook the *haricots verts* until just tender (about 3–4 minutes), transfer with a slotted spoon to a bowl of ice water, then drain. In a large pot of boiling water, cook the *edamame* for 4 minutes, drain in a colander, then rinse under cold water (if you're using *edamame* in pods, shell them into a bowl and discard the pods). In a heavy 2 to 4 quart saucepan, combine the onion, garlic, bay leaf, rosemary, salt, pepper, and oil, and cook over moderately low heat, stirring, until softened (about 3 minutes). Add the carrot and celery, and continue to cook, stirring, until softened (about 3 minutes). Add the white beans and stock, cover, and simmer for 10 minutes, stirring occasionally. Add the *haricots verts* and *edamame* and simmer, uncovered, until heated through (about 2–3 minutes). Add the butter, parsley, and chervil, stir gently until the butter is melted, discard the bay leaf and rosemary sprigs, and serve immediately.

WEEK IV-2

THAI PINEAPPLE-SHRIMP FRIED RICE

Back to simple—this light dish is easily prepared.

YIELD: 4 SERVINGS

1 20-ounce can unsweetened pineapple tidbits, in own juice

4 scallions, sliced

1 handful chopped fresh cilantro

¹/₂ teaspoon minced canned Thai chili peppers (available in Oriental markets or the ethnic section of grocery stores)

1 cup uncooked jasmine rice

1 pound broccoli florets

3 tablespoons sesame oil

1¹/₂ pounds fresh shrimp, cleaned and deveined

2 cloves garlic, minced or crushed

2 tablespoons fish sauce

2 tablespoons soy sauce

1 teaspoon honey

Additional fresh cilantro sprigs for garnish

In a small bowl, combine the pineapple and juice with the scallions, chopped cilantro, and chili paste, and set aside. Cook the rice according to package directions and set aside. Steam the broccoli until tender-crisp and set aside. In a large skillet or wok, heat the oil and sauté the shrimp and garlic until shrimp are just pink (about 2–3 minutes), remove from skillet, and do not drain. In the same skillet, add the fish sauce, soy sauce, and honey, mix in the rice, stir to coat evenly, add the pineapple mixture, and heat through to combine the flavors. Add the shrimp and broccoli, mix well, heat through, and serve immediately, garnished with the cilantro sprigs.

BERTOLLI RISOTTO WITH SHRIMP

This wonderful rice dish is a little high in carbohydrates but is a nice change of pace for people who enjoy the energizing effects of a high-carbohydrate meal. True risotto is made with white rice; brown rice, however, provides more nutrition with a similar taste but a different texture and longer cooking time, so choose according to the dictates of mood and schedule.

YIELD: 6 SERVINGS

4–5 cups chicken broth

2 tablespoons olive oil

2 tablespoons diced red onion

1 $1/4$ cups uncooked white or brown rice (see variation)

$1/3$ cup dry white wine

1 pound shrimp, shelled and deveined

1 cup frozen or fresh peas

1 teaspoon julienned lemon rind

1 tablespoon lemon juice

Salt and pepper to taste

Finely chopped fresh basil for garnish

Bring the broth to a slow simmer on the stove and keep it hot while you cook. In a large saucepan over low heat, heat 1 tablespoon of the oil, cook the onion, stirring frequently, until tender (about 5 minutes), add the rice, and stir to coat with oil. Add the wine, heat to boiling, and stir over high heat until almost evaporated. Add 1 cup of the hot broth, stir until absorbed, and continue adding broth about $1/2$ cup at a time, stirring constantly, with each portion absorbed before adding the next. With the last $1/2$ cup, add the shrimp, peas, and lemon rind, and cook, uncovered, stirring

constantly, until the broth is absorbed, the rice is tender, moist, and creamy, and the shrimp are pink. Stir in the lemon juice and remaining 1 tablespoon of oil. Season with salt and pepper as desired, garnish with the basil, and serve.

Variation: If you choose brown rice, you can achieve the right texture and consistency by using the following cooking method: After sautéing the onion, add the rice, wine, and 3 cups of the chicken broth, bring to a slow simmer, cover, and allow the rice to cook. When the rice is nearly done, add more broth if necessary and the rest of the ingredients, cook until the shrimp are just pink, and then finish using the rest of the instructions above.

WEEK IV-3

GRANDMA'S HOMEMADE VEGETABLE-BEEF SOUP

Who can resist a recipe from Grandma?

YIELD: 8–12 SERVINGS

A splash of olive oil

1 $1/2$ pounds top round beef, trimmed of fat and diced into $1/2$-inch pieces

2 cups water

3 cups tomato sauce

4 cups beef stock or bouillon

1 $1/2$ teaspoons dried oregano

1 teaspoon chili powder

2 bay leaves

$1/4$ teaspoon ground black pepper

$1/2$ cup uncooked barley

1 $1/2$ cups diced root vegetables (rutabagas, turnips, or parsnips are great)

1 $1/2$ cups diced carrots

1 large white onion, diced

1 $1/2$ cups diced fresh green beans

In a nonstick heavy saucepan, heat the oil over medium heat, then add the beef and stir-fry until it turns brown (about 4 minutes). Stir-fry only a little meat at a time so it browns nicely instead of steaming. Add the water, tomato sauce, stock, spices, and barley, bring to a simmer, cover, and simmer, stirring occasionally, for 30 minutes. Add the root vegetables, carrots, onion, and green beans, return to a simmer, cover, and simmer, stirring occasionally, until the vegetables are tender (about 30 minutes). Serve with Northern Cornbread (recipe follows) for a complete meal.

SILKY BLACKENED PEPPERS AND ONIONS

This savory blend is delicious with scrambled eggs, on grilled chicken, or as a simple side dish.

YIELD: 4 SERVINGS

A splash of olive oil

3 large bell peppers (green, red, and yellow), cored, seeded, and cut into $\frac{1}{2}$-inch slices

1 large white onion, peeled, cut into $\frac{1}{4}$-inch slices

A sprinkle of kosher salt

In a heavy saucepan that has a lid, heat the oil on medium-high heat, add the vegetables, and sauté, stirring occasionally, until they start to darken (about 5 minutes). Reduce heat to low, cover tightly, and cook, stirring occasionally, until they are very dark, very soft, and slightly sweet (about 20 minutes or more). Sprinkle with the salt and serve.

SAVORY CELERY

Celery is often relegated to a garnish or a behind-the-scenes flavoring for soups and broths—but prepared the right way, celery is delicious as a side dish with dinner. Alkalinizing too!

YIELD: 4 SERVINGS

2 celery clusters, including leaves

2 tablespoons butter

2 tablespoons olive oil

Salt and pepper to taste

Separate the celery ribs, trim the ends and any blemishes, and cut each rib into 1-inch pieces. Chop the leaves and set aside. Melt the butter and olive oil together in a large skillet over medium-high heat, and sauté the celery pieces (not the leaves), stirring often. Reduce heat to medium and cook celery until tender when pierced (about 8 minutes). Add the chopped celery leaves, sprinkle with salt and pepper as desired, and serve.

WEEK IV-4

Tip: Before going to work in the morning, mix together the following meat loaf recipe's ingredients,

press into the baking dish, cover tightly, and refrigerate; in the evening, scrub a few yams and bake them with the meat loaf while you relax over a glass of wine or play with your kids, and then serve dinner with a crisp green salad. Meal-in-a-flash!

MEAT LOAF

Meat loaf—love it, or hate it? I think you'll love this one. I really enjoy a rich brown gravy over meat loaf; use one of the broth recipes in this book as a gravy base if you have time (see pages 268–270).

YIELD: 6–8 SERVINGS

1 pound extra-lean ground beef

$\frac{1}{2}$ pound ground veal stew meat

$\frac{1}{2}$ pound ground pork shoulder

1 tablespoon olive oil

1 medium onion, finely chopped

1 large clove garlic, finely chopped

$\frac{1}{4}$ cup finely chopped fresh parsley

1 egg, lightly beaten

1 teaspoon salt

$\frac{1}{2}$ teaspoon freshly ground pepper

$\frac{1}{4}$ teaspoon ground allspice

$\frac{1}{2}$ teaspoon dried thyme

1 bay leaf

Preheat oven to 350°F. Put the meats in a large mixing bowl. Heat the oil in a pan and sauté the onion and garlic until soft and transparent (about 5 minutes). Add all other ingredients except the bay leaf, and mix thoroughly with your hands. Pack the mixture into a 1-quart loaf pan, lay the bay leaf on top, and bake on the middle rack in the oven for $1\frac{1}{2}$ hours. Leave the loaf in the pan and keep it warm for 20 minutes before slicing so it doesn't crumble easily.

NORTHERN CORNBREAD

A fine, slightly sweet cornbread with a sturdy, smooth texture. I enjoy it with a little fruit-only jam and a bowl of thick soup.

YIELD: 6 SERVINGS

1 cup Kamut flour or spelt flour

1 cup organic stone-ground cornmeal

1 tablespoon nonaluminum baking powder

¹/₂ teaspoon salt

1 cup soy milk

¹/₄ cup honey or rice syrup

2 eggs, beaten

¹/₃ cup butter, melted

Preheat oven to 400°F. Butter an iron skillet or 8x8x2-inch baking pan. In a large bowl, stir together the flour, cornmeal, baking powder, and salt. In a medium-sized bowl, beat together the milk, honey, eggs, and butter. Stir the liquid ingredients into the dry ingredients until just blended, pour into the prepared pan, and bake until the top is slightly golden (about 25–30 minutes)—don't overbake or it will be dry.

WEEK IV-5

STAR ANISE PORK

Don't even *think* about changing this recipe! This dream dish is the most succulent pork I've ever enjoyed. You can purchase star anise at a gourmet cooking store or Oriental market—don't substitute! Adapted from another of my favorite cooking magazines, *Food and Wine*, which suggests serving it over *pappardelle* noodles; however, people on a wheat-free diet can serve it over mashed potatoes or brown rice. You'll want to savor every spoonful of the delicious gravy.

YIELD: 6 SERVINGS

¹/₂ cup chicken stock

¹/₄ cup dry sherry

¹/₄ cup soy sauce

2 tablespoons light-brown sugar

2 whole star anise pods, crushed

2 cloves garlic, minced

¹/₄ teaspoon Chinese five-spice powder

1 3-pound boneless pork shoulder, tied

Salt and freshly ground pepper to taste

1 tablespoon olive oil

2 tablespoons coarsely chopped fresh cilantro for garnish

In a small bowl, mix the stock, sherry, soy sauce, sugar, star anise, garlic, and five-spice powder. Season the pork as desired with salt and pepper. Heat the oil in a large, enameled, cast-iron casserole pot, add the pork, and cook over moderate heat, turning occasionally,

until browned all over (about 15 minutes). Add the sauce mixture and bring to a boil, scraping up any browned bits from the bottom of the pot. Cover tightly and cook over low heat until very tender (about 3 hours), turning the roast every 30 minutes. Remove the pork and boil the sauce until it is reduced to 1 cup (about 5 minutes). Remove the strings from the pork, pull the pork into long shreds, return it to the pot, and stir to mix with the sauce. Garnish with the cilantro and serve.

Note: You can also braise this pork in a Crock-Pot. I recommend low heat for 4–5 hours, depending on your unit—do not overcook, or the pork will be dry.

WEEK IV-6

PAN-ROASTED PORK CHOPS IN BOURBON SAUCE

This recipe is reconfigured from one of my f avorite cooking magazines, Cuisine.

YIELD: 4 SERVINGS

Brine

¹/₂ cup kosher salt

¹/₂ cup brown sugar

2 cups hot water

6 cups ice water

Chops

4 1"-thick pork chops

Pepper to taste

A sprinkle of gluten-free flour

2 tablespoons olive oil

1 tablespoon chopped fresh garlic

1 tablespoon chopped shallot

¹/₃ cup bourbon

1 ¹/₂ cups chicken broth

2 tablespoons brown sugar

1 tablespoon apple-cider vinegar

2 tablespoons heavy cream (optional)

In a 1-gallon sealable freezer bag, dissolve the salt and sugar completely in the hot water, then add the ice water. Add the pork chops, seal the bag, and refrigerate for 1-2 hours. Preheat oven to 425°F. Dry the chops, season with pepper as desired, and dust lightly with flour. In an oven-proof pan, brown the chops in the oil over medium-high heat. Cover, roast the pork in the oven for about 10 minutes, and remove the chops to a plate. In the pan, sauté the garlic and shallot in 1 tablespoon of the pork drippings over medium-high heat until soft. Deglaze the pan with the bourbon and chicken broth, add the sugar and vinegar, and cook until the liquid is reduced by half. Add the cream and chops to the pan, cook the chops for 2 minutes on each side while the sauce thickens, and serve.

WEEK IV-7

CURRIED CHICKPEAS AND KALE

Our local CSA members loved this recipe! The aroma wafting through the house while this dish simmers will draw everyone to the table (including the neighbors). Serve over brown rice for a rich meal, or serve as a soup and sop up the broth with gluten-free bread.

YIELD: 4 SERVINGS

2 tablespoons olive oil

1 1/2 cups chopped onions

4 cloves garlic, crushed

1/2 teaspoon cumin powder

3 cups chopped kale (thoroughly cleaned)

1 1/2 tablespoons curry powder

1 teaspoon ground ginger

1 teaspoon ground coriander

1 1/2 cups chicken broth or vegetable broth

3 cups cooked, drained chickpeas (garbanzo beans)

1 cup chopped canned tomatoes

1/4 teaspoon salt (optional)

Combine all ingredients in a Crock-Pot and cook on high for 4 hours; or, combine all ingredients in a casserole dish and bake in the oven at 325°F for 4 hours.

GREEN BEANS WITH MUSTARD

Green beans take on a new personality with mustard. For even more of that personality, try sautéing a few chopped mustard greens and adding them to the beans.

YIELD: 4 SERVINGS

1 pound green beans, trimmed

2 teaspoons olive oil

2 teaspoons dijon mustard

Salt and pepper to taste

Cook the green beans in a pot of boiling water for 3–4 minutes, drain in a colander, and pat dry. Heat the oil in a skillet over moderately high heat, add the beans and mustard, and season with salt and pepper as desired. Sauté, stirring, until heated through (about 3–4 minutes), and serve.

WEEK IV-8

Is it Christmas yet? I don't know what time of the year you are reading this, but whenever the holidays approach, you will need some goodies for you and the family. Of course, you can try these recipes at any time of year . . .

CAROL'S FRUITCAKE

Forget all the fruitcake jokes—they were made by people who haven't tried this recipe. Although it uses a little candied fruit, the sugar content is at a minimum. This fruitcake will become a tradition for your family as well.

YIELD: 3 LOAVES

3 cups white spelt flour

2 teaspoons cinnamon

1/2 teaspoon allspice

1/2 teaspoon ground cloves

1/2 teaspoon nutmeg

2 teaspoons nonaluminum baking powder

2 cups (1 pound) mixed candied fruit

1 cup dried Bing cherries

1 pound dark raisins

1/2 cup dried cranberries

1 1/2 cups pitted dates, cut into large pieces

2 cups pecan halves

1/2 cup whole almonds

1 cup whole Brazil nuts

4 eggs

1 cup fruit-concentrate sweetener, brown-rice syrup, or honey

1 cup almond milk

1/4 cup molasses

3/4 cup melted butter

1/2 cup peach brandy or other flavored brandy (optional)

Grease 3 loaf pans and line with waxed paper or foil. Sift the flour with the spices and baking powder into a large mixing bowl, add the candied fruit, dried fruits, and nuts, and mix until all the pieces are coated. Beat the eggs until foamy, and then continue beating while you gradually add the fruit sweetener, almond milk, molasses, and butter. Pour over the floured fruit mixture, stir until well blended, and divide the batter among the loaf pans, filling them 2/3 to 3/4 full. Bake at 275°F for 1 1/2 to 2 hours (a tester inserted into the center should come out clean) and cool. Remove the cakes from the pans to a plate, pour the brandy over them, wrap them in towels or other cloths, and refrigerate, allowing the brandy to permeate the cakes for a few days. Remove the cloths, wrap the cakes in plastic wrap, and refrigerate (they will keep for several weeks).

CHOCOLATE-COVERED APRICOTS

Chocolate is not inherently evil. Although your consumption of refined sugar should be kept to a minimum, life should be savored, and chocolate should be enjoyed—in small amounts! (This recipe does contain cream and butter, so if you are truly allergic to dairy, you'll have to pass.)

YIELD: 30 IRRESISTIBLE APRICOTS

2 cups whipping cream

1/2 cup unsalted butter

1 1/2 pounds bittersweet chocolate, finely chopped

30 dried apricots

Bring the whipping cream and butter to a boil, pour the hot liquid over the chocolate, and let stand 3–5 minutes. Gently stir with a rubber spatula or wooden spoon just to mix. The *ganache* should be satiny and smooth with a minimum of air bubbles. Let it cool to the point that you can touch it without being burned, and then dip each apricot into it, coating the lower half only and allowing excess to drip off. Place the apricots on a buttered cookie sheet and let them firm up in the refrigerator before serving. Fabulous and beautiful!

WEEK IV-9

More goodies!

DARK SECRETS

These cookies are reminiscent of fruitcake but a little richer. Really, really good!

YIELD: 12 BARS

1/3 cup chopped pecans

2 1/2 cups chopped dates

1/3 cup white spelt flour or Kamut flour

1/2 teaspoon nonaluminum baking powder

1/3 cup chopped walnuts

2 tablespoons melted butter

3 large egg yolks

1/2 teaspoon vanilla

In a bowl, combine the pecans, dates, flour, baking powder, walnuts, and melted butter. Add the egg yolks and vanilla and mix thoroughly. Spread the batter in a buttered 8-inch pan, bake at 300°F for 25 minutes, cool, and cut into bars.

MOLASSES BUTTER COOKIES

These will remind you of Russian tea cakes or Mexican wedding cakes—but this recipe uses no sugar other than the powder on top, and no wheat, so you can enjoy the buttery goodness without the guilt.

YIELD: APPROXIMATELY 24 COOKIES

1 cup butter

1/4 cup molasses

2 cups white spelt flour or Kamut flour

2 cups very finely chopped walnuts

A dusting of powdered sugar

In a mixer bowl, beat the butter for 30 seconds, add the molasses, beat until fluffy, add the flour, and beat at low speed until well blended. Stir in the nuts. Shape the dough into 1-tablespoon balls, place on an ungreased baking sheet, and bake at 325°F for 20 minutes. Remove to a wire rack, cool, and sprinkle lightly with powdered sugar.

WEEK IV-10

MUFFALATA SPREAD

This spread is wonderful on wheat-free bread or crackers (check the selection at your local health food store or purchase a wheat-free bread mix).

YIELD: APPROXIMATELY 3 CUPS

10 pepperoncini peppers

4 ounces mild cherry peppers

1/4 cup pitted black olives (Greek or Italian)

¹/₄ cup pitted green olives
¹/₂ cup minced red bell pepper
¹/₂ cup artichoke hearts, drained
5 tablespoons capers
4 cloves garlic, minced
5 tablespoons minced shallots or onions
2 cups olive oil
Tabasco sauce to taste (optional)

Chop the first 9 ingredients in a food processor or by hand. Add the oil and mix. Add Tabasco sauce as desired and mix. Serve at room temperature.

MISO-SAKE SALMON

How appropriate to end our time together with one of the original Wings recipes! You'll love this delicious salmon dish, served with your favorite rice pilaf and vegetables or a crunchy salad.

YIELD: 2 SERVINGS

1 tablespoon miso
¹/₄ teaspoon sugar
¹/₂ bunch scallions, chopped
¹/₂ cup sake
10 ounces salmon, divided into 2 pieces
1 tablespoon lemon juice
1 tablespoon butter

Mix the miso, sugar, scallions, and 1 tablespoon of the sake, smear it all over the salmon, and marinate in the refrigerator for at least 2 hours. Place the salmon in an ovenproof pan, pour the remaining sake around it, and broil in the oven for approximately 10 minutes (cooking time depends on the thickness of the fish). Remove from the oven and transfer the salmon to a plate, leaving the sauce in the pan. Place the pan over medium heat, add the lemon juice, reduce the sauce by half, add the butter, and stir to mix. Pour the sauce over the fish, and serve.

RECIPE NOTES

Resource Guide

To my readers:

I am so excited about my new web-enabled tool, MyProConnect, which allows my clients to receive direct counseling through my website. MyProConnect, a web-based software application for the health, wellness, and nutrition professions, enables clients to exchange, store, track, and present information about their health and wellness directly to me. It also allows clients to communicate with me about daily food intake, supplements, exercise, and much more via a PC or wireless device. This tool answers the call of today's increasingly health-conscious society and allows me to be connected to my clients.

Through MyProConnect, I become your personal nutrition coach and your Wings accountability partner! Visit me online today at www.flywithwings.com/pnc.html, click on the link MyProConnect, and start your personalized program!

—Carol

CONTACTING YOUR PERSONAL WINGS NUTRITIONIST

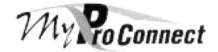

Powered by ProNex, Inc.
*Connecting the Healthcare Professional
with the Individual*

Personal Online Consultation

Want to schedule a personal online consultation with Carol? Go to the website www.flywithwings.com/pnc.html, click on MyProConnect, and get started today! Enroll for one session, or let Carol be your accountability partner, and enroll module by module.

FINDING A HOLISTIC PHYSICIAN OR NUTRITIONIST

- To locate a holistically trained physician in your area, log on to the following websites:

  The American Association of Naturopathic Physicians, www.naturopathic.org

  American College for Advancement in Medicine, www.acam.org

- To locate a nutritionist in your area, log on to the following websites:

  National Association of Nutrition Professionals, www.nanp.org

  International and American Associations of Clinical Nutritionists, www.iaacn.org

BASE SUPPLEMENT PROGRAM

As you proceed through the Wings Program, you will see why supplements are essential. I recommend that you start with the base supplement program outlined below, and then customize your supplement list as you learn more about your particular requirements.

- Wings Breakfast Drink: daily as described in the Wings food plan
- VRP Optimum 6, a multivitamin-mineral supplement: 6 capsules per day, divided between breakfast and lunch or dinner
- Carlson Fish Oil: 2–4 softgel capsules per day
- Juice Plus+, for extra antioxidant nutrition (important for everyone!): 2 capsules Orchard Blend each A.M., 2 capsules Garden Blend each P.M.
- VRP Advanced Essential Minerals: 4 capsules each P.M.

Supplement Ordering Information

- Wings Breakfast Drink, VRP Optimum 6, and all other physician-formulated, pharmaceutical-grade VRP products: www.flywithwings.com or 1-866-999-4647 (1-866-99WINGS)
- All Juice Plus+ products: www.JuicePlus.com
- You may purchase Carlson Fish Oil from your local health food store or directly from Wings.

pH STRIPS AND ALLERGY TESTING

Remember that allergy tests are available by prescription only and require a blood draw.

- Perque Laboratories, www.perque.com or 800-525-7372
- Great Smokies Diagnostic Laboratories, www.gsdl.com

WINGS: WEIGHT SUCCESS FOR A LIFETIME

Several other products and services to help you succeed in your quest for health may be ordered or accessed through Wings at www.flywithwings.com or 1-866-999-4647 (1-866-99WINGS).

Wings Videotapes

Every lesson in the Wings Program has been videotaped, along with additional information about the practical application of the principles being presented, in a series that corresponds with Modules I, II, III, and IV of this workbook. Each module is accompanied by the Wings Student Manual for that series of lessons. Due to the large amount of information presented in this workbook, I strongly recommend that readers purchase the relevant videotapes prior to beginning each module. For more information on the videotape series, go to the Wings website or call the Wings office.

Other Books by Carol Simontacchi

- *Your Fat Is Not Your Fault* (New York, NY: Jeremy P. Tarcher/Penguin, 1998)
- *The Crazy Makers: How the Food Industry Is Destroying Our Brains and Harming Our Children* (New York, NY: Jeremy P. Tarcher/Penguin, 2000)
- *A Woman's Guide to a Healthy Heart* (New York, NY: Contemporary Books, 2004)
- *Natural Alternatives to Vioxx and Celebrex* (Garden City, NY: Square One Publishers, 2005)

ADDITIONAL PRODUCT RECOMMENDATIONS

I highly recommend the following supplements, although there are many fine products on the market that are not listed here. These products can be purchased from your local health food store, or through the Wings website.

- Thyroid support: Enzymatic Therapy Thyroid and L-Tyrosine Complex
- Hormonal support: VRP HerBalance I (for PMS), VRP HerBalance II (for menopause), HerBalance Cream (progesterone cream)
- Stress relief: Enzymatic Therapy Rhodiola Energy, Eclectic Institute Relaxation Support, Enzymatic Therapy Adrenal Stress-End, VRP Adaptaphase I and Adaptaphase II
- To increase metabolism: Country Life DHEA, Enzymatic Therapy DHEA, VRP ThermoAMP, VRP Metabolic Support Formula
- To reduce sugar cravings and stabilize blood sugar: VRP Gymnema Sylvestre, VRP Carbohydrate Metabolism Support
- To reduce synthesis of fats from carbohydrates and inhibit appetite: VRP Garcinia Cambogia
- To break a strong sugar addiction: Sugar Stop gum

Note: If you have been diagnosed with a medical condition, suspect that you have a medical problem, or are under a physician's care, please consult your physician before using any of these recommended products.

Leave this form blank in the workbook—make copies for your use.

Name: _____

Date:

FOODS	TIME	SUPPLEMENTS	TIME	COMMENTS
1st Meal:				
2nd Meal:				
Snack:				
3rd Meal:				
Snack:				

Date:

FOODS	TIME	SUPPLEMENTS	TIME	COMMENTS
1st Meal:				
2nd Meal:				
Snack:				
3rd Meal:				
Snack:				

Date:

FOODS	TIME	SUPPLEMENTS	TIME	COMMENTS
1st Meal:				
2nd Meal:				
Snack:				
3rd Meal:				
Snack:				

Date:

FOODS	TIME	SUPPLEMENTS	TIME	COMMENTS
1st Meal:				
2nd Meal:				
Snack:				
3rd Meal:				
Snack:				

Wings: Weight Success for a Lifetime™
1633C Periwinkle Way • Sanibel, Florida 33957 • Phone: 239-472-4499
Toll Free: 866.99WINGS • Fax: 239-472-6815 • www.flywithwings.com

APPENDIX 2 · Exercise Diary

Leave this form blank in the workbook—make copies for your use.

Name: _____   Date: _____

As described in Lesson II-10, design your own exercise program (preferably, in consultation with a personal trainer) based on your time limitations, interests, starting fitness level, and so on, gradually building up to burning 2,500 calories per week. Use the charts in Lesson II-10 and the following form to plan your exercise program and record your achievements.

Exercise goal(s): _____

_____

Exercise(s) I enjoy:_____

Week #　　　 Activity	Intensity	Duration	Calories Burned
Monday			
Tuesday			
Wednesday			
Thursday			
Friday			
Saturday			
Sunday			
		Total Week's Calories Burned	_____

Week #　　　 Activity	Intensity	Duration	Calories Burned
Monday			
Tuesday			
Wednesday			
Thursday			
Friday			
Saturday			
Sunday			
		Total Week's Calories Burned	_____

Week #　　　 Activity	Intensity	Duration	Calories Burned
Monday			
Tuesday			
Wednesday			
Thursday			
Friday			
Saturday			
Sunday			
		Total Week's Calories Burned	_____

APPENDIX 3 • pH Testing Form

Leave this form blank in the workbook—make copies for your use.

Name: _____

Testing your internal pH is simple—and important! (See Lesson I-1.) Upon awakening in the morning, or after having slept for at least five hours, briefly dip a strip of pH testing paper in your urine stream. The dampened strip will change color immediately. Compare its color to the chart on the pH paper's package, and record the pH number on this form. For your own reference, there is also space to note any changes in your eating program or anything unusual in your life (such as extra stress) that may affect your pH.

Day/Date	pH	Notes	Day/Date	pH	Notes

Wings: Weight Success for a Lifetime™
1633C Periwinkle Way • Sanibel, Florida 33957 • Phone: 239-472-4499
Toll Free: 866.99WINGS • Fax: 239-472-6815 • www.flywithwings.com

Leave this form blank in the workbook—make copies for your use.

Name: _____

Starting with Lesson I-1, use this form as described in the text to record your height, weight, and girth measurements, and also your BMI value (refer to BMI chart in Appendix 4b). Remember, do not measure and record these data any more frequently than every four weeks!

	Date:	Date:	Date:	Date:	Date:	Date:
Height						
Weight						
Chest						
Waist						
Hips						
R. Thigh						
L. Thigh						
BMI						

	Date:	Date:	Date:	Date:	Date:	Date:
Height						
Weight						
Chest						
Waist						
Hips						
R. Thigh						
L. Thigh						
BMI						

Wings: Weight Success for a Lifetime™
1633C Periwinkle Way • Sanibel, Florida 33957 • Phone: 239-472-4499
Toll Free: 866.99WINGS • Fax: 239-472-6815 • www.flywithwings.com

Find your height in the left-most column, move to the right in that row to find your weight in pounds (or the weight closest to it), and move up that column to find your BMI value at the top. *Example: A person 65 inches tall who weighs 170 pounds has an approximate BMI value of 28.*

BODY MASS INDEX (BMI)																
19	20	21	22	23	24	25	26	27	28	29	30	31	32	33	34	35
HEIGHT																
58" — 91	96	100	105	110	115	119	124	129	134	138	143	148	153	158	162	167
59" — 94	99	104	109	114	119	124	128	133	138	143	148	153	158	163	168	173
60" — 97	102	107	112	118	123	128	133	138	143	148	153	158	163	168	174	179
61" — 100	106	111	116	122	127	132	137	143	148	153	158	164	169	174	180	185
62" — 104	109	115	120	126	131	136	142	147	153	158	164	169	175	180	186	191
63" — 107	113	118	124	130	135	141	146	152	158	163	169	175	180	186	191	197
64" — 110	116	122	128	134	140	145	151	157	163	169	174	180	186	192	197	204
65" — 114	120	126	132	138	144	150	156	162	168	174	180	186	192	198	204	210
66" — 118	124	130	136	142	148	155	161	167	173	179	186	192	198	204	210	216
67" — 121	127	134	140	146	153	159	166	172	178	185	191	198	204	211	217	223
68" — 125	131	138	144	151	158	164	171	177	184	190	197	203	210	216	223	230
69" — 128	135	142	149	155	162	169	176	182	189	196	203	209	216	223	230	236
70" — 132	139	146	153	160	167	174	181	188	195	202	209	216	222	229	236	243
71" — 136	143	150	157	165	172	179	186	193	200	208	215	222	229	236	243	250
72" — 140	147	154	162	169	177	184	191	199	206	213	221	228	235	242	250	258
73" — 144	151	159	166	174	182	189	197	204	212	219	227	235	242	250	257	265
74" — 148	155	163	171	179	186	194	202	210	218	225	233	241	249	256	264	272
75" — 152	160	168	176	184	192	200	208	216	224	232	240	248	256	264	272	279
76" — 156	164	172	180	189	197	205	213	221	230	238	246	254	263	271	279	287

APPENDIX 4b · Body Mass Index (BMI) (continued)

HEIGHT	BODY MASS INDEX (BMI)																		
	36	37	38	39	40	41	42	43	44	45	46	47	48	49	50	51	52	53	54
58"	172	177	181	186	191	196	201	205	210	215	220	224	229	234	239	244	248	253	258
59"	178	183	188	193	198	203	208	212	217	222	227	232	237	242	247	252	257	262	267
60"	184	189	194	199	204	209	215	220	225	230	235	240	245	250	255	261	266	271	276
61"	190	195	201	206	211	217	222	227	232	238	243	248	254	259	264	269	275	280	285
62"	196	202	207	213	218	224	229	235	240	246	251	256	262	267	273	278	284	289	295
63"	203	208	214	220	225	231	237	242	248	254	259	265	270	278	282	287	293	299	304
64"	209	215	221	227	232	238	244	250	256	262	267	273	279	285	291	296	302	308	314
65"	216	222	228	234	240	246	252	258	264	270	276	282	288	294	300	306	312	318	324
66"	223	229	235	241	247	253	260	266	272	278	284	291	297	303	309	315	322	328	334
67"	230	236	242	249	255	261	268	274	280	287	293	299	306	312	319	325	331	338	344
68"	236	243	249	256	262	269	276	282	289	295	302	308	315	322	328	335	341	348	354
69"	243	250	257	263	270	277	284	291	297	304	311	318	324	331	338	345	351	358	365
70"	250	257	264	271	278	285	292	299	306	313	320	327	334	341	348	355	362	369	376
71"	257	265	272	279	286	293	301	308	315	322	329	338	343	351	358	365	372	379	386
72"	265	272	279	287	294	302	309	316	324	331	338	346	353	361	368	375	383	390	397
73"	272	280	288	295	302	310	318	325	333	340	348	355	363	371	378	386	393	401	408
74"	280	287	295	303	311	319	326	334	342	350	358	365	373	381	389	396	404	412	420
75"	287	295	303	311	319	327	335	343	351	359	367	375	383	391	399	407	415	423	431
76"	295	304	312	320	328	336	344	353	361	369	377	385	394	402	410	418	426	435	443

APPENDIX 5 · Pulse Test

Leave this form blank in the workbook—make copies for your use.

Name: _____

How to Use this Form

Use this form along with the instructions in Lesson I-10 for Dr. Coca's pulse test. (Special thanks to my friend, Suzanne, for help designing this form!)

For the First Three Days

Take and record your pulse count upon arising, before and after each meal as indicated on the form below, and before retiring for the night.

DAY 1 • Pulse upon arising _____   (take this pulse lying down, but take every other pulse sitting up)

Breakfast: Pulse before _____   Pulse 30 min after _____   Pulse 60 min after _____   Pulse 90 min after _____

Foods eaten: _____

Lunch: Pulse before _____   Pulse 30 min after _____   Pulse 60 min after _____   Pulse 90 min after _____

Foods eaten: _____

Snack: Pulse before _____   Pulse 30 min after _____   Pulse 60 min after _____   Pulse 90 min after _____

Foods eaten: _____

Dinner: Pulse before _____   Pulse 30 min after _____   Pulse 60 min after _____   Pulse 90 min after _____

Foods eaten: _____

Snack: Pulse before _____   Pulse 30 min after _____   Pulse 60 min after _____   Pulse 90 min after _____

Foods eaten: _____

DAY 1 • Pulse before retiring _____

DAY 2 • Pulse upon arising _____   (take this pulse lying down, but take every other pulse sitting up)

Breakfast: Pulse before _____   Pulse 30 min after _____   Pulse 60 min after _____   Pulse 90 min after _____

Foods eaten: _____

Lunch: Pulse before _____   Pulse 30 min after _____   Pulse 60 min after _____   Pulse 90 min after _____

Foods eaten: _____

Snack: Pulse before _____   Pulse 30 min after _____   Pulse 60 min after _____   Pulse 90 min after _____

Foods eaten: _____

Dinner: Pulse before _____   Pulse 30 min after _____   Pulse 60 min after _____   Pulse 90 min after _____

Foods eaten: _____

Snack: Pulse before _____   Pulse 30 min after _____   Pulse 60 min after _____   Pulse 90 min after _____

Foods eaten: _____

DAY 2 • Pulse before retiring _____

APPENDIX 5 · **Pulse Test** (continued)

DAY 3 • Pulse upon arising _____   (take this pulse lying down, but take every other pulse sitting up)

Breakfast: Pulse before _____   Pulse 30 min after _____   Pulse 60 min after _____   Pulse 90 min after _____

Foods eaten: _____

Lunch: Pulse before _____   Pulse 30 min after _____   Pulse 60 min after _____   Pulse 90 min after _____

Foods eaten: _____

Snack: Pulse before _____   Pulse 30 min after _____   Pulse 60 min after _____   Pulse 90 min after _____

Foods eaten: _____

Dinner: Pulse before _____   Pulse 30 min after _____   Pulse 60 min after _____   Pulse 90 min after _____

Foods eaten: _____

Snack: Pulse before _____   Pulse 30 min after _____   Pulse 60 min after _____   Pulse 90 min after _____

Foods eaten: _____

DAY 3 • Pulse before retiring _____

Upon finishing Day 3, record the following information:

▪ Normal maximum pulse rate: _____ (at most, 12 points above lowest rate)

▪ Low pulse rate: _____ (As allergens are eliminated, the low pulse will go down and finally settle at a "real" low.)

▪ Foods that produced a high pulse count (over the normal maximum pulse rate): _____

_____

▪ Foods that did not produce a high pulse count: _____

_____

▪ Possible environmental allergens: _____

_____

APPENDIX 5 · **Pulse Test** (continued)

After the First Three Days

Test a single food every hour, for as many days as it takes to test all the foods you eat. Take and record your pulse count upon arising and before and after eating, as indicated on the form below.

DAY _____

Pulse upon arising _____ (take this pulse lying down, but take every other pulse sitting up)

Food #1 _____ Pulse before _____ Pulse 30 min after _____

Food #2 _____ Pulse before _____ Pulse 30 min after _____

Food #3 _____ Pulse before _____ Pulse 30 min after _____

Food #4 _____ Pulse before _____ Pulse 30 min after _____

Food #5 _____ Pulse before _____ Pulse 30 min after _____

Food #6 _____ Pulse before _____ Pulse 30 min after _____

Food #7 _____ Pulse before _____ Pulse 30 min after _____

Food #8 _____ Pulse before _____ Pulse 30 min after _____

Food #9 _____ Pulse before _____ Pulse 30 min after _____

Food #10 _____ Pulse before _____ Pulse 30 min after _____

Food #11 _____ Pulse before _____ Pulse 30 min after _____

Food #12 _____ Pulse before _____ Pulse 30 min after _____

Record the following information at the end of each hourly testing day:

- Normal maximum pulse rate: _____ (at most, 12 points above lowest rate)

- Low pulse rate: _____

- The difference between the highest and lowest pulse rate: _____
  (There may be a succession of these, as the pulse continues to go down
  and finally settles at a "real" low.)

- Foods that produced a high pulse count (over the normal maximum pulse rate): _____

- Foods that did not produce a high pulse count: _____

- Possible environmental allergens _____

Wings: Weight Success for a Lifetime™
1633C Periwinkle Way • Sanibel, Florida 33957 • Phone: 239-472-4499
Toll Free: 866.99WINGS • Fax: 239-472-6815 • www.flywithwings.com

Index

About the Author

Carol Simontacchi, C.C.N., M.S., is a certified clinical nutritionist and the author of a number of books on nutrition, including *Your Fat Is Not Your Fault, The Crazy Makers: How the Food Industry Is Destroying Our Brains and Harming Our Children,* and *A Woman's Guide to a Healthy Heart.* She is a contributing writer for the *Healthy Hearts* newsletter, published online on eDiets.com.

Ms. Simontacchi earned her Master of Science Degree from Columbia Pacific University, and obtained her certification as a clinical nutritionist through the Clinical Nutritionist Certification Board. She is also a professional member of the International and American Associations of Clinical Nutritionists. She has served on the Education Committee of the National Nutritional Foods Association, and has served as the President of the Society of Certified Nutritionists.

Ms. Simontacchi, a highly sought-after lecturer, has appeared on numerous national, regional, and local radio and TV shows. Her work has been featured in *Newsday, First for Women, Woman's Day,* and other popular publications. Ms. Simontacchi currently lives with her family in Florida.

Printed in the USA
CPSIA information can be obtained
at www.ICGtesting.com
JSHW060043150824
68134JS00031B/2625

9 781683 366867